THE DOMESTIC RABBIT

Also of interest from Blackwell Science

DISEASES OF DOMESTIC RABBITS
Library of Veterinary Practice
Lieve Okerman
0-632-02254-X

THE DOMESTIC RABBIT

Fifth Edition

J. C. SANDFORD

MA (CANTAB)
Life President of the British Rabbit Council
Formerly Chairman of the British Rabbit Council
and Founder of the Commercial Rabbit Association
Honorary Life Member of the British Commercial Rabbit Association

**Blackwell
Science**

Blackwell Science Ltd
Editorial Offices:
Osney Mead, Oxford OX2 0EL
25 John Street, London WC1N 2BL
23 Ainslie Place, Edinburgh EH3 6AJ
238 Main Street, Cambridge
  Massachusetts 02142, USA
54 University Street, Carlton
  Victoria 3053, Australia

Other Editorial Offices:
Arnette Blackwell SA
  224, Boulevard Saint Germain
  75007 Paris, France

Blackwell Wissenschafts-Verlag GmbH
  Kurfürstendamm 57
  10707 Berlin, Germany

  Zehetnergasse 6
  A-1140 Wien, Austria

First published in 1957 by
Crosby Lockwood & Son Ltd
Third edition 1979 published by
Granada Publishing
Fourth edition 1986 published by
Collins Professional and Technical Books
Fifth edition 1996 published by
Blackwell Science

Set in 10½/12½ pt Times
by Avocet Typeset, Brill, Aylesbury, Bucks
Printed in Great Britain at the Alden Press
Limited, Oxford and Northampton.
Bound by Hartnolls Ltd., Bodmin, Cornwall.

DISTRIBUTORS

Marston Book Services Ltd
PO Box 269
Abingdon
Oxon OX14 4YN
(*Orders:* Tel: 01235 465500
        Fax: 01235 465555)

USA
Blackwell Science, Inc.
238 Main Street
Cambridge, MA 02142
(*Orders:* Tel: 800 215-1000
        617 876-7000
        Fax: 617 492-5263)

Canada
Copp Clark, Ltd
2775 Matheson Blvd East
Mississauga, Ontario
Canada, L4W 4P7
(*Orders:* Tel: 800 263-4374
        905 238-6074)

Australia
Blackwell Science Pty Ltd
54 University Street
Carlton, Victoria 3053
(*Orders:* Tel: 03 9347-0300
        Fax: 03 9349-3016)

A catalogue record for this title
is available from the British Library

ISBN 0–632–03894–2

Library of Congress
Cataloging-in-Publication Data

Sandford, J. C. (John Cecil)
    The domestic rabbit/J.C. Sandford.
    — 5th ed.
      p.   cm.
    Includes bibliographical references
    (p.   ) and index.
    ISBN 0–632–03894–2 (alk. paper)
    1. Rabbits   I. Title
SF453.S33   1996   95-42725
636'.9322—dc20   CIP

Contents

Foreword

Timid, inquisitive and clever, the domestic rabbit responds readily to the affections of its owner and is Britain's favourite garden pet, being topped only by the dog and cat in the popularity pecking order.

The charming nursery-book concept of Peter Rabbit and his cabbage-patch friends, and that rascally but lovable Bugs Bunny, encourages the idea that the rabbit is the easiest animal in the world to keep – after all, it does not bark or indeed make any unpleasant noise; it does not have to be taken for walks; and can be fed and housed inexpensively.

If all this sounds idyllic and idiotically easy, I must warn you that it is not. If you want to keep your rabbits healthy and value their quality of life, it is worth taking a little time and trouble to study the subject thoroughly before setting out for the pet shop or your nearest rabbit breeder. Even if you already have rabbits, the best way to make progress is to listen to the experts. Some will give you good advice, others not – so it is also essential to read as much as you can. Again, not every book gives the right advice, in fact some can be dangerously misleading when it comes to advice on feeding and housing.

As editor of the rabbit magazine *Fur & Feather* I am always being asked, 'Can you recommend a really good book on rabbit keeping?' Well, here it is! Long recognised by 'the Fancy' as the rabbit keeper's bible, John Sandford's new edition of *The Domestic Rabbit* is beyond a shadow of a doubt the best and most comprehensive book on rabbit-keeping ever published.

The author covers the value of the rabbit as both pet and companion, or as a highly-prized exhibition animal bred in a range of colours, shapes and patterns to an exacting standard of perfection. Every fact that is of interest to the rabbit-keeper is included. There is also reference to the rabbit's valuable use in the commercial world.

Like many traditional rabbit-keepers, I was brought up in wartime when the need to breed rabbits for flesh and fur was a basic necessity; millions of Britons took up rabbit-keeping as a means of supplementing their meagre meat ration; many kept Angoras for their wool, or used rabbit pelts to make gloves and other garments. The British Rabbit Council (BRC) under its Secretary John Sandford (later to be its

Chairman and then Life President) showed us the basic rules of rabbit husbandry as well as encouraged us to take up one or more of the many breeds that already existed, or were in the process of being created. Thus began the post-war boom of the 'rabbit show' where BRC members exhibited their best animals at events up and down the country. British stock soon gained an enviable reputation world-wide and many top quality animals were subsequently exported to other countries.

Fifty years on, 'the Fancy' has changed considerably; during that time the BRC was joined by the British Commercial Rabbit Association (BCRA). The former governs the exhibition side of the rabbit fancy and is responsible for the introduction of new breeds whilst offering a great deal of advice via its county advisors, free leaflets, etc., to all rabbit keepers. The BRC's original aim 'to encourage the production, marketing and consumption of the products of the rabbit (i.e. fur, wool and flesh)' was removed in recent years at the request of its members, but these aims are of course recognised by the BCRA.

Recently the BRC set up a committee to study the health and welfare of the rabbit and the author has devoted a new chapter to this subject in his book, as well as increasing his already extensive coverage of diseases.

The first edition of *The Domestic Rabbit* was published in 1957 and was followed by subsequent revisions, the last one being in 1986. They are a unique guide to the history of the rabbit and its every-changing 'Fancy'. Now we have the Fifth Edition from Europe's most distinguished rabbit expert. Completely revised and with new chapters – the one on the house rabbit will delight many modern rabbit keepers – the book contains colour photographs of 47 breeds.

A previous Editor of *Fur & Feather* once wrote: 'I would not be without *The Domestic Rabbit*. Whatever its price, I would save up a long time to buy it. The truth is that the book is the most comprehensive work on rabbit keeping ever written. It is also far and away the best. "Complete" is the word for it. Fanciers have never had a book comparable to it.'

No matter how many times you pick up this book, you will learn something new. Everything you want to know, or will ever need to know, on the subject of the rabbit is within the pages of this excellent book. I cannot recommend it highly enough.

Patricia Gaskin
Editor of *Fur & Feather*

Preface

Since the first edition of this book was published almost forty years ago there have been many changes in rabbit husbandry worldwide. Some of these changes have been of benefit to the rabbit and rabbit husbandry, whilst others have not. In order to reflect these many changes, this fifth edition of the book has been extensively revised and is now substantially larger, with three new chapters and 47 colour photographs.

In the last few decades, great developments have occurred within the commercial rabbit industry which currently produces over a million tonnes of rabbit meat per year throughout the world. Modern technology has been introduced and many units involved in the production of rabbit meat have greatly increased in size. Countries, such as China, which previously have not been known for their commercial use of the rabbit are now producing both rabbit meat and angora wool.

At the other extreme of rabbit keeping, there has been the emergence of the companion rabbit, also known in France as the apartment rabbit and in America as the house rabbit. Companion rabbits are distinct from pet rabbits and there is now a greater understanding of the beneficial relationship that can develop between man and rabbit. Particular emphasis is placed on the companion animal in this text and also on the welfare of the domestic rabbit.

In the last twenty years, much work has been dedicated to the welfare of the rabbit. This work, when conducted correctly, has led to advances in the understanding of the rabbit's needs. However, whilst most animal welfare organisations do much good there are those that may be doing harm as a result of their lack of understanding of the true needs of the animal. Rabbit keeping enthusiasts, of necessity, pay the greatest attention to the welfare of their animals and it is hoped that others also concerned with the welfare of the rabbit will learn as much as possible about the animal.

One area where there have been advances in rabbit husbandry is in the attempt to use the rabbit as a food source in those third world countries where food is so badly needed. A small section of this book deals with this use of the rabbit. The rabbit can provide a high quality protein food for man and as such can be of great importance in developing countries. Those countries that have started to investigate the use of the rabbit in this way have met with a good deal of success.

The rabbit has always been what might be termed as the 'Cinderella' of the livestock exhibiting world. However, the increasing awareness that rabbit keeping can bring both enjoyment and a reduction in the stress of everyday life, coupled with the changes occurring in the larger animal exhibiting world, may go some way towards changing this. There is, quite apart from the pleasure which domestic rabbit keeping on a small scale brings to the owner, a great deal of mental relaxation to be derived from the hobby. This psychological value is increased by the many social activities which are part and parcel of the rabbit fancy.

In this country, although the exhibition side of rabbit keeping has remained basically the same since the late 1940s, some changes have occurred. The nature of shows has changed somewhat with an increasing number of female exhibitors and a more active social side to rabbit exhibiting. Also, there has been an acceleration in the number of new breeds introduced and established and as a result a decline in popularity of a number of older breeds. The fifth edition contains details of sixteen new breeds and for the first time includes colour photographs of 47 breeds that are covered in the book. Unfortunately illustrations could not be found, despite much effort, for the rare breeds of Beige or Isabella, Blanc de Hotot, Blanc de Termonde, Deilenaar, Pointed Beveren and Squirrel.

One of the reasons for writing the first edition of this book all those years ago was for use as a text for the national examinations in rabbit husbandry. Whilst the national examination board has since disbanded it is still important that people involved in the keeping of domestic rabbits do not limit their knowledge to their specific area of interest. Rabbit keeping has many sides and all rabbit keepers have something to offer to their counterparts. It is for this reason that this book attempts to cover as many aspects of rabbit husbandry as possible.

John Sandford

THE AUTHOR

John Sandford died in April 1995. His passion for the rabbit began as a boy when he visited his local livestock market and met a rabbit breeder from Hampton Wick named Christopher Wren. Chris Wren was one of the great rabbit men of his day, having created the Chinchilla Giganta. When the boy asked, 'Will you teach me about rabbits?' the reply was, 'Come and see me next Saturday'. John Sandford duly arrived at the Wren rabbitry and was given his first lesson. Clean out all the hutches' (and there were plenty of them), 'Then report back to me'. This exercise was repeated each Saturday until Mr Wren was satisfied that the next lesson – handling the rabbit – could begin. Wren was a good teacher, perhaps recognising that John Sandford's interest in the domestic rabbit was to become legendary.

After a period in the Indian army John Sandford went to Magdalen College, Cambridge to study agriculture.

In 1950 John Sandford became the Secretary of the British Rabbit Council. Three years later myxomatosis arrived in this country and he was appointed by the Minister of Agriculture to serve on a myxomatosis advisory committee. He also fought many cases on members' behalfs to enforce the provisions of the Allotments Act, and helped to draw up the Pet Act. He also liaised with government departments and research organisations worldwide. John Sandford remained Secretary of the British Rabbit Council until 1965, and then became its Chairman until major heart surgery forced him to retire in 1973. He returned in 1985 to assist the BRC in an advisory capacity and in 1994 was elected its Life President. Although suffering poor health, John Sandford completed his revision of *The Domestic Rabbit* in April 1995. He died one week later, whilst holidaying in France.

Acknowledgements

Grateful thanks are extended to all the various institutes, libraries and individuals worldwide who gave the author valuable help with research for this book. Special thanks go to Mrs Joyce Potter for her support and help with research and proof-reading; the British Rabbit Council and Eric and Pat Gaskin of *Fur & Feather* for the provision of breed photographs; Ken Lettington, president of the British Rabbit Council, and John Self for technical advice; and finally to all those within the Fancy who gave their help and advice during the latter stages of publication after the untimely death of the author.

Chapter 1

History and Aspects of the Rabbit

THE EARLIEST RECORDS

The first records in the history of man's relationship with the rabbit start with the Phoenicians at the end of the second millennium BC. They gave the name Spain to the country where the rabbit originated and where they found rabbits so widespread. The rabbit did not spread quickly as it did in later centuries, for eight hundred years later, none of the Greek writers mention the rabbit, which indicates that it had not reached the eastern Mediterranean by then. No further records occur until the second century BC, when some mention of it in Corsica is made by Polybius.

The next, and certainly the most important, text is that of Varro (116–27 BC) who in his eightieth year wrote his treatise on farming, *De Re Rustica*. In the book, he speaks of what 'is still called by its ancient name of hare-warren' (leporarium). He says 'Everyone knows, too, that if you put in but a few hares of both sexes, the warren will swarm with them in a short time, so prolific is this quadruped ... often when a litter has not long been born, they are found to have others inside them.' And again 'There is also the recent fashion, now general, of fattening them – by taking them from the warren, shutting them up in cages, and fattening them in confinement.' There can be no doubt from this description that the Romans kept rabbits in warrens and also in cages. It seems certain that some of the details given of hares during those times, really applied to the rabbit and not the hare.

Pliny the Elder (c. 23-79 AD), wrote 'There is also a species of hare, in Spain, which is called cuniculus; it is extremely prolific, and produces famine in the Balearic islands, by destroying the harvests', and 'It is well known that the inhabitants of the Balearic islands begged of the late Emperor Augustus the aid of a number of soldiers, to prevent the too rapid increase of these animals.'

DOMESTICATION

Charles Darwin, writing in 1888 believed that the writings of Confucius (551–479 BC) indicated that the rabbit was probably domesticated in China at this time, but most authorities have considered this to be incorrect. However, Chen Yaowang

1

(1984) takes the view that the present domestic rabbit originated from the native wild white rabbit of China, also *Oryctolagus cuniculus*, and that the domestication of the rabbit began in the Han dynasty (220–202 BC). But this suggestion is opposed to the views of other Chinese scientists who consider the domestic rabbit in China was introduced as the wild (domestic?) rabbit from Europe, via the Silk Road during relatively modern times.

It is often suggested that the first true domestication of the rabbit took place in medieval France and that it was not the Romans who first domesticated the rabbit. The grounds for this belief are that selection from a warren for killing, by the Romans, would work in favour of the perpetuation of wild characteristics, that is, when the animals were caught up for fattening, the wildest would remain and those most likely to be tamed would be caught and eaten. There is, however, another hypothesis. The Romans were aware that the rabbits bred in relative captivity and if they put them, as Varro says, in cages, and young were born therein as must surely have happened, after a period the Romans might very easily have continued to keep them in cages for breeding, thus reaching the usual definition of a stage of domestication.

Certainly the start at least of the domestication of the rabbit, then, began some 2000 years ago; it is, thus, one of the last species of common animals to be domest-icated. Others have been domesticated at least five times longer.

Even before domestication began, man started to move rabbits from one place to another where they became established. He has continued as the great distributor of the rabbit to the present time. Whether the Romans brought the rabbit to Britain 2000 years or so ago has often been the subject of debate. There is no question that they brought many of the other food animals and birds which they greatly appreciated. The pheasant, the quail, the edible dormouse and others were certainly so brought in. It is probable then that they brought the first rabbits to England. If they did the rabbits did not survive, which is not surprising with the range of carnivorous animals then in Britain. It was not until the Norman Conquest that the animals became established in England, after a long presence in warrens (or preserves) in France.

There was very probably some natural spread of the Spanish rabbits into Southern France, but almost certainly man also brought rabbits into France. Since Roman times, the pleasures of hunting have driven men to release rabbits on their estates, often in enclosed warrens, and this has accounted for much of its spread. The same process still occurs today. For this purpose it is probable that the original wild stock was procured. Domesticated animals would have been too valuable to use in this way.

The completion of the domestication process occurred in the 5th or 6th century and very probably it was the French medieval monastic establishments that were responsible. They were also responsible for the early spread of the domesticated animal. The domestication stage spread over a number of centuries. There is a belief that it was only the wild rabbits that escaped from warrens, but it is probable that at a quite early date there was also the introduction into the warrens of the domesticated types. There are records of movements of domestic rabbits as early as the 6th century.

The speed with which the domestication of apparently wild rabbits can be accomplished at the present time, may of course be that it is done with apparently wild, but really feral, stock. It is sometimes suggested that it is extremely difficult to obtain fully 'tamed' rabbits by handling and selection from apparently wild rabbits. It has, however, relatively frequently, been done, and a year or two with several generations, usually suffices. The reverse is of course also true. If domestic rabbits are allowed total freedom (but usually protection and assistance is also necessary in the beginning), they will revert relatively quickly to the characteristics of the wild type.

Domestication has a number of effects. Whilst the animals become less shy and timid, the longer term physical effects include:

- usually an increase in weight up to as much as five times the weight of the wild animal;
- a reduction in brain weight, eye size, and proportion of dry skeleton to liveweight, of over 20% compared with the wild animal of the same weight;
- a considerably larger proportionate reduction in heart size.

These are, of course, all features not essential to survival when the animals are otherwise protected. There are also increases in fecundity and in fertility over a lengthened breeding season. More apparent however are the changes which, usually, occur in bodily conformation.

The rabbit was introduced into England by the Normans, probably during the 12th century. Certainly towards the end of the 14th century they featured in the laws of the country. That the wild rabbit had become fairly widespread by the 15th century in England is indicated by the fact that some 4000 'conies' were part of the feast celebrating the appointment of the Archbishop of York and Chancellor of England in 1465.

From at least as early as the 12th century, domestic rabbits were being transported from country to country in some parts of Europe; records show animals being sent from France to Germany and almost certainly other countries. Whatever the source, by the 16th century there were different domestic types or colours of rabbits in England, some of which had certainly originated here.

EARLY HOUSING

By the end of the Middle Ages domesticated rabbits were widely spread. Georgii Agricola in the mid 16th century gives details of different colours of rabbits which were being kept in Germany. Thomas Tusser, writing his *A hundreth good points of husbandrie* in 1557, says in the list of work for January, 'Let Doe go to buck, with Conie good luck, Spare Labour nor monie, store borough (i.e. warren) with conie.' There can be little doubt that he is making a distinction between rabbits kept confined in cages of some sort and rabbits in the warren. By the 17th century some domestic rabbit keeping had become established in England and elsewhere.

In 1600 a translation of a French book was published which discusses rabbits in detail. It refers to the French situation but it becomes clear that the warren was not to be confused with rabbits running wild in a wood, and also that a 'clapper' (i.e. French clapier or rabbitry of hutches) was necessary for the proper conduct of the warren by re-stocking, and the fattening of rabbits. The clapper would consist of 'certaine small lodgings paved with boards', and the book appears to be the first to recommend post-partum mating.

Gervase Markham, a most prolific writer on agricultural matters in the early part of the 17th century, has in several books much to say about rabbits, both wild and tame. In *A Way to Get Wealth* (1631) he writes that 'The female or Doe Conies are wonderful in their increase, and bring forth young ones every month: Therefore, when you keep them tame in Boxes, you must observe them, and as soone as they have kindled, to put them to the Buck. The boxes, in which you shall keep your tame Conies, would be made of thin Wainscot-board, some two feet square, and one foot high; with a lesser room in which the Conie may lodge and kindle ... and thus you may make boxe upon boxe in different stories.'

His directions for the choice of bucks is explicit. 'As for the choice of these tame rich Conies, you shall not, as in other Cattel, look not to their shape, but to their richness.' Size was important but the silver colour (richness), with fur 'thicke, deepe, smooth and shining' was paramount. After the silver 'a blacke coat without silver hairs, though it be not reckoned a rich coat, yet it is to be preferred before a white, a pyde, a yellow, a dun or a grey'. The best rabbits were worth five times as much as others, and the best skins eight or ten times other skins, fetching as much as 2 shillings or more.

Mortimer (in 1707) remarked that 'many make great Profit of them by keeping of them in Hutches near great Towns, ... for the tame Rabbets must lie dry, and warm, or else they will not Breed in Winter, which is the chief time of their Profit.' He also mentions most unusually 'the White Shock Turky Rabbet' by which he means the Angora.

Although the rabbit court and rabbit pit had been in existence for very many years it was at this time beginning to be realised that there were greater profits to be made by keeping rabbits in hutches rather than in pits.

Any number of agricultural books were written in the 18th century, most of which included some details of rabbits, both in warrens and in hutches. Without fail they enlarged upon the profits to be made. It must however be said that quite often they were copied one from another, indeed in some cases word for word, a situation that sometimes exists today.

Thus in 1771 *The Country Gentleman and Farmer's Treasury of Useful Knowledge* was written by an unknown author, to the title of which was added 'To which are added a curious Treatise on the Breeding and Management of Wild and Tame Conies'. This item was entirely a copy of the words of Gervase Markham on tame rabbits, written 140 years before.

It is somewhat singular that it is difficult to find at this time much mention of Angoras or their wool in England. It is peculiar because the Angora and its culture must have been known, for in 1789 there was published in Dresden a book of some 114 pages which dealt in detail with Angora keeping. It records that in 1777 the 'English Silkhaired Rabbit' (one of the names by which the Angora was then known) was taken from England to Germany where they were found to be very useful. In a fairly short period they were exported from Dresden to Vienna, Prague, Bayreuth and Holland. The author adds that Angoras were to be found in France, Italy, Denmark and England.

In England although warrens had been increasing in number slowly from the 14th century by the 18th and 19th centuries a great increase in warrening as a commercial activity took place. It was generally considered that poor quality land invariably paid better with rabbits than any other crop. Some details of warrens in the early 19th century give profits of some £518 a year on a total expenditure of £332. These costs are fascinating compared with today: annual rent of farm, £250, full time warrener £31 (including rent and two cows), three killers for 12 weeks, including cost of board, £20.8s.

Whilst many were much in favour of warrens opposition occurred because of its dreary appearance, the impossibility of growing trees, the impossibility of all field sports in the area, the encouragement of poachers and, on moral grounds, that the system used less labour than other forms of farming!

Rabbit dung was very highly prized as a fertiliser. There are records of farmers in Buckinghamshire who were so anxious to get it that they would transport it from London where it was 'sold so cheap as about 6d a bushel' (about 1.25 cubic feet)! This would mean that the price per ton would be at least equivalent to some four weeks wages of a labourer at that time. The manure seems to have contributed quite a lot to the profits made from the domestic rabbit.

During the second half of the 19th century what could be called a split between the warren and hutch rabbit keeping occurred. There was a definite movement to small-scale rabbit keeping in hutches. The cottage economy became the subject of much agricultural writing. From this time on, with increasing frequency, small handbooks were published encouraging the keeping of rabbits on a small scale. Some of them, towards the end of the period, were very good, and included an excellent colour plate *Book of the Rabbit* (1881). But others were very poor indeed with advice which certainly meant that little success would attend the enterprise. In very many cases, general farming books contained sections devoted to rabbit keeping. But almost without exception these books had one thing in common – they all treated the subject by linking together meat rabbits, children's pets, the simplicity of rabbit keeping and the fancy rabbit. It was solely a home or cottage economy with some overtones of the rabbit fancy.

In the 1880s and 1890s in England, agriculture was in a very poor state. Attempts were being made by the Government to exterminate the wild rabbit on agricultural land and the Ground Game Act of 1880 was introduced, which gave all occupiers a right to kill rabbits on their land. One result of the legislation, however, was that fears grew that the supply of rabbit meat would greatly diminish and in just a few years the price increased by 50%.

This gave rise to a great deal of discussion on the subject of rabbits as food and how they should be kept in the future, and two books, which had a great influence, were published. These were: *Rabbits as a Food Supply*, by G.F. Morant, 1883; and *Rabbits for Profit and Rabbits for Powder*, by R.J. Lloyd-Price, 1884. Both dealt with hutch-bred rabbits, although Lloyd-Price added a section on 'shooting warrens'.

Morant's book led to his name being given to a particular type of rabbit keeping by the use of a movable ark with a wire-meshed floor, through which the rabbits could graze, with a wooden roof and sides except for part of the front. It could be used for growing stock or, with a nest box, as a breeding hutch. The Morant hutch was moved usually twice per day over grass. This system, sometimes with modifications was still used occasionally until the 1950s. It was also the system mainly used in large-scale farming in the CIS in the late 1920s.

Lloyd-Price firmly believed that if his hutch system of rabbit farming 'had been more thoroughly explained … the notion would not have been so prevalent that rabbit farming upon a large scale was, as poultry farming is admitted to have been, bound to fail'. That the idea of large-scale rabbit farming, in hutches, became something of a fashion is indicated by these books being reprinted several times at short intervals. Within 15 years, however, there was very little large-scale commercial rabbit farming with this or any other system.

THE BELGIAN HARE BOOM

There is perhaps some link between these writers and the subsequent Belgian Hare 'boom' in America, for both authors wrote in one way or another of Belgian Hares, and there is little doubt that this information was communicated to America which started off the Belgian Hare craze.

The American Belgian Hare boom which started in the 1890s is of interest in the history of the domestic rabbit, for it was the first instance in which modern forms of advertising rabbit farming played an important part in the rapidity and extent of the spread of that craze. It also introduced new selling techniques; for example, the seller offering to buy back animals produced and hence seemingly guaranteeing a profit to the purchaser. And it gave great impetus to the rabbit fancy in America, linking this with commercial rabbit farms.

Belgian Hare farms established in such places as Minnesota, caused uproar amongst farmers in the North-West, resulting in petitions to Congress demanding action and claiming rabbits to be of doubtful food value but without doubt a menace to agriculture. A situation repeated often in other countries. Finally the craze developed to such an extent, that a buyer from America established the highest prices ever paid for a rabbit in Britain. The then enormous sum of £600 was paid for a single Belgian Hare buck, this being the equivalent at the present time, to a sum of over £27 000!

The Belgian Hare boom is noticeable also because despite the fact that it was probably one of the worst breeds that could have been selected for meat production, it was the one selected. The confusion which existed between the Belgian Hare of England and the large Belgian Hare of Belgium (certainly much better for meat production) and the Brown Hare contributed to this situation.

The Belgian Hare craze collapsed in less than 20 years and closed down when 'the public at large learnt that the Belgian Hare was indeed a rabbit like all others, causing the animal to be condemned and execrated' as remarked by a senior US Department of Agriculture official in the first US Department of Agriculture Farmers Bulletin dealing with the domestic rabbit.

It is interesting also that one of the leading Belgian Hare breeders in England, Ernest Wilkins, was so encouraged by the interest in its commercial use, that he wrote a book entitled *The Belgian Hare – The Business Rabbit of the World*. The first edition was published in 1896 and the second in 1901. The book is now rare and few were sold. Perhaps because only those engaged in the sale of Belgian Hares to the American market could believe the title!

The numerous failures that occurred during this affair – as so frequently since – clearly illustrate again how ignorance, coupled often with avarice, and often also the problem of disease, have caused such a high rate of failure in the rabbit world. It was also the clearest possible indication that no livestock industry can be based solely upon the sale of livestock to other breeders. Whilst the Belgian Hare boom was such a disaster, it certainly helped to establish the present very widespread rabbit fancy in America.

INTRODUCTION OF THE RABBIT INTO VARIOUS COUNTRIES

The first attempt to introduce the rabbit into Australia using domestic animals was in 1788, with some five domestic rabbits. There followed several other importations which did not establish themselves. It was only when a consignment of 24 wild rabbits were shipped from England in 1859, to stock a farm near Geelong, Victoria, for sport, that it became firmly established. The speed with which it spread was astonishing. By 1880, 20 years later, the rabbits had moved a distance of some 300 miles. In the next six years they moved over 350 miles.

In New Zealand, many early introductions, the first in the very early 1800s and all probably of domestic or recently feral types, were unsuccessful. In the 1860s however, introductions of wild animals took a similar course to the explosive spread in Australia.

In many other countries the wild rabbit was established by introduction, including such diverse places as Chile, the Swedish Island of Gotland and parts of Norway, Lower Egypt, Uganda in Africa and very many others. In the last century or so, rabbits (mostly domestic) have been introduced into literally hundreds of islands where they have often become established as feral and have often reached plague proportions.

At the start of the Belgian Hare boom, previously discussed, a lighthouse keeper in the islands off the Washington coast, purchased some to add to his income by selling them in the Seattle markets. A new lighthouse keeper simply let all the domestic animals loose, when they became feral, until 1924 when the Navy Department requested assistance to exterminate them as they were causing such damage.

These and many similar cases prompted a ban on the importation of domestic rabbits into various countries. For example, South Africa imposed a ban on imports in the early 1920s, although at that time there were numbers of domestic rabbits in the country. The ban was lifted a few years later when a very small but thriving rabbit industry was established and the government even went so far as to authorise a small amount of research on the domestic rabbit. A second ban was later imposed and it was not until the end of the 1970s that this ban was lifted again. The same sort of ban with the illogical reasoning behind it was imposed in many countries.

ADAPTABILITY OF THE RABBIT

A study of the introductions which have been made almost world wide indicates two important features. The first is the enormous adaptability of the rabbit, both wild and domestic, which can exist in conditions ranging from the tropical to the Arctic on an exceptionally wide and varied diet. This adaptability has important implications for those who are interested in the use of the rabbit for the benefit of man.

The second point is something of a paradox. It is that the domesticated animals have on many occasions only managed to survive with the aid of man until they have established a firm foothold in their new environment. In other cases domestic rabbits have been able, in apparently exceptional circumstances, to establish themselves in areas which would not at first sight seem promising.

Notwithstanding the knowledge that true domestic stock usually have great difficulty in establishing themselves in the wild, resistance to domestic rabbit farming, not only in Australia and New Zealand, but in other countries, where there are far less bitter memories, has been based on the totally mistaken belief that if some domestic rabbits were allowed to become feral they would survive happily, return to the truly wild state, and, often remaining as giant rabbits, become an even greater danger.

The damage and loss to agriculture and forestry throughout much of the world is caused not only by the food that the rabbit consumes, but by its destruction of young trees and the damage that occurs through its burrowing. The first plague of rabbits was, as mentioned above, in the Balearics, when the occupants were almost driven out of their country by rabbit damage to their harvests. Since then, some 2000 years ago, there have been innumerable others. The costs of the wild rabbit in different parts of the world are incalculable but astronomical. They run into very many millions of pounds each year. For example, the additional annual value in 1953 of the sheep wool and meat crop in Australia, attributable solely to the reduction of the wild rabbit by myxomatosis, was estimated to be of the order of £35 000 000. Again, when myxomatosis entered the UK, it was welcomed with delight by the majority of the farming community. Estimate of the yearly cost to farming and forestry varied from a minimum of £50 million to over £100 million or more per annum at today's values.

REASONS FOR KEEPING RABBITS

As there has been for at least 150 years, there exists an interacting relationship between wild, pet, exhibition and commercial rabbits. There has also been an odd relationship between the rabbit farmer and the rabbit fancier. Some may change from one to the other and some may be both, but this is unusual in the UK where there has always existed a coldness between them.

That the fancier has maintained a wide gene pool cannot be doubted, and this must be of benefit to the rabbit world in general. To many rabbit fanciers it often seems somehow wrong to utilise the domestic for meat production. There are today a greater number of fanciers throughout the world who select breeding stock for non utilitarian characteristics than there are meat, fur or wool producers, and this has unquestionably influenced the development of a purely utilitarian industry.

The philosophies and aims of the rabbit farmer and the rabbit fancier are completely different. The commercial producer must be concerned to produce the largest number possible of animals of a uniform good quality, for meat or wool or fur, at the lowest possible overall cost. The rabbit fancier on the other hand is concerned with the production of single individuals which resemble to the highest degree possible a somewhat arbitrary exhibition standard. A number of characteristics of this standard are obtained by processes which involve but little certainty.

What has always been necessary for the establishment of the intensive (or indeed semi-intensive) commercial production of rabbit meat has been the development of pure meat type rabbits, with no concessions whatsoever being made to the exhibition requirements or mentality. Exactly the same problem has occurred in the field of Angora wool production. Indeed in this case it is true to say that some of the best exhibition characteristics are positively opposed to important commercial requirements.

THE WAR YEARS

It is in times of war, protracted ones at least, or other times of scarcity of food, that the rabbit is utilised most. This of course, is due to its ability to produce meat from foods that cannot be easily utilised for other animals or man, the rapidity with which that meat can be produced and the fact that people who do not normally produce food can do so with relatively little training and space.

The 1914–18 war produced a great increase in rabbit keeping in many countries. In the UK, great efforts were made and the number of rabbit keepers for meat for local consumption, increased by an estimated 15 times. Quite a few of these later became fanciers.

Rabbit keeping during the 1939–45 war increased to an even greater extent. When the possibilities of war became apparent, considerable thought was given to domestic food production. Rabbits featured quite largely in these deliberations and reports were made to the Minister of Agriculture concerning the actions which should be taken some time before war became imminent.

It was decided that government action would have to be limited to widespread encouragement and training and possibly a small allotment of feeding stuffs which were not entirely satisfactory for other animals. Rabbits would have to exist on green foods, waste from the home and any foods that the home producer could grow himself. Some prior organisation took place and soon after the war started officials were appointed to encourage rabbit breeding.

The numbers of rabbit breeders claiming rations for breeding does increased until well over 100 000, mostly in one or other of the 3000 rabbit breeding clubs which sprang up, were involved. The actual number of breeders was, however, very substantially more than this, for very many breeders did not think much of bran, even as a supplement and did not claim it, or had insufficient breeding does.

Bran rationing ended in July 1953, the number of claimants having dropped a good deal. Some bureaucratic circles considered this an indication of a steady decline in rabbit keeping. It was nothing of the sort. Much other evidence indicated quite the reverse. A survey conducted then, showed well over three-quarters of a million rabbit breeders in the UK still kept breeding stock.

The same encouragement of rabbit keeping for meat has occurred in all countries subjected to war and other periods of food scarcity. The current attempts to encourage the use of the rabbit in Third World countries is a classic example. It might be mentioned that some 40 years ago attempts to do this were made through what were then known as Empire Livestock Officers. Some of the present domesticated stocks of rabbits in many countries of the old Empire are in fact a legacy of that period.

THE OSTEND RABBIT

Whilst there had been an industry based on the warren rabbit for a considerable period, a rabbit industry based on the hutched domestic rabbit can only be said to have started spasmodically in the UK in the early part of the19th century. In France the rabbit industry started up slightly later but of course that industry continued with far fewer interruptions than the English, and has progressed infinitely further.

The commencement of any industry is difficult to establish accurately and certainly rabbit husbandry, merging as it does over a long period with a cottage economy type of rabbit keeping, is particularly difficult. Furthermore commercial rabbit farming started at greatly different periods in different countries. In the first years of the 19th century there were reports of one or two large farmers near London, with 1500 to 2000 hutched does each. These had by 1815 stopped production. Most of the supplies of rabbit meat came from the country, the animals being kept in small cages in huts. There were, however, a number of smaller producers actually in London. It was apparently the custom to feed cereals to a great extent and disease did not appear to be a problem. From the middle of the century increasing numbers of domestic rabbits (mostly carcases) came from the Continent. Estimates between 350 000 and 500 000 per week have been given, but these figures are almost certainly too high, although an average of 5 million per year of 'tames' were recorded at Leadenhall market in London alone in the early 1900s.

During the last quarter of the 19th century, the term Ostend rabbit became synonymous with the best quality of domestic rabbit ('tame' as it was always called) and a particular method of dressing the carcase for display. At the same time increasing amounts of wild rabbit meat were also being imported from Australia and New Zealand which all prevented any large-scale increases in domestic rabbit farming.

RABBIT FUR AND WOOL INDUSTRIES

The 1920s saw attempts to start both a rabbit fur and a rabbit wool industry. By 1920 the Fur Board Ltd. had been established. It was the first true co-operative and its members sent in their dried rabbit pelts and received immediately a percentage of the market value. After the skins had been sold, the surplus was divided amongst the members. By 1930, the membership of the Fur Board had increased to slightly over 3000 members. The size of the Angora wool industry is difficult to estimate, but a census in 1928 established that there were a minimum of 1300 Angora breeders and a minimum of over 100 000 breeding Angoras, not including animals kept solely for wool. That domestic rabbit meat, at this time, was still in demand is shown by the import and market sales figures. These show a total of all rabbit meat of the order of 30 000 tonnes per year, probably one third of this being domestic rabbit.

During the 1920s, both the fur industry and the wool industry developed to a fair extent, and in some cases thriving enterprises were established. Prices of as much as 10 shillings each for the best skins were obtained, this being equivalent to about one quarter of a week's wage for an agricultural worker. The meat, of course, was sold on the meat markets. By the end of the 1920s it seemed that at last a rabbit industry would develop. However, in the early 1930s enormous numbers of Russian furs (not many rabbit) came into the country, the great depression occurred and the fur market collapsed. Angora wool producers suffered no better. This was the situation by 1939.

The interest in rabbit husbandry during the 1939–45 war and the knowledge of American rabbit farming practices, generated an interest among a number of mostly ex-servicemen (and women), and some slight movement was made in rabbit keeping for profit. It was, however, the advent of myxomatosis in 1953, with the almost immediate fall in the quantities of hatting fur available and the thought that rabbit meat would need to be replaced, which was probably the most significant stimulant to encouraging attempts at large-scale rabbit farming.

Rabbit fur was the sole material used in the manufacture of bowler hats and the hatting fur industry was a very substantial one, using many millions of skins from English and Australian wild rabbits and millions more from Europe, which included considerable numbers of domestic skins. Some influential members of the industry encouraged in several ways the development of the new industry.

In the case of the Angora, there were only very small-scale enterprises, mostly producing wool for home use or as a cottage industry. In the 1980s there was a surge in interest with the importation of German Angoras of commercial type. Until then there were no Angoras other than exhibition type, which however, produced a very fine type of wool in modest amounts.

The first large-scale farm, based to some extent on the American wire-floor self cleaning system, fairly short litter intervals, but above all pelleted specially designed feeding stuffs, was started in the south of England in 1957. It grew to a unit of some 600 breeding does, using the services of a geneticist and a statistician to control the breeding systems, in order to establish specialist hybrid lines. It was supported by a consortium of a major feeding stuffs manufacturer, the largest meat (and grocery) retailer in the country and an extensive agricultural estate. It was fairly successful but after some years, on change of management a part was sold and the remainder closed down, after a total life of some 15 years. Similar enterprises, on a smaller scale were also established.

RABBIT ASSOCIATIONS

In 1960 the British Rabbit Council founded the Commercial Rabbit Association (CRA), whose members then started to attempt to organise and establish an industry. It collected and published information and commenced an accredited breeders scheme in an attempt to improve the general stock of commercial rabbits and to try to prevent dishonest dealers from selling poor animals at high prices. The CRA brought together everyone with interests in a commercial rabbit industry. The members included producers of meat animals and breeding stock, manufacturers of feeding stuffs, cages and equipment, medicines and disinfectant, veterinarians, rabbit processors, meat retailers and so on. The majority of members were small-scale breeders, with probably, on average, less than 30 breeding does and usually most of them had insufficient capital. Many failed.

Although the previous attempts by national bodies to form co-operatives had failed (for example the National Utility Rabbit Club in 1910 to 1921 and the Fur Board), the CRA after a few years encouraged the formation of rabbit producer groups. These groups were never formal co-operatives but consisted of producers within usually an area of about 30 miles radius. In many cases they acted as bulk buying agents for their members and as collecting points for the rabbits for processing from the smaller producer. The producer group also acted as a forum for discussion and instruction, particularly for the newcomer to the industry. The success of each group depended almost invariably on two or three persons (and in some cases only one) and usually the demands upon their time meant that they retired and the group eventually failed. At one time there were as many as 60 groups in the country. Almost all the groups had ceased to exist by the 1980s but one or two still remain.

There are today some well-established profitable rabbit farms, but, they are the exception. At most at any one time in the UK, there are probably about 1500 commercial rabbit meat producers of which at most 100 establishments could be called professional rabbit farms. In the 1970s the rabbit industry earned itself the nickname of 'the eighteen month industry' as a reflection that the majority of people who went into rabbit farming for profit, left within eighteen months or so. There were several reasons for these failures.

Possibly the most important was that the majority of the entrants to the industry were completely untrained in any form of livestock production. They were often led to believe that rabbit farming was very easy. The literature of unscrupulous dealers in stock proclaimed (and in some cases still today proclaim) that 'Anyone can make money by breeding rabbits,' and 'It's so simple anyone can be successful'. Totally unbelievable by anyone with the slightest knowledge of rabbit husbandry, the exaggerations and falsehoods told by some dealers are unfortunately often very successful.

An example of one major breeder/dealer's advertisement claimed that his 219 best does produced an average of 123 young each in one year, whilst on average his best 216 and his worst 216 does together produced on average 91.5 young each in one year. It is improbable that the very best does produced as many as 50 young per year. Furthermore, it was claimed that each square foot of rabbit housing would produce over six times as much profit per square foot as the Ministry of Agriculture figures showed was the highest profit per square feet for broiler chicken production. An even more exaggerated claim.

Many people investigating rabbit farming saw what appeared to be very profitable enterprises. It did not occur to them that this was often because the proprietors were selling breeding stock to newcomers at very high prices which they were unable to get later for their own animals. Another major reason was that the newcomer was sold poor quality and diseased animals to establish his or her farm. With such animals there was no possibility that a profit could be made. The problem of disease, which in many cases was considerable, was not easily met by people of limited or no knowledge or experience. The final major reason was the difficulty of marketing their produce which is always sold to rabbit processors. The sales income they obtained did not allow a sufficient margin over costs. In some cases this was due to insufficient production – the average weaners sold per doe in many cases reached less than 40. Food costs were high and winter production, when animals were always in demand, was poor.

The very frequent failures have caused further problems to a rabbit industry in the UK. The knowledge that these failures occur is passed on to those people who would be able to make a success of rabbit farming. Because of the failure rate, they decide not to enter the industry.

Rabbit has not been a popular meat in the UK in recent years, although there are some signs that the attitude to it is changing. There is certainly a smaller per capita consumption than anywhere else in Europe. In Italy for example, the amount consumed per head of population per year is approximately 80 times the amount in the UK. In other countries it is of a similar order.

The attitude towards animals in the UK (particularly those that are not totally recognised as producers of food) militates against the use of the rabbit as meat. The effect of what might be called the 'cuddly bunny' syndrome, at least in England, on the development of the commercial rabbit industry has been unquantifiable but great. The idea of the clever, pretty, little rabbit as a friendly, rascally but lovable character, has very frequently become implanted into the mind first of the child and then of the adult. The nursery bunny doll, beloved of so many children at an age when they are most impressionable is one of the most popular of all children's toys. Strangely, in other countries where to a large extent the rabbit is recognised in the same way, the effect on the meat rabbit market appears to be minimal.

Allied to this there is the situation which occurs as a result of the pet rabbit. This phenomenon started in the Victorian era but continues today. A surprising percentage of entrants into the commercial rabbit industry, albeit on a small scale, do so in the certain knowledge that ' young boys keep rabbits. Obviously therefore it is very easy.' Commercial rabbit farming is not easy and requires talents, knowledge and expertise, and if the sole background of a new entrant is the knowledge of pet keeping, his failure in rabbit farming is certainly partly explained.

The rabbit husbandry world, whether including the fancier and the farmer or not, is given to the formation of associations. In all countries where rabbit breeding is conducted, there are usually national associations for both the exhibition and commercial sides of rabbit husbandry. The fancy national associations, older by far than the commercial associations, often have affiliated to them breed specialist societies which promote their particular breeds of rabbits, and clubs or groups of rabbit breeders in the same area, often with the addition of agricultural societies.

It is fairly common in all countries, that, certainly until the associations become strong enough, there are break away groups, and thus two almost identical bodies are formed. This inevitably leads to a weakening of the interests of all concerned with the inevitable result that costs are increased, and the effectiveness of the organisations is greatly diminished. This, in fact, is what occurred in 1980, with the break away from the Commercial Rabbit Association of the larger rabbit farmers, to form the British Rabbit Federation. After a period of nine years, wiser councils prevailed and the two bodies merged to form the British Commercial Rabbit Association. Almost invariably, all national bodies are under funded.

There are two supra, or multi-national bodies for rabbits. One is the World Rabbit Science Association. The WRSA was founded for professional breeders and scientists. The other, EEAC (in English the European Federation for Aviculture and Rabbit Breeding) was founded over 60 years ago for the exhibition breeders of poultry, pigeons and rabbits.

Apart from associations of rabbit breeders there are, or in many cases have been, other types of establishments of importance. These include research and teaching establishments, both official and commercial.

HISTORY OF THE RABBIT

This then is a very brief introduction to the history of the rabbit. The different aspects which the rabbit has presented over the years, to a great variety of people and an understanding of the existence of these different aspects of the rabbit lead to a fuller understanding of the animal and its life. These different lines running through its long history can best be summarised as follows:

- the original rabbit in Spain which the Phoenicians knew, certainly different in many respects to the wild/feral rabbit in the modern world;
- the rabbit of the Romans, raised in their leporaria and almost certainly, partly if not substantially domesticated and in one form or another taken elsewhere;
- the rabbit in medieval France, there left to remain wild or feral and from other stock to become fully domesticated;
- the rabbit of the warrens, for certainly 600 years providing food and substantial profits, but the countryside in which it lived with a burden of loss;
- the rabbit for sport, being hunted for a thousand years or more and in more recent times one of the main small game animals of the world;
- the rabbit taken by man to so many places where it has most often survived and caused plagues of quite remarkable proportions;
- the rabbit of great variety, developed constantly into new breeds and colours which in many cases themselves become changed and are sometimes lost;
- the rabbit of natural history, the subject of much study by the great naturalists and scientists of the past, and present, Agricola, Aldrovandi, Gesner, Darwin, Leeuwenhoek and thousands of others;
- the rabbit of genetics, the animal used a great deal for the elucidation of the Mendelian laws of inheritance, by the early geneticists Castle, Nachtsheim, Punnet, Crewe and so many others;
- the rabbit of science with its two-fold role, its numerous uses in the study of biological phenomena and disease and its role in the preparation and testing of medicines for use by man;
- the rabbit of the rabbit farmer, with a great number of different types of industry worldwide and its three main products, the meat, the fur, and wool;
- the rabbit of the fancier, worldwide, which, for the last 200 years or so, has been bred by dedicated men and women to produce more and more perfect specimens of the different varieties of rabbits with a passion that builds into intense rivalry in the exhibition world;
- the rabbit of the agricultural farmer and almost invariably his great enemy, the creator of enormous damage to crops and forests, and to be destroyed at all times and in any possible way;
- the rabbit of the child, the hero of innumerable children's books, cartoons, films and videos and from early Victorian times, a beloved pet and the third most popular in England;
- the rabbit so well known to man, for in both its wild and domestic form it is better known than any other animal throughout the world.

Chapter 2

Breeds and Varieties

THE EVOLUTION OF NEW BREEDS

All domestic rabbits throughout the world are the same species, *Oryctolagus cuniculus*. The domestic rabbit is the same species as the wild rabbit, and the different characteristics of all domestic breeds arise through either mutations or by a combination of different inherited characteristics. Selection thereafter modifies the breed or colour variety by an increase or decrease of the modifying genes.

The term 'breed' can be used in a number of different ways, but in the rabbit world it is a group of animals, or populations, which resemble each other more than they do other breeds. Closely coupled with the term breed is the term 'variety'. Consider for example the Chinchilla Giganta and the Chinchilla. Whilst there are other differences, one could say that the most important feature which distinguished these two breeds, is size. In the case of Dutch or English, it is the pattern. In the case of Rex it is the coat.

VARIETIES

The term variety relates to a colour. Thus the Dutch breed has eight different colour varieties. Difficulties however arise in some cases where there are more than two levels of breed or variety. For example, the Rex is a breed having a number of different colour varieties. But the Otter Rex, which is a variety of Rex, has four colours. In some cases therefore the terms are used differently. Some people consider that the Black Rex, for example, is a breed and not a colour variety.

Breeds and varieties are not static. They evolve by selective breeding often at a remarkably rapid rate. Some breeds change over a period of say 40 years, to such an extent that they might not be considered to be the same breed. Furthermore the same breed, perhaps originating separately in two different countries, or being taken from one country to another, may subsequently vary to such an extent that they become recognisably different breeds.

Different breeds are produced and evolve for purely utilitarian purposes or for exhibition and competition. In many cases in the past, those that have been produced for one purpose have often changed to the other, usually from the utilitarian to the fancy. Attempts to produce breeds, or more accurately strains or families, having the best utilitarian characteristics, in particular for the production of meat, have lagged far behind the search for new fancy rabbits. France with, certainly after the war, the largest rabbit industry in the world, has been the leader in this field, followed perhaps by Italy and Spain. In many countries it has been greatly neglected. In the UK it has rested almost entirely with the individual farmer to attempt to improve his own stock by judicious breeding.

On the other hand the increase of fancy breeds has been great. Although the fur breeds started on the basis that they would be of utilitarian value they are now, in the UK, almost solely confined to exhibition purposes.

Prior to 1850, apart from Silvers and occasionally pure colours, the rabbits were usually more or less spotted or patterned and by 1850 the English pattern (Butterfly smut) had gained some form of formal description of excellence or standard, although this pattern then for a time fell from popularity. Colour was not however of much importance, either to the rabbit farmers (or feeders as they were then known, to distinguish them from warreners), or to the fancier. The Lop, with its very enlarged ears and weight, was *par excellence* the fancy exhibit. As Delamer, the leading fancy writer at the time said in 1854, 'Flat Lops are the most unnatural, and therefore the most perfect and valuable rabbits in a fancier's estimation'.

The proliferation of breeds, particularly the fur breeds, in England during the 1920s occurred for several reasons. The main one was the growing interest in the establishment of a fur industry using rabbits. This brought about the importation of Chinchillas from France, from which the Sables were derived, and the Rex following their first discovery in 1919. There was also at this time the synthesis of new breeds. Experimental work at Cambridge to establish the colour of a rabbit homozygous for self, brown and dilution by H. Onslow prior to 1913 (when it was first exhibited in London) produced the Lilac known originally as the Cambridge Blue. Pickard attempting to emulate the wild Silver Fox, produced the Silver Fox rabbit. The Sables, originally rejects produced in litters of Chinchillas, were developed in response to the fur trade's desire for a rabbit the fur of which resembled as closely as possible the fur of the wild Sable.

INTRODUCTION OF NEW BREEDS

The introduction of new breeds occurs in waves of fashion. Thus immediately the Rex breeds were available, considerable numbers were imported into England and most other breeds were 'rexed', producing what amounted to new breeds. The novelty of a new breed has an important influence on its early spread. There has been a marked increase in the smaller breeds, particularly those but recently imported into the UK. The number of new breeds and colours developed and recognised in this country has accelerated at an ever increasing speed, the degree of which is illustrated in Table 2.1.

Table 2.1 shows the number of separate breeds and the total of colour varieties for all the breeds that were recognised and standardised, with a formal written description, and were being bred, even if only to a very limited extent. There were some other varieties which were created and bred but not recognised by the standards authorities. At different dates there were also breeds and varieties (not included) which had previously been recognised and bred but which had become extinct.

Table 2.1 A comparison of the number of breeds and varieties of the domestic rabbit in the UK over the past 150 years

Year	Fancy		Normal Fur*		Rex*		Total	
	Breeds	Varieties	Breeds	Varieties	Breeds	Varieties	Breeds	Varieties
1850	4	10 colours	–	–	–	4	10	
1900	11	42	–	–	–	–	11	42
1950	13	71	15	43	4	42	32	156
1995	22	264	30	113	8	154	61	531

*includes Satin

In 1850 (and almost certainly in 1800) there was the Angora, two classes of tame rabbits – Small Variety and Large Variety – and the Lop, of which there were four types depending on the fall of ear – Half Lop, Oar Lop, Horn Lop and Flat Lop (i.e. the present English Lop form). In total there were ten colours rarely pure and most often spotted or broken. Distinct colour varieties were only recognised in the Lop in exhibitions and these totalled nine altogether.

This, then, is a brief history of the growth of the breeds and varieties in the UK. The same situation has been very similar in many other countries although probably fewer breeds have been developed. The total identifiable breeds throughout Europe (if one uses the definition of breed given above) approaches 200 (with innumerable colour varieties) and the number throughout the world is in excess of that.

THE ORIGIN OF BREEDS

A breed may be produced in one of three ways. A mutation may occur. That is to say, the mechanism which controls the inherited characters producing a particular colour or type of fur etc., may be changed, thus producing an entirely new character. The second method is by the combination of characters existing in two or more breeds. The third system is by selection for particular characteristics carried to such a degree that a strain differing greatly from the original stock is produced. All these ways, and variations of them, have been used or have occurred in the production of the present breeds and varieties of domestic rabbits.

Examples of mutations are the Rex and the Satins. The first Rex was found, in 1919, by M. Caillon, a French peasant of the district of Sarthe, in a litter out of an ordinary grey-haired doe and the second in a subsequent litter from the same doe. Fortunately one animal was a buck and the other a doe, and shortly after first breeding these animals together, M. Caillon handed some stock to a priest, Abbe Gillet, who perpetuated the breed. There are two further interesting features in this matter. The very first Rexes did not breed true, in that there was great variation in the length of the guard hairs in siblings. In the same litter animals with the length of the guard hairs reduced to the length of the undercoat were born with others in which the length of the guard hairs was such as to seem as though the animals were normal coated specimens. By repeatedly breeding only those which appeared to be Rex, i.e. those with fully reduced guard hairs was the breed made true breeding. This selection appears to have eliminated all modifying genes which had any effect on long hair.

The first Rexes were exhibited at the Paris International Show in 1924. It was not, however, until two years later that stock was distributed, and some were imported into this country in 1927. These original Rexes were Castors, but very soon, by amalgamating the Chinchilla colour with the Rex coat, the Chinchilla Rex was produced, and then many other colours were combined with the Rex coat. Since its introduction more than 50 different varieties or colours in standard Rex (i.e. excluding rough-coated and miniature) have been produced and standardised.

It should perhaps be added that the Gillet mutation was not the only one. Three further Rex mutations occurred, and that at least two are not the same as the original mutation is shown by the fact that when animals of the different mutations are bred together they do not produce Rex-coated young until the second generation.

A second mutation of a coat character is the Satin. In this mutation, the scales of the hair are smoothed and the central hollow cells of the hair fibre eliminated, thus producing a considerable sheen on the hair fibre. This mutation occurred in America, and Satins were imported into this country during the late 1940s. The Satin coat has also been combined with a number of colours and patterns.

It can be seen that when a mutation occurs, the original form taken by the mutation is combined with existing breeds to form new breeds or varieties. The method of producing a breed by selection can be illustrated by the cases of the New Zealand Red and the Netherland Dwarf. The New Zealand Red was produced in America, largely with the aid of the Belgian Hare and the Golden Fawn. It was imported into this country in 1916, and since that time certain breed characteristics have been selected as the ideal. In its country of origin, different breed characteristics were preferred. The New Zealand Red in the USA has been selected to produce an animal which differs considerably from the animal produced by selection in this country. For example, in America the adult breed weight is between 4.5 and 5 kg. In this country it weighs about 3.5 kg. The type or conformation and fur character also differ. Similarly the South African Red was produced from the New Zealand Red by changing the qualities of its coat to a very soft fur as opposed to that of the British version of the New Zealand Red, which is harsh.

The Polish rabbit, one of the early fancy breeds produced in England, was exported to Holland many years ago. The Dutch breeder selected this breed towards a standard differing materially from that in England. Thus a distinctly different breed was produced, and in fact re-imported into this country since the late 1940s. As the Dutch Polish and the English Polish differed so markedly from each other the imported Polish was renamed Netherland Dwarf. Now both breeds exist in this country side by side.

BREED STANDARDS

A breed standard is a detailed description of the characteristics of the ideal specimen of the breed, in which the importance of the different characteristics is shown by the number of points (out of 100) allotted to each. Thus from the breed standard the breeder can picture the ideal specimen, and can judge its quality from an exhibition point of view.

Many breed standards, for example those for the Dutch and the English, have been in existence for over 100 years. Others, for example those drawn up by one of the parents of the British Rabbit Council, are 60 to 70 years old whilst during the last five years eight new breeds have been standardised. Standards were produced by the particular National Specialist Club catering for the respective breeds, and all are recognised and supported by the British Rabbit Council, which publishes them. At the present time the standards are revised, if necessary, every five years, but remain static during each period. There was a change in 1994 when the British Rabbit Council established a Breed Standards Committee which, after a great deal of consultation with breeders, approves all new standards. In many countries of the world a similar arrangement exists, but the European Association for Aviculture and Rabbit Keeping, founded in 1938, after years of discussion obtained the agreement of 14 of its 15 members (in 1980) to a universal standard for each breed. The exception was the UK. Now, however, the Breed Standards Committee works with much consideration for these European standards.

In the case of breeds produced primarily for exhibition purposes, the standards bear little or no relation to the economically valuable characteristics of the rabbit, whereas in the fur breeds, which were produced to some extent for their high quality pelts, greater attention was paid to the commercial qualities of the animal. For example, in the Netherland Dwarf, a breed of no value for meat or fur production, type is allotted 65 points, colour 15, coat 10, and condition 10, whilst for Rex, the best pelt producers, the points are 20 for type, 40 for colour, and 40 for coat.

THE CLASSIFICATION OF BREEDS

The breeds of domestic rabbit in Great Britain, are, rather arbitrarily, divided into two groups – fancy breeds and fur breeds. The fur group is further divided into the normal fur breeds (that is, those breeds in which the coat consists of an undercoat and projecting guard hairs), the Rex breeds (in which the guard hairs are shortened and do not appear above the level of the undercoat), and the Satin breeds (in which the hair fibres are altered from the normal structure and the coat has a pronounced sheen). In each of these four sections, a number of breeds, some with colour varieties, are to be found. In the Rex group, all Rexes being basically the same – except for the rough-coated and the miniature Rex – the different colours are grouped according to their general colour group. Thus there are Self Rexes, in which the colour is uniform, or nearly so, over the entire body; Shaded Rexes, in which there is a darker saddle shading to a lighter colour on the flanks; Agouti Rexes, in which the hairs are banded with different colours; Tan Pattern Rexes, in which the animals have self-coloured backs and light-coloured bellies; and finally, Marked and Other Varieties. To this classification of the smooth-coated Rexes must be added the rough-coated Rexes – the Astrex, in which the coat is waved, and the Opossum Rex, in which the guard hairs are extended over the undercoat, curled parallel to the body, and the Miniature Rex which of course is much smaller than the standard Rexes.

In the Satin group standards have been drawn up for over 50 colours or patterns, although a number of colours either do not exist at the present time, or are in the experimental stage.

The same breed is sometimes produced in different countries at different times without any importation having been made. In the same way a breed may be produced in the same country on a number of different occasions and in fact by using different breeds to produce the same result. For example, although the Polish was originally imported from Belgium (as a food rabbit), it was again produced from several different strains or breeds of small albino rabbits which had originally occurred in this country. At one time albinos from Dutch marked animals were sometimes used and the early Polish were similar in type to early Dutch.

There is often a great expansion of one particular breed and then it loses its popularity until it may cease to be bred in the country. This has happened to quite a number of breeds, particularly the fur breeds. A classification of all breeds which are or have been recognised, including extinct or very rare ones, is given in Table 2.2.

Table 2.2   Breed classification, colours and weights. The weights given are the mid weight between the upper and lower limits in the standard or the ideal weight given for the adult animal.

Breed	Colour varieties	Weight (kg)	Notes
Fancy breeds			
Angora	White and 12 other colours	3	Although there are French and German Angoras, these are not currently recognised in the UK
Belgian Hare	Single colour	3.8	A black hare has been produced but not recognised
Dutch	Black, Blue, Chocolate, Brown Grey, Pale Grey, Steel Grey, Tortoiseshell, Yellow	2.1	
Dutch Tri-colour	Black, Blue, Chocolate	2.1	The colours are all banded with orange
English	Black, Blue, Tortoiseshell Chocolate, Grey	3.2	
Flemish Giant	Single colour	5.2	Large as possible, but size important
Giant Papillon	A patterned white rabbit with all colours recognised	6	As large as possible
Harlequin (Magpie)	Black, Blue, Brown, Lilac	3.2	The colours are banded with orange. In the case of the Magpies, which are the same as the Harlequin, the orange is replaced with white
Himalayan	Black, Blue, Chocolate, Lilac	2	The colours are restricted to the extremities
Lop – Cashmere	The same as the Dwarf Lop	2	Long coated variety of Dwarf Lop
Lop – Dwarf	24 colours are recognised	2	

Breed	Colour varieties	Weight (kg)	Notes
Lop – English	Any colour	–	As large as possible but not out of proportion
Lop – French	15 colours are recognised	5	As large as possible
Lop – German	All recognised colours and butterfly pattern	3.2	
Lop – Meissner	All self colours (except white), evenly silvered	3.6	
Lop – Miniature	All recognised colours	1.5	The newest variety, standardised – 1994
Netherland Dwarf	5 self colours, 6 shaded, 5 Agouti patterned, 7 tan patterned and 4 other varieties of colour	1	In addition to colours specified, any other colour which conforms to a recognised breed is accepted
Polish	5 self colours, 2 shaded self colours, 5 Agouti patterned, 10 tan patterned, 4 other varieties and 4 colours of Himalayan	1	In addition to those colours listed any other variety which follows the normal pattern is accepted. The White may be Red- or Blue-eyed
Rhinelander	A white rabbit with pattern of black and yellow	4.1	Very few are bred at the present time
Silver	Grey, Blue, Fawn, Brown	2.7	Weight not laid down in the standard
Tan	Black, Blue, Chocolate, Lilac	2	
Thrianta	Single colour	2.4	A brilliant golden orange

Normal fur breeds

Breed	Colour varieties	Weight (kg)	Notes
Alaska	Single colour	3.6	Black only
Argente	Champagne	3.6	
	Clair	–	Became extinct, now recreated, but not recognised
	Bleu	2.7	
	Creme	2.3	
	Noir	–	Became extinct, now recreated, but not recognised
	Brun	2.7	
Beaver	Brown – (resembling real beaver)	3.5	Early French breed now extinct there. Remade in UK in 1920s, also now extinct here
Beige	Single colour	2.5	Now extinct, but see Isabella.
Beveren	Blue, White, Black, Brown, Lilac	3.6	Black Beveren originally called Sitka
Blanc de Bouscat	White	6.5	Rare on Continent, very rare in UK
Blanc de Hotot	White with black eye circles	4.2	Very popular on Continent. Not well known in UK. Has been produced as Rex and as Dwarf

Table 2.2 *continued*

Breed	Colour varieties	Weight (kg)	Notes
Blanc de Termonde	White	4.5	Well known on Continent. Rare if not now extinct in UK
Blue Imperial (Imperial)	Blue	3	First true fur breed produced in England early 20th century. Now extinct
Brabancon – Blue	Single colour	–	Now extinct. Introduced to assist in improving Beverens
British Giant	White, Black, Blue, Dark Steel Grey, Brown Grey	over 5.6	First produced in 1940s, ceased to be recognised 1956, re-established 1980s
Californian	Black, Chocolate, Blue, Lilac	4.1	Second commercial meat breed imported from the USA in 1960s
Chifox	All colours	4	As large as possible. The fur was some 6 cm in length. Now extinct
Chinchilla	Single colour	2.75	
Chinchilla Giganta	Single colour	4.65	Created in 1918–21 by Chris Wren
Deilenaar	Rich Chestnut with black ticking	3	Not well known
Fox	Black, (Silver) Blue, Chocolate, Lilac	2.8	Early name of Black was Silver Fox, which it is sometimes still called
Glavcot	Silver, Golden	2.5 .	The Silver was first produced, now extinct. The Golden was re-created after 40 years in 1976 but still rare
Havana	Dark Chocolate	2.7	One of the earliest fur breeds
Isabella	Light sandy colour	2.6	Rare re-introduction of Beige
Lilac	Pink shade of dove grey	2.8	
New Zealand Red	Reddish gold	2.6	First of the New Zealands. The White was produced in the USA for meat production and has had worldwide success. The Black and Blue were derived for exhibition from the White
New Zealand Black	Black	4.75	
New Zealand Blue	Blue	4.75	
New Zealand White	White	4.75	
Nubian	Single colour	2.5	The first true black rabbit in UK, became extinct and has now been replaced by the Alaska
Perlfee	Greyish blue	2.7	Three shades permitted
Perle de Hal	Single colour	2.3	Correctly Gris Perle de Hal. Now extinct in UK
Pointed Beveren (Pointed Fox)	Colour black, with blue undercolour, moderately ticked with white-tipped hairs	3.6	Was originally created in 1920s, but became extinct. Re-created in 1980s

Breed	Colour varieties	Weight (kg)	Notes
Sable – Marten	Light, Medium, Dark	2.7	Three different shades of rich deep sepia on saddle, shading off to the flanks, with ticking on flanks, chest and legs
Sable – Siamese	Light, Medium, Dark	2.7	As Marten Sable, but no ticking
Sallander	Single colour	3.75	Introduced in early 1990s and standardised in 1994. Identical to Thuringer except for colour
Siberian	Black, Blue, Brown, Lilac	2.7	Created in 1920s from self English for use as a fur breed
Sitka	Black	–	Extinct – was forerunner of Black Beveren
Smoke Pearl	Marten, Siamese	2.7	Smoke coloured saddle shading to pearl grey on flanks. Martens well ticked with white hairs, from which Siamese are totally free
Squirrel	Single colour	2.7	Originally produced in England, but became extinct in 1930s. Re-created in late 1980s
Sussex	Gold, Cream	3.4	Recent creation in England
Swiss Fox	Black, Blue, Havana, White	2.8	Fur should be 5 to 6 cm long
Thuringer	Single colour	3.75	A yellow ochre general colour, has sooty coloured shadings, which fade towards the upper part of the body
Vienna Blue	Single colour	4.5	One of the most popular fur breeds on the Continent. First standardised in UK in 1994. Four other colours recognised abroad

Rex breeds

The Rex varieties are grouped into colours or patterns. Apart from the Mini-Rex (which has an ideal weight between 1.4 and 1.8 kg) the weight range of all adult Rex is between 2.7 and 3.6 kg.

Group	Colour varieties	Notes
Self Rex	Black, Blue, Ermine, Havana, Lilac, Nutria	
Shaded Rex	Orange Buff, Seal, Siamese Sable, Smoke Pearl Siamese, Smoke Pearl Marten, Tortoiseshell	
Tan Pattern Rex	Fawn, Fox – Black, Blue, Chocolate, Lilac – Marten Sable, Marten Seal, Orange, Otter – Black, Blue, Chocolate, Lilac – Tan – Black, Blue, Chocolate, Lilac	

Table 2.2 *continued*

Breed	Colour varieties	Notes
Agouti Rex	Castor, Chinchilla, Cinnamon, Lynx, Opal	
Other varieties of Rex	Dalmatian	May be bi-colour, i.e. white with pattern of one colour, or tri-colour, white with patches of two colours. In both cases colour may only be black, blue, brown, orange or fawn
	Dutch, English, Harlequin	These three varieties should resemble as closely as possible the normal varieties in colour and markings, but with Rex coat and type
	Himalayan	Markings to be Dark Seal, Blue or Chocolate
	Silver Seal	Colour is jet black with silvering over whole body
Satin Rex	Any colour or pattern	Smooth coated: as Rex with satin sheen. Rough-coated: satin sheen with wave or curl
Rough Coated Rex	Astrex	As normal Rex but with tight curls over the whole body, in any recognised Rex colour. Now very rare if not extinct
	Opossum Rex	Whole body covered with white tipped curled hairs carried at right angles to body. Any colour recognised. Now very rare if not extinct
Miniature Rex	All recognised Rex Colours	Ideal weight of 1.4 to 1.8 kg. The newest addition to the Rex family, being first recognised in 1990

Satin breeds

Varieties of Satin differ only in colour. The weight lies between 2.7 and 3.6 kg. Whilst the following standards have been recognised, in some cases few or no exhibits of certain colours have been bred at the present time.

Breed	Colour varieties
Argente	Champagne, Bleu, Brun, Creme
Beige	Single colour
Black	Single colour
Blue	Single colour
Bronze	Single colour
Brown	Single colour
Castor	Single colour
Chinchilla	Single colour
Cinnamon	Single colour
Fawn	Single colour

Breed	Colour varieties
Fox	Black, Blue, Chocolate, Lilac
Havana	Single colour
Himalayan	Black, Blue
Ivory	Single colour
Lilac	Single colour
Lynx	Single colour
Marten Sable	Light, Medium, Dark
Opal	Single colour
Orange	Single colour
Seal point	Single colour
Siamese Sable	Light, Medium and Dark
Smoke Pearl	Marten, Siamese
Sooty Fawn	Single colour
Squirrel	Single colour
Others	Any not included above: the Satin standard for coat and type with the colour or pattern as the normal haired variety or Rex variety

THE INTRODUCTION OF FOREIGN BREEDS

It is certain that domestic rabbits were imported (and indeed exported) from this country as early as the beginning of the 18th century. The Angora was certainly exported to several countries. During the early part of the 19th century, two varieties of which there is definite knowledge are the Polish and the early type of Dutch, albeit at that time not known by those names. In general there were no further introductions until the New Zealand Red was brought in and established. In the second decade of the 20th century there developed an interest in fur farming and the Blue Beveren was introduced, followed shortly afterwards by the Chinchilla. In the 1920s, the first Rex entered the country, and on a much smaller scale the Perle de Hal (or by its correct name Gris Perle de Hal) which unfortunately later became extinct.

The late 1940s and 1950s saw the introduction for the first time for many years, of some new breeds. The first of these was the Netherland Dwarf from Holland, followed by the Satin from America. Both were imported for exhibition purposes. Later, some impetus was given to the introduction of foreign breeds by the development of the commercial rabbit industry, and the New Zealand White and Californian – the two important early growth breeds for commercial purposes – came from America and the Danish and French Lops originally from Scandinavia and France. The Blanc de Bouscat (France), the Blanc de Hotot (France) and the Blanc de Termonde (Belgium) were also imported for commercial meat production. The demand for these breeds, by the developers of strains of meat rabbits, was great, and these three latter breeds became spoilt by mixing with other breeds.

All the breeds brought in for the improvement of meat rabbits became exhibition animals, of varying degrees of popularity. The three white Land Race rabbits, i.e. the Blanc de Bouscat, de Hotot and de Termonde, indicate again the way in which commercial strains develop in similar ways at separate times and in separate places. Following these commercial breeds came more exhibition animals, the Rhinelander, the Thuringer and the Alaska from Germany, and the Dwarf Lop from Holland. The Giant Rabbit, of purely British origin, was again recognised as an exhibition breed having ceased to exist for a number of years, but this time was considered a fur breed, rather than as originally a fancy breed.

The 1970s and early 1980s also saw the introduction of more new breeds, such as the Meissner Lop, which is not so heavily built as the French Lop; the Thrianta, a brilliant orange breed of medium size; the Deilenaar (which itself has a history of only forty or so years, having been produced from crosses involving the Belgian Hare, the New Zealand Red and the Chinchilla), the Perlfee, the Isabella and a delightful small Swiss Fox, which has long thick fur and is produced in several colours. In the early 1990s came the Vienna Blue, the Sallander, the Giant Papillon and the Miniature Lop.

In different countries at different times there have always been changes in fashions amongst different breeds, and this will doubtless continue. New breeds will arise and will move from country to country. Their popularity will rise and fall and some will sadly become extinct, although at any time, given sufficient time any of the extinct breeds can be re-created, even though the best possible specimens may take a great deal longer. The small breeds such as the Netherland Dwarf and the Dwarf Lops have increased considerably in the past few years and there is little doubt that the Miniature Lop will prove as popular.

THE BREEDS

The following notes on the different breeds which are currently found in this country will give an idea of the immense variety that exists. A major point, however, should be made. A very definite split has been made between populations (for they cannot in some senses be called breeds) that are used for intensive commercial rabbit meat production, and the exhibition breeds of rabbit. The exhibition breeds are, by definition, bred for 'fancy' points, that is to say, colour, texture of fur, pattern, conformation, or as it should be called, type, which are not usually allied to meat qualities. Commercial meat rabbits are selected to provide good quality meat in a good carcase in large numbers per doe and at an economic rate, i.e. fast growth with good food conversion. The fur texture of a meat rabbit is unimportant. What is wanted is a fast-growing young rabbit, with good resistance to disease, and does and bucks which will produce a very large number of such young per year, all of them doing this on the least possible amount of food. Gone is the time when high quality fur was also produced (this can in general only be done from mature animals), except in the case of a relatively few, almost DIY, enthusiasts. Thus, in the section that follows, when the animal is said to be suitable as a fur producer, it relates to this type of operation only. Again, because in general the standardised breeds are used for exhibition, the notes refer to animals kept for this purpose.

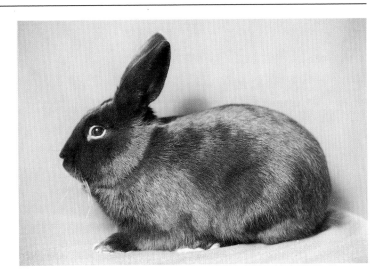

Fig. 2.1
Alaska

The Alaska

The present Alaska rabbit, which weighs between 3.2 and 4 kg was introduced from Belgium in 1972 and after. This same breed existed in France in the 1920s, but, there, then weighed only 2 kg. An identical breed existed in the UK (sometimes called the Nubian and weighing about 2.5 kg) but became extinct in the 1930s. The Nubian itself had an interesting career being one of the few rabbits adopted by the Self Coloured Rabbit Club, a competitor of the national British Fur Rabbit Society. After the SCRC ceased to exist the breed, being at that time very popular was immediately adopted by the BFRS in 1928. The Alaska has intensely black, silky fur and is a stocky, compact breed. It is a good example of the production of the same breed in different places at different times. This also accounts for the various opinions expressed as to its origin. It has been said that it was first an English breed and taken to the continent as the Nubian. Other opinions are that it was first created in Germany in the late 1920s by crosses of Himalayan (continental type) and Argentes. Certainly in the 1930s in France – where it was usually considered to have arisen from melanistic specimens of large type Himalayans – it had great popularity for use in producing Black Rex. Whatever its origin it always seems to arrive at the same lustrous black colour and to be an increasingly popular exhibition animal.

The Angora (Fig. 2.2)

The Angora is one of the oldest known breeds of domestic rabbit, and has been kept for its wool for some hundreds of years. Prior to the present universal name of Angora, it had a number of others. It was at the beginning of the 18th century spoken of as the White Shock Turkey rabbit, and later as the English Silk Rabbit. Its export was then prohibited. However, it was taken to France (irregularly) as early as the 1720s and was later exported from England to several countries during the late 18th Century.

The Angora is the only breed from which wool for spinning can be obtained. Until the mid-1920s the major world supply was produced in France, but at that time Eastern European and Japanese production became extensive; production in China

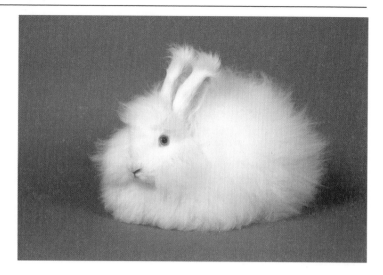

Fig. 2.2
Angora

increased to very large proportions and did much to cause chaos in world Angora wool markets. In this country too there was a certain amount of production, but at the present time there is little, and that on a very small scale.

The English Angora has a much finer coat and is smaller than its Continental counterparts, weighing on average about 2.75 kg as against 3.6 kg or more for the French Angora or slightly over 4 kg for the larger German Angora. The wool yield of the English variety is substantially less than the others. A good yield for the English Angora would be about 350 g per year, whilst that of both French and German Angoras would be three or even more times that figure.

The Angora undoubtedly requires more attention than other breeds, for it needs to be groomed fairly frequently to ensure that the coat does not matt. The breed is recognised in white and twelve different colours, but the majority of Angoras bred are white – i.e. albinos. As a breed the Angora has considerable exhibition success and often achieves supreme honours at shows.

The Argentes (Fig. 2.3)

The Argente Champagne, the oldest and largest of the four Argente varieties, is certainly the oldest fur breed in the world. It existed in France in the early 17th century and was said to have been brought there by the Portuguese sailors who found it in Indo-China. The truth of this is impossible now to establish but such fanciful stories are very common (and usually quite untrue) when the origin of breeds is discussed. Certainly the breed has been kept for its fur, particularly in the Champagne area of France for at least three centuries. During the early 1900s sales of these pelts were held in France and prices up to the equivalent of £15 at today's values per pelt were obtained. It is often suggested that the Argente Champagne was first produced from Silver Greys, the silvering then being greatly intensified.

The Argente Champagne was introduced into England during 1919, when it became very popular. The undercolour of the fur is a dark slate blue, for the Argente Champagne is genetically a black rabbit. The silvering, which appears at the first moult, is due to loss of pigment in the tips of the undercoat, the guard hairs being

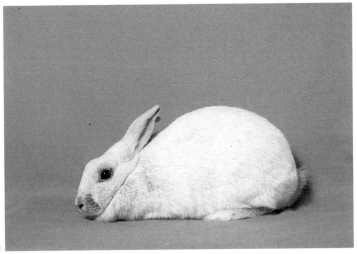

Fig. 2.3
Argente Champagne

unaffected and remaining black. The physiological action producing the loss of the pigment in the hair fibres is incompletely understood. The Champagne is the largest of the Argentes, weighing approximately 3.6 kg and were certainly the most satisfactory from a pelt production point of view, although the pelts were never greatly sought after by the furrier in this country.

The Argente Bleu is smaller than the Champagne, weighing about 2.7 kg. The undercolour of the fur is lavender blue, for the variety is genetically a blue rabbit (that is, a dilute black), and the breed carries, of course, the same silvering factors as all the Argentes.

The Argente Brun is very similar in type and weight to the Argente Bleu. It was introduced into England in the early 1920s from the Continent where it had been bred for many years. It made little progress and became extinct, but was recreated by H. D. H. Dowle during 1939–41. By crossing Argente Cremes (which genetically are silvered yellows) with Argente Bleus, silvered Agoutis were produced. These were mated with normal-coated Havana rabbits and produced silvered blacks (known previously as Argente Noir) which, when mated amongst themselves, gave Argente Bruns. Argente Bruns are, of course, silvered browns. At a later stage Brown Beverens were introduced to improve the length and colour of the coat.

The last variety is the Argente Creme. This variety is the smallest of the group, weighing approximately 2.25 kg, and is a silvered yellow, the undercolour being orange, top colour creamy white, the whole interspersed with longer orange hairs.

The Beige or Isabella

During the late 1920s the Beige was produced in England. This was towards the end of the great interest in fur farming and the decline which then occurred meant that only the very best of the fur breeds survived. The Beige did not. However, the breed was exported to the continent and now occurs, under that name in several countries. In Holland, for example, the standard was registered in 1940. Subsequently it was imported back into this country in the 1980s and renamed Isabella. It has been re-established on several occasions in other countries.

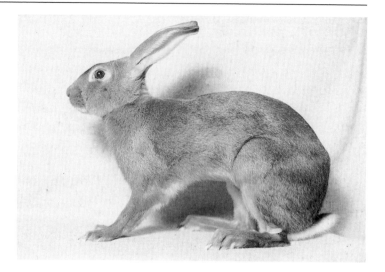

Fig. 2.4
Belgian Hare

The Belgian Hare (Fig. 2.4)

The Belgian Hare is one of the early fancy breeds, having been brought from Belgium in 1874, although at that time it was nothing like the animal of today. It is true to say that the early importations can be considered as being the raw material from which the English breeder produced what is now known as the exhibition Belgian Hare. The best Belgian Hares anywhere in the world have descended from that early English improvement. It was, strangely, at one time used a fair amount for meat production, and during the last war as a cross with other breeds for the same purpose.

The breed was exported to America from both Belgium and, mainly, from England at the end of the 19th century and then produced the Belgian Hare boom, one of the more astonishing phenomenons of the rabbit world. Genetically it is of the wild Agouti colour, much modified by additional genes to give it a rich deep red of a tan or chestnut shade.

The breed has been selected always for extreme length, fineness and gracefulness, and compares very well with a wild hare rather than a rabbit, a fact which has led many to believe that it is a hare, which of course it is not. The myth that it can be crossed with a wild hare is equally erroneous and the idea that it was the result of a rabbit and hare cross – the Leprid – has long since been disproved.

The actual origin of the Belgian Hare is obscure, although there is a good deal of evidence to show that it was selected from an old breed known as the Patagonian, which has been extinct for nearly a hundred years. The Patagonian was also the progenitor of the Flemish Giant in this country, although both breeds, today, differ very greatly from the original and each other.

The Beveren (Fig. 2.5)

The Blue Beveren originated in Belgium, in the district of that name, in the 1890s. It is thought that it was produced from crosses of the St. Nicolas Giant and the Vienna Blue, both of which, although fairly common on the Continent, were not found in this country until the import of the Vienna Blue. There were in fact two types of Beveren

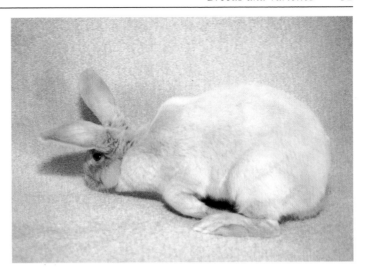

Fig. 2.5
Blue Beveren

imported into this country in 1915, one being a small blue rabbit of about the type of a Dutch, weighing about 2.25 kg, known as the Brabancon type, whilst the other, the Blue Vienna derivative, was the breed which was first named the Giant Blue Beveren.

The Brabancon rabbit was an extremely old breed kept widely in the province of Brabant in Belgium. It obviously carried some Dutch genes for it often showed patches of white. It was also said to have been the progenitor of the Dutch Rabbit, for animals with much more emphasised Dutch pattern were certainly brought to this country long before its association with the Beveren. It is even suggested that the true origin of the typical Dutch rabbit was the improvement of some early heavily patterned Brabancon by early fanciers in England. The St. Nicolas Blue (also a very ancient breed) obviously had Brabancon genes in it, for the Blue Beveren and the St. Nicolas Blue, whilst being regarded as being very closely linked if not the same breed, were distinguished from each other because, certainly in the early specimens, there were white markings in the St. Nicolas Blue. This entanglement of breeds illustrates clearly how different breeds arise in some case from the mixing of others.

The Blue Beveren is genetically a blue rabbit, that is, a dilute black. The Black Beveren (originally known as the Sitka) was produced in 1919 by a cross with a black rabbit of unknown breed. The White Beveren, which differs from nearly all the other white breeds of rabbit in being a blue-eyed white (following the genetical pattern of the Vienna White), was produced some years later. The original White Beverens were, however, albinos, and not blue-eyed. It was not until some ten years later that the Brown Beveren was first exhibited.

The Beveren was one of the first and major fur breeds. It has a coat which is silky, dense, and lustrous, and is between 25 and 30 mm in length. The Blue Beveren was the mainstay of the early fur industry, the pelts fetching good prices, whilst as a table rabbit the breed was good, the desired weight of an adult being not less than 3.6 kg.

The Blanc de Bouscat (Fig. 2.6), the Blanc de Hotot, and the Blanc de Termonde

These three continental breeds were introduced into the country largely at the

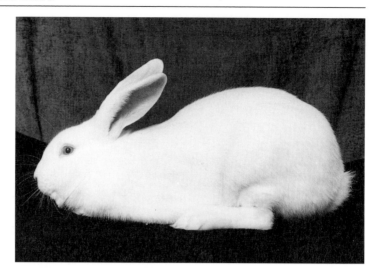

Fig. 2.6
Blanc de Bouscat

instigation of commercial rabbit farmers attempting to produce new strains. The first two came from France, the third from Belgium. The Blanc de Bouscat is well known in France, in which it originated by crosses of Flemish Giant, Argente and Angora. Albinos from the crosses were selected and the breed was first standardised in 1924, although it was being shown for at least 15 years before. It is a large rabbit with minimum weights for adult bucks of 5.0 kg and for adult does 5.5 kg. The length of the coat is long, being 35 to 40 mm with excellent properties. It is still not well known in England, although it was standardised in the late 1960s.

The Blanc de Hotot is also a French breed and is even older than the Blanc de Bouscat, having been produced in 1902. Its origin is certainly Dutch and/or English, for all markings except eye circles are suppressed. It is not so popular in France as the Blanc de Bouscat, but in other countries where the pattern has been imposed on dwarfs and rex, these are very popular. The breed is somewhat smaller than the Blanc de Bouscat, with an ideal weight of 4 to 4.5 kg. It also was standardised in England in the late 1960s.

The Blanc de Termonde is of Belgian origin, having been produced from Flemish Giants with the introduction of probably Beverens to improve the coat characteristics. They were not standardised in France until 1928, and are no longer recognised there. They were standardised in this country in the late 1960s. There are very few if any existing in the UK. The weight is the same as the Blanc de Hotot.

British Giants (Fig. 2.7)

'Giant' rabbits are bred in many parts of the world. Because the Flemish Giant world would not accept other colours than the steel grey of the Flemish Giant, in the late 1940s a British Giant Rabbit Club was established by breeders who brought in other colours of Flemish Giants from America. They believed, and there is some evidence that it may be so, that the steel-grey Flemish in the country were linked to small size. It is certainly true that on the Continent there was a very widespread belief that any inbreeding of Flemish Giants would very quickly lead to much reduced size, and the Flemish Giant stock in this country at that time were much inbred.

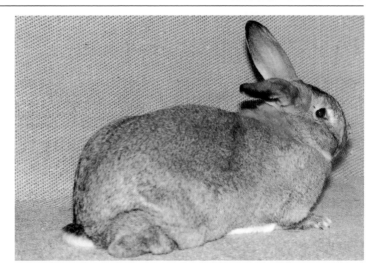

Fig. 2.7
British Giant
(Brown Grey)

The British Giant Club and its members were successful for some six or seven years, when the club was disbanded. A new Club started and the breed was again recognised in 1981 with a standard calling for adult bucks weighing not less than 5.6 kg and adult does not less than 6.1 kg. Up to 1995 five separate colour varieties were recognised.

The Californian (Fig. 2.8)

The first introduction of the Californian into Great Britain took place in 1958, but it was not until 1960 that substantial numbers were imported. In that year over 400 Californians arrived, largely due to the interests of commercial rabbit farmers, the breed having been developed in America for its commercially desirable characteristics. It was first developed there (in the early 1920s) by crosses of New Zealand White and Himalayan with the further introduction of Chinchilla. The purpose was a good meat rabbit with good fur qualities. It did not become too well known in America for some 15 years after its original development. It is today possibly the second most important meat producing rabbit throughout the world.

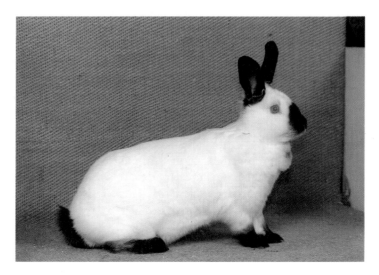

Fig. 2.8
Californian

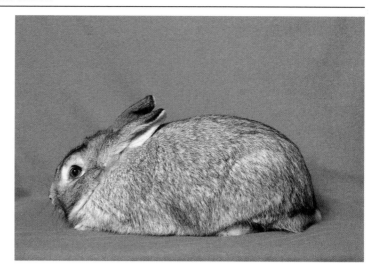

Fig. 2.9
Chinchilla

In essence the Californian is a Himalayan pointed white land breed which, since its introduction as a commercial variety, has proved a popular fancy rabbit. It is recognised in four colours, Normal (black points), Chocolate, Blue and Lilac, the last three colours having been produced in this country. Adults weigh between 3.5 and 4.75 kg.

The Chinchilla (Fig. 2.9)

The first Chinchillas were exhibited in France in 1913 by J. J. Dybowski, who claimed that they were produced by crosses of wild rabbits with Blue Beverens and Himalayans. As the colour of the Chinchilla is due to a mutation, however, in which the yellow of the wild Agouti pattern is suppressed, its place being taken by pearl, M. Dybowski's claim is open to considerable doubt. However, he was certainly the originator of the breed and most of the importations into this country were from him, the first arriving in 1919. Within a very short period it became one of the most widely kept of all breeds.

The original strains of the Chinchilla were very impure, and produced many non-Chinchilla animals, for example, the Sable breeds, both Marten and Siamese with their various shades, the Silver Fox, the Squirrel and through the Sables, the Smoke Pearls. A number of other breeds were used in efforts to improve the Chinchilla, and this gave rise both to undesirable recessives which still appear, such as 'woollies' (resulting from the use of Angoras to improve coat) and 'ghosts', and to further breeds. For example, by using the Black Tan to improve ticking, the Silver Fox was produced. Even the specimens normally discarded were used in some cases, for the Chifox, a breed with a coat of about 65 mm or more in length was produced from the woollies from the Chinchilla. In fact the Chifox carried, at the start, the Chinchilla colour and a silky coat which resembled the wild fox rather than the Angora from which it was derived, hence the name. The original breeder and developer was T. Leaver of Kent, but although this breed achieved some early success, it eventually lost its popularity and is now no longer seen.

The Chinchilla, as a fur breed for the production of pelts, has seen several booms.

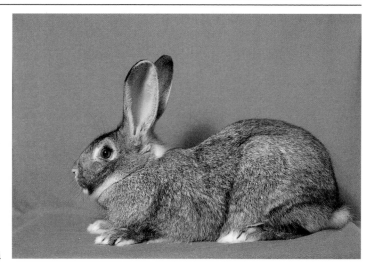

Fig. 2.10
Chinchilla Giganta

At one time, the early pelt of the rabbit at a month old fetched good prices, and during the 1920s many relatively large fur producers specialised with this breed. In colour the Chinchilla closely resembles the real Chinchilla lanigera from Chile and Peru, the pelts of which are the most expensive in the world. It is not surprising therefore that the pelts of the Chinchilla rabbit, which are impossible to imitate with dyes, usually fetched a better price than other normal fur-breed skins. The Chinchilla had a further advantage from a pelting point of view in that the intermediate coat, taken when the rabbit is from four to five months of age, is of value, whereas this is not the case with other breeds. The Chinchilla is also a popular and attractive exhibition breed. It weighs between 2.5 and 3 kg.

The Chinchilla Giganta (Fig. 2.10)

The intention in the production of the Chinchilla Giganta in the early 1920s by Chris Wren, was to produce a large, graceful rabbit, with good meat qualities, and a good pelt with Chinchilla colouring. That this has succeeded is shown by the fact that many authorities considered the breed to be the ideal meat and fur breed, and the most valuable normal fur breed from a commercial point of view. The colour is very similar to the Chinchilla, although being perhaps rather darker. The coat is also usually rather less silky, but pelts of excellent size are produced, and meat qualities and growth rate are excellent. The weight must not exceed about 5 kg. Genetically the colour is the same as the Chinchilla, that is, wild Agouti colour with the yellow replaced by pearl grey.

The Deilenaar

This breed is a mixture of Belgian Hare, Chinchilla and New Zealand Red, which breeds were used in its composition just before the 1939–45 war in Holland. It was first standardised there in 1940 and in England in the late 1980s. Its weight lies between 2.5 and 3.5 kg.

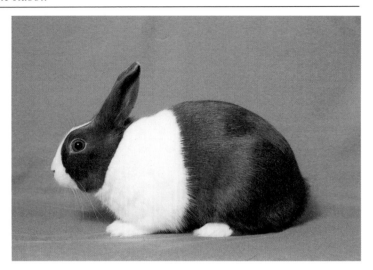

Fig. 2.11
Dutch

The Dutch (Fig. 2.11)

The Dutch rabbit, together with the English, were until recently, when they were overtaken by the dwarf breeds, the most popular of the fancy breeds. The origin of the breed is again rather obscure, but there is little doubt that their immediate progenitors originated in Holland or Belgium. As early as the 1830s there were exports of rabbits, both live and as carcases to this country from Ostend and Antwerp, and these included what were known as 'little Brabancons'. These animals were almost certainly the early Dutch breed, and selection for the particular pattern of today's Dutch was started by the early English fanciers.

The popularity of both the Dutch and English should not lead one to suppose that they are 'easier' to breed than other breeds, for this is certainly not the case. The only advantages which might be claimed in the exhibition world is that they can be examined to a certain extent for quality when in the nest and the mis-marked specimens rejected, and they can be shown at a relatively very early age. Furthermore, as with all marked varieties, their show life is very long, some exhibits winning consistently for several years, almost an impossibility with other breeds.

The genetical constitution of the Dutch rabbit is most complicated and not as yet entirely proven. There is little doubt, however, that it is controlled by several factors which are not linked together, and consequently when other breeds are crossed with Dutch, traces of the Dutch pattern are liable to be exceedingly difficult to eradicate.

There are eight different colours of Dutch: Black, Blue, (these two being the most popular), Chocolate, Tortoiseshell, Pale Grey, Brown Grey, Steel Grey and Yellow. The breed, weighing under 2.25 kg, was used in many crosses with larger breeds, for meat production during the 1939–45 war. It had good meat properties, although on the small side. It has also been used to a fair extent for work in laboratories and has always been a popular choice as a foster mother.

The Tri-colour Dutch, known also on the Continent, was imported into this country in the late 1960s. Its origin is unknown but was said to have been produced from crosses between Dutch and other breeds. It is sometimes suggested that the Harlequins resulted from these Tri-coloured Dutch. This is not so. The Tri-colour arose from crosses between Harlequin and Dutch, the confusion having arisen because the Harlequin was produced from Tortoiseshell Dutch.

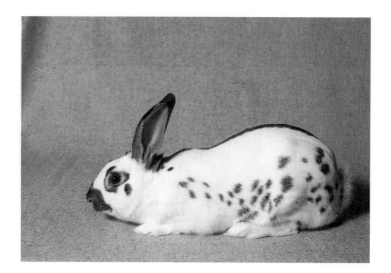

Fig. 2.12
English

The English (Fig. 2.12)

The English breed is one of the oldest fancy breeds, although for some reason, after being popular in the early part of the 19th century, it appeared to become relatively unknown from the 1850s until towards the end of the century. J. Rogers, writing in 1849, gives the following description of what were obviously the earliest Blue and Black English:

> What is termed the 'blue butterfly smut' was for some time considered the most valuable of fancy rabbits; it is thus named on account of having bluish or lead-coloured spots on either side of the nose, considered as having some resemblance to the spread wings of a butterfly ... A black and white rabbit may also have the face marked in a similar manner, constituting a 'black butterfly smut' .... But a good fancy rabbit must likewise have other marks ... and there ought to be dark stripes on both sides of the body in front, passing backwards to meet the saddle, and uniting on the top of the shoulders, at the part called the withers in a horse; these stripes form what is termed the 'chain'.

Following this reference, no further mention of the English rabbit is found until the Blacks were reintroduced in the 1880s, followed by the Tortoiseshell some years later, and then the Blues, Chocolates, and Greys, these being the five colours recognised. The genetics of the English rabbit have been closely studied and are an excellent example of a breed which is exhibited only in the heterozygous state (see Chapter 5). Apart from its great popularity as an exhibition breed, the English is often used as a foster doe, having, as a breed, excellent maternal characteristics.

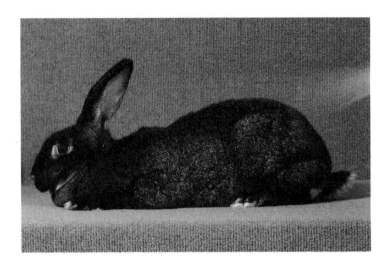

Fig. 2.13
Flemish Giant

The Flemish (Fig 2.13)

The Flemish, or Flemish Giant, is (apart from the British Giant) the largest breed of rabbit recognised in this country. The adult bucks should not weigh less than 4.9 kg, nor the adult does less than 5.4 kg. In shows, however, animals under these weights but over six months of age are catered for by 'Intermediate classes'. Flemish of 6.3 kg or more are of good size at the present time, although specimens up to 9.5 kg have been exhibited in the past.

Although the Flemish Giant existed on the continent before the origin of it in England, it was a very sandy coloured animal and the breed in its present form can be considered to be of entirely English origin. There is evidence to suggest that it is descended from the Patagonian, with the introduction of some other blood, principally Silver Grey. The fancier who undoubtedly produced the present form of the Flemish Giant was Chris Wren.

The steel-grey colour of the Flemish (the only colour recognised in this country) is a combination of the genes for dominant black and normal extension of black, with the Agouti pattern. Although this is the basic genetic constitution to give the dark steel-grey colour, there are also modifying factors which affect it. In other countries many other colours are recognised and the weights are almost invariably a good deal higher.

The Foxes (Fig. 2.14)

Genetically a chinchillated (a term indicating removal of yellow colour) black and tan, the Silver Fox – now sometimes incorrectly known as a Black Fox – was produced by the introduction of the Tan into the Chinchilla, the object being the improvement of the ticking in the latter breed. The first specimens of the Silver Fox were exhibited in 1926 and these were shortly followed by Blue Foxes, Chocolate Foxes and Lilac Foxes. Originally the breed did not gain a great deal of popularity, but became one of the most popular of the normal fur breeds. Although a most attractive rabbit, the pelts were never in great demand, for with the usual methods of manufacture, much of the attractive ticking was removed when the flanks were cut back. The weight of the breed is between 2.5 to 3.1 kg.

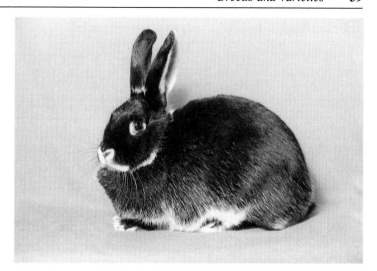

Fig. 2.14
Silver Fox

The Giant Papillon (Fig. 2.15)

The Giant Papillon is the French large version of the English of this country although with patches on the flanks rather than a chain and weighing usually 5.5 to 6 kg, although larger specimens are found. In many countries the English patterns are found, and the Giant Papillon arose from these. In the same way in Germany a very similar breed exists, as it does in Holland, where it is called the Lotharinger, of which a 2.5 kg version is also bred. The Giant Papillon was standardised in England in 1994 and all recognised colours are admissible.

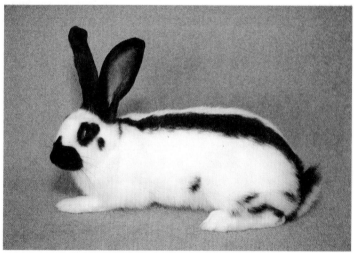

Fig. 2.15
Giant Papillon

The Glavcots (Fig. 2.16)

The original Glavcot was the Silver, from which the Golden later derived. Strangely no standard was ever created for the Silver, but the Golden was standardised in 1934, although it had then been in existence for seven or more years. Both breeds became extinct shortly after the standard was first published for the Golden, but with the use of Siberian, Havana and Beveren crosses, the Golden Glavcot has been recreated and was first shown in 1976. The breed weighs some 2.5 kg.

The Harlequin (Fig. 2.17)

The Harlequin, a chequered marked breed, was originally known as the Japanese, a name it retains in most other countries. The name was changed to its present one, in a burst of patriotic fervour, during the 1939–45 war. The breed originated in France during the 1880s, and according to M. Meslay, the leading authority at the time, was produced from Tortoiseshell Dutch. A few years later Harlequins were imported into this country. The skins, being marked as a checkerboard, had little value, except for novelty items, and although the breed had some little vogue during the 1939–45 war as a meat producer, it had little commercial value and was always an exhibition breed.

The inheritance of the Harlequin banding is due to a recessive gene, which, when associated with the Agouti colour, prevents the development of ticking. The Harlequin factor is an epistatic character, that is to say, when it is combined with the Agouti, the Self, or the Tan pattern factors, it will produce the same result, the epistatic gene hiding the appearance of the others.

There are eight colours of Harlequin, (or Magpies, as the variety in which the golden orange or fawn is replaced by white is called). These are: black and golden orange (or white), blue and golden fawn (or white), brown and golden orange (or white), and lilac and golden fawn (or white).

The Havana (Fig. 2.18)

The Havana was first produced in Holland in 1898 from a cross between a black and white scrub rabbit and an unknown sire. They were first called Ingensche Venoraoz (Fire-eye from Ingen) after the name of the village, near Utrecht, in Holland, and the fact that the eye glows ruby-red. At about the same time another Havana, lacking the purple sheen of the first was produced, again in Holland, and was shown in 1902. A third Havana, the French Havana, was produced in France by a cross between a wild rabbit and a Himalayan. It is this strain which occurs in France.

The original Havana, that being the type now in this country, originally had a number of names on the Continent, including the name Beaver. This name was then given to the rabbit produced in the 1920s in this country, from a cross of Havana and Beveren. After spreading fairly rapidly through Europe, the first of the Havanas were imported here in 1908 and the first class for the breed was guaranteed at the Crystal Palace Show in 1910. Since that time they have remained an attractive and popular exhibition breed.

The Havana has given rise to several other distinct breeds. There is the Feh de Marbourg which originated in Germany, and has widely spread, which itself gave rise to the Perlefee, now in this country. The Gris Perle de Hal was produced about 1910 from apparently pure Havana crosses. Litters produced some silvered young, and these bred true. Although he was urged to introduce several blue breeds the originator never did, but he did breed back from time to time to Havanas to prevent too great inbreeding.

The rich dark chocolate-coloured fur of the Havana makes it very attractive to the furrier from whom there was usually a good demand, although the breed was rather on the small side for the best grade of pelt, weighing approximately 2.7 kg.

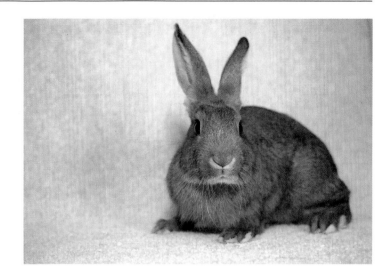

Fig. 2.16
Golden Glavcot

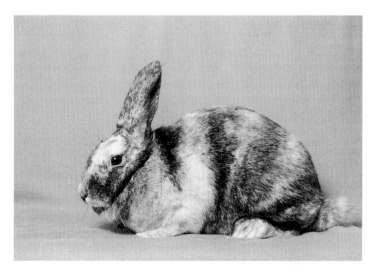

Fig. 2.17
Harlequin

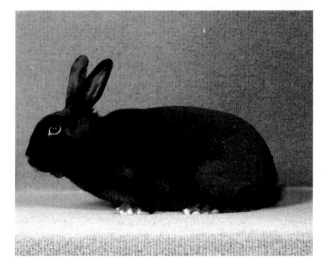

Fig. 2.18
Havana

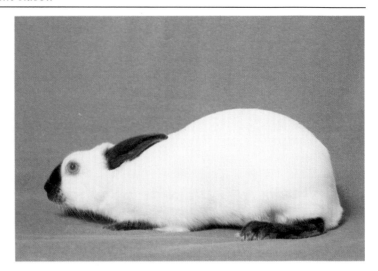

Fig. 2.19
Himalayan

The Himalayan (Fig. 2.19)

The Himalayan is one of the oldest fancy breeds. Its name bears no relation to the mountains of that name, although it was popularly but quite wrongly supposed that they originated in this area. The breed is also known as 'the Russian' on the Continent and was at one time, both in this country and elsewhere, known as the Chinese. It is possible that it originated in the East, for it was popular in that area. It is more likely that it has occurred in a number of places at different times. The fur of this breed was at one time considered to be valuable and enormous numbers were bred in Europe (including the CIS, Poland and Germany), in Egypt from which one of its names, the 'Egyptian Smut', was derived, and elsewhere. Today, although used to some extent for laboratory work, the breed is almost entirely an exhibition animal. It makes an excellent pet, being very docile.

The Himalayan is genetically an albino with the extremities, i.e. ears, nose, tail and feet, coloured either black, blue, chocolate or lilac. The factor causing the development of the Himalayan colouring, rather than a true albino, is a gene in the series of factors controlling the development of colour. The Himalayan factor is dominant to true albino, but recessive to all other genes in this series. The actual development of pigment in the fur of the extremities is due to a temperature difference. Dark patches of fur can be developed in other areas, if these areas are subjected to cold treatment, such as bathing regularly with cold water during growth. Himalayans in the nest show no colour development, which begins only after the animal leaves the nest and is not fully developed until a number of weeks later. The Himalayan appears in many other countries, where, however, there are often two varieties, one about the same as the English breed (2 kg), the other usually a good deal larger, weighing some 4 to 4.5 kg.

The Lilac (Fig. 2.20)

The Lilac has been produced in a number of places at different times. It was first produced by H. Onslow in Cambridge in 1910 (being exhibited in London in 1913).

By the same time it had also been produced by a Miss Illingworth, who called it the Essex Lavender. Subsequently it was again created by the geneticist Professor R. C. Punnett at Cambridge in 1922. A Blue Beveren (a dilute black) was mated to an Havana (a brown, recessive to black). All the progeny were black in appearance, but carried the factors for the recessive brown and dilution. On mating these black rabbits together, blacks, blues, browns and lilacs were produced in the ratio of 9:3:3:1, the lilac rabbits being dilute browns. The original name given to the breed was 'Cambridge Blue' but this was later changed to Lilac.

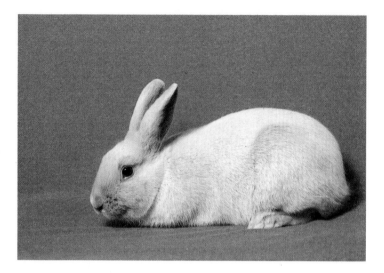

Fig. 2.20
Lilac

In the same way Lilacs were produced on the Continent at about the same time and were then given the names Gouda (from the district in which they were first produced) or Marburger or Marbourg (from the district in which they were next produced). The name was then changed in Holland to Gouwenaar.

The fur is a most pleasing dove grey, and usually of very good quality from the furriers point of view. It is therefore curious that it did not become popular in the fur trade. The breed weighs approximately 3 kg, is one of the more docile of breeds, but in recent years has achieved only moderate popularity.

The Lop family (Figs 2.21– 2.24)

The English Lop has the distinction of being the oldest breed to be exhibited anywhere in the world. There are it is true older breeds, but these were not used by fanciers until later. The specimen Lops of 150 or more years ago were very different from those of the present day. The ear length, width, shape and texture are the features for which the fancier breeds, and some considerable success has been achieved in this direction, for ear spans of up to 68 cm or even more is attainable. The breed, at one time certainly the most popular of all fancy rabbits, has now lost much of its popularity. It is essentially an exhibition breed and, after its origin in England, has spread to almost all countries of the world where exhibition rabbits exist. At one time it was considered imperative to keep the animals in a very warm atmosphere as it was thought that this would improve the ears. A bakery was thought to be ideal! This idea is quite erroneous, and the practice should be strongly condemned.

The English Lop was the first of all Lops and from the English Lop crossed with Giant breeds on the Continent, such as the Flemish and Normandy (with selection for shorter ears), was produced the French Lop. From the French Lop other breeds were produced, for example, the German Lop and the Dwarf Lop. The Danish Lop which was imported into the UK for commercial purposes is very similar to the French Lop, but no longer exists as a separate breed in this country. These Continental Lops, which are all short-eared Lops, were at first produced not so much as fancy breeds but as meat producing breeds, for they were all of a very suitable type and produced excellent carcases.

The French Lop, which has ears far shorter than its English counterpart, is a massive, almost cubic animal, and the standard calls for the largest weight possible. A good weight would be 5.5 kg. The French Lop was first introduced to the UK to improve the qualities of meat-producing strains of rabbits, largely due to its excellent carcase type, but also to other characteristics. Later, in 1965 the first French Lop for exhibition purposes was imported by Meg Brown. Today in the UK it is a popular exhibition breed. The German Lop is smaller than the French Lop weighing about 3.2 kg.

The Dwarf Lop, certainly one of the most popular of all exhibition rabbits, has an ideal weight of 1.9 kg. and was derived from the French Lop by Dutch fanciers. Although not represented in the UK there is another example of a smaller Lop, derived from the German Lop by German fanciers which has an ideal weight of 3 to 3.5 kg. The Dwarf Lop was first produced in Holland in the 1950s, was first introduced to the UK in 1968 and was standardised in 1976. There have been subsequent importations. The popularity of the Dwarf Lop as an exhibition breed is exceeded today only by the Netherland Dwarf.

In the early 1980s, in several parts of the country, a long-haired variety of Dwarf Lops appeared. By some these were considered useless, but some enterprising breeders developed them, using the silkier coated types and eventually in the mid 1980s had these recognised as the Cashmere Lop. From the original size Cashmere, there has arisen a Giant Cashmere Lop, but this, as yet, has not been officially recognised. Today an even smaller Lop, the Miniature Lop, having an ideal weight of 1.5 kg and a maximum permissible weight of 1.6 kg, has been produced.

Fanciers in Holland, since they created the Dwarf Lop, have continued to attempt to reduce their size, whilst in the UK, the size of most original strains of Dwarf Lop has tended to increase. However, some fanciers of Dwarf Lops in the UK persisted in their efforts to reduce the size of the Dwarf Lop and thus two distinct groups are present. In the early 1990s some Dwarf Lops (miniature) were introduced from Holland and thus the new Miniature Lop was established, the standard being recognised in 1994.

The last member of the Lop family is the Meissner Lop, which was produced in Germany by crossing continental Lops with silvered breeds during the late 1920s and the early 1930s. The weights in different countries vary, but in the UK the standard weight is approximately between 3 and 4 kg. The silvering resembles that of the Silver rather than the Argente.

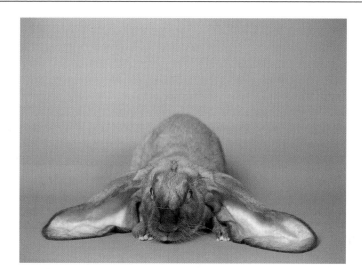

Fig. 2.21
English Lop

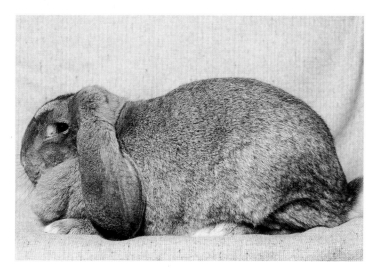

Fig. 2.22
French Lop

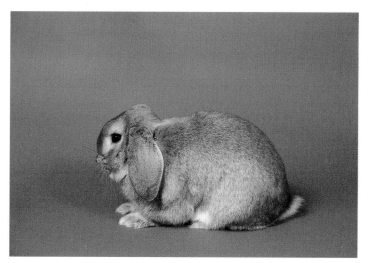

Fig. 2.23
Dwarf Lop

The Netherland Dwarf (Fig. 2.25)

The Netherland Dwarf was developed in Holland from the Polish rabbit imported from England in the late 19th and early 20th centuries, but the selection of the breeding stock was such that there is now little similarity between the two breeds except for size.

Their development as separate breeds started prior to the 1939–45 war but was interrupted by the German occupation of Holland. It was not until 1950 that Netherland Dwarfs were introduced into the UK. Since that time they have become very popular and now they are one of the most popular of fancy breeds. They have now been produced in a number of colours including sable, black, brown, smoke pearl and even chinchilla.The Dwarf, as it tends to be called, is entirely an exhibition rabbit and undoubtedly makes an excellent pet for a small child being cobby and compact, and so small as to be easily handled. The breed suffered initially from poor breeding characteristics, but this problem has been overcome to some extent. It does in some cases suffer more from malocclusion of the teeth than many other breeds. The maximum weight is 1.13 kg as an adult. It should perhaps be noted that this breed is known as 'Polish' in most parts of Europe.

The New Zealand Red (Fig. 2.26)

The New Zealand Red was one of the first utility breeds developed in America. There was at some time a good deal of controversy as to whether it originated from some imports, in 1909, of animals from New Zealand, they in turn being derived from wild stock, or whether they were developed from Golden Fawn 'sports' from Flemish Giants crossed with Belgian Hares. The latter is almost certainly correct.

The breed was imported into this country in 1916, although prior to this date a very similar breed, known as the Old English Red, had been standardised by an organisation known as the National Self-Coloured Rabbit Club. The same breed, although differing in some ways, was and is known in France as the Fauve de Bourgogne, and in Italy as the Fulvo di Burgogna. The Thrianta is a very similar breed.

These various breeds, or rather variations of the same breed, have been selected by breeders in the different countries to different ideals, until they differ considerably in some cases, although remaining basically the same breed. The genetical constitution of the New Zealand Red includes a gene for the elimination of all black pigment from the Agouti colouring which thus gives a complete extension of the yellow colour. There are doubtless a number of modifying genes to produce the bright reddish-buff colour. Although developed in America as a utility rabbit for the production of young meat, the breed in the UK has been selected away from this standard and the fur being harsh is of little value.

It is interesting to note that a different emphasis again in France has led to a markedly different animal in the Fauve de Bourgogne which is a larger 4.5 kg against 3.6 kg for the New Zealand Red, and which has a dense and lustrous coat as opposed to the harsh coat of the New Zealand Red.

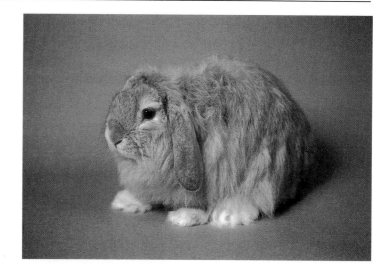

Fig. 2.24
Cashmere Lop

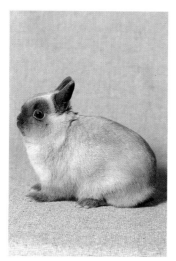

Fig. 2.25
Netherland Dwarf

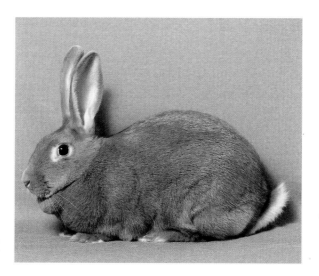

Fig. 2.26
New Zealand Red

The New Zealand White (Fig. 2.27), Black and Blue

The New Zealand White although originally very similar to the New Zealand Red in America differs markedly from the New Zealand Red of this country. It is a much larger animal, weighing 4 to 5.4 kg compared with the 3.6 kg of the Red in the UK. It has become the most popular breed for young meat production in many parts of the world. Its spread throughout the world has greatly exceeded that of any other breed. It is undoubtedly the most suitable breed for meat production. It has very rapid growth characteristics, and will produce a 1.3 to 2 .5 kg rabbit at 8 to 10 weeks of age. The feeding of both the mother and young for this production must, however, be good. Furthermore the breed has excellent meat type with considerable fleshing of the hindquarters and back, and also has excellent breeding qualities.

The New Zealand White was imported into England after the 1939–45 war and has become fairly popular as an exhibition animal. It is also a most useful laboratory animal. It is an albino as opposed to the White Beveren which is a blue-eyed white.

Recognised in the late 1960s as a further variety was the New Zealand Black which resembles, except for colour, the New Zealand White in every way. A further development was the New Zealand Blue which again, is in size and conformation identical to the white.

The Perlfee (Fig. 2.28)

This is a little known rabbit even in its country of origin, which is Germany. It is a derivative of the Feh de Marbourg (another German breed which itself is a derivative from the Havana). It was standardised in the UK in the late 1980s. It is a small breed usually weighing as an adult in the region of 2.5 kg. The basic colour is a grey blue, and whilst three different shades are permissible, the medium shade is preferred. In the UK, as with others, for some reason it has not achieved much popularity.

The Pointed Beveren

The Pointed Beveren is another breed which was established in the 1920s. It was standardised in 1928, but became extinct in the 1930s. It was originally known as the Pointed Fox, its name being changed to Pointed Beveren in 1931. In the early part of its history 'an exceptionally bright future' was predicted for it, but in company with many of the then newer fur breeds it lost its admirers until the late 1980s when it was re-created. Originally only black and blue versions were permitted, but now there are four, brown and lilac being added. In type and weight it is the same as the Beveren. It differs from the Beverens by having white-tipped hairs over all the body.

The Polish (Fig. 2.29)

The Polish is a neat, compact and sprightly rabbit weighing between 1.1 and 1.4 kg. Its origin is unknown but it is probable that it was first bred from Dutch or Himalayan rabbits in Belgium. Some Polish were certainly produced in this way in England during the 1860s and 1870s, but prior to that the breed was introduced from Belgium where it was produced as a rabbit for the gourmet. At this time it was larger than at present, weighing between 1.6 and 2 kg.

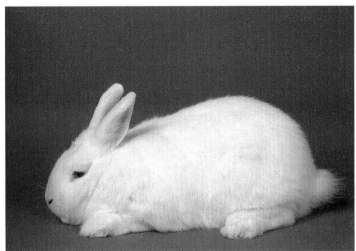

Fig. 2.27
New Zealand White

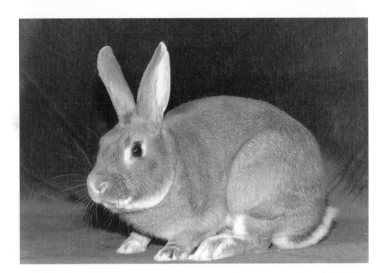

Fig. 2.28
Perlfee

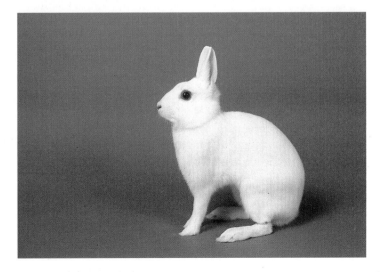

Fig. 2.29
Polish

Although today no one would consider the Polish a utility animal, in the early 1900s they were in great demand on the Continent, particularly in Belgium, and in the UK as an epicurean luxury, the rabbits for this purpose being fed largely on milk and meal.

The Red-Eyed White Polish is of course an albino, whilst the Blue-Eyed White carries the factor for Vienna White. Although from time to time coloured Polish have always appeared, they were not recognised until the 1950s, since when numerous colours and patterns have been produced.

The Rex breeds (Figs 2.30–2.36)

A description of the origin of the Rexes has been given earlier in this chapter. Following their introduction into this country (as the Castor Rex in 1927), many of the normal furred breeds were used to produce colour Rexes. The combination of any colour with the Rex coat is, of course, a fairly simple matter, although the improvement of the colour Rex so produced may take some time.

The Rex character consists of a shortening of the guard hairs until they lie below or level with the undercoat, thus producing an exquisite, plush-like coat, some 12.5 mm in length, with a velvet touch. In some cases guard hairs do project, and are considered a fault of the breed.

Rex furs were the most valuable rabbit furs commercially, and the carcases were also suitable for the meat trade. The best qualities of Rex furs usually brought as much as double the price obtained for the normal furred pelts. Not all colours were, however, in demand. The Chinchilla Rex and the Havana Rex pelts were almost always wanted, but some of the other pelts, the Orange Rex for example, although a most popular exhibition variety, had a lower value. The Rex fur is only at its best when the animal is mature, and it is therefore necessary to keep the Rexes a minimum of six to seven months, and more usually eight months, before pelting. The adult Rex will weigh between 2.7 and 3.6 kg, and thus the carcase weight of the Rex when pelted will be about 1.8 kg or slightly more.

The early Rexes were of weak constitution, and suffered considerably from various ailments. Indeed, it was thought by many that the character arose through disease. This, of course, is completely incorrect, and today the Rexes are constitutionally as sound and hardy as the other breeds.

The above refers to the standard smooth-coated Rexes, although there are three other types, the Mini Rex, the Astrex and the Opossum Rex.

The Astrex, evolved during 1932–34, has a Rex coat which is tightly waved over the entire body. At present there are very few, if any, to be seen but in the past there were some cases in which the waving was assisted, at least, by artificial means, a practice greatly frowned upon by the exhibiting world. The Astrex had little commercial value for the curling would not often stand up to dressing. Astrex were recognised in all colours, although ermine, black, lilac and Havana were the most common.

The Black Rex is of a lustrous blue-black (being self-coloured) with slate-blue undercolour. They were a most useful colour for furriery work, for they invariably matched well. It is one of the most popular of all Rexes.

The Blue Rex was one of the earliest colours, although the colour has been greatly

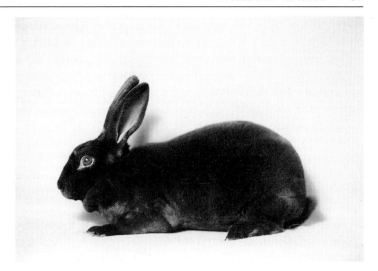

Fig. 2.30
Black Rex

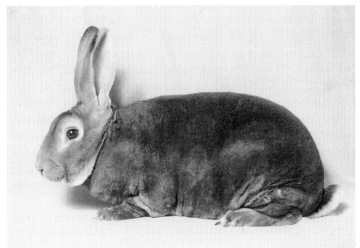

Fig. 2.31
Castor Rex

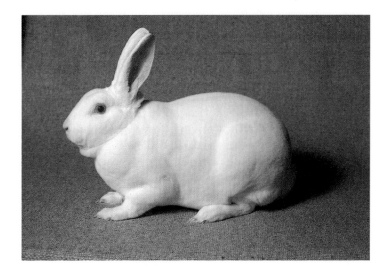

Fig. 2.32
Ermine Rex

improved, usually by crossing with Blue Beverens. The blue is a clear bright medium shade (not lavender) and again the pelts usually matched fairly well.

The Castor Rex was, of course, the original Rex, being an Agouti with a dark rich chestnut-brown colour, the intermediate colour being rich orange on a dark slate-blue undercolour. The variety has changed considerably from the original, and in fact has been remade on a number of occasions. For some reason it was never one of the furriers popular colours.

The Chinchilla Rex was undoubtedly the most popular colour for fur work, although perhaps more difficult to match well. The pelts, when of good quality, certainly fetched the best prices of any. The colour is a dark-slate base, over which is a near-white intermediate colour, the top colour being lightly tipped with black and white giving a sparkling, chinchillated wavy effect. It should perhaps be added that the Chinchilla Rex is one of the most difficult of the Rexes to produce in the highest quality.

The Cinnamon Rex is an Agouti Rex, the top colour being bright golden tan, the intermediate colour a light orange, clearly defined on a blue undercolour. The belly is of course white on a blue undercolour. They are uncommon. Genetically the variety is a brown Agouti.

The Dalmatian Rex was one of the last Rex to be imported to this country. It has a white fur covered with small coloured patches which are self- or bi-coloured.

The Dutch Rex is a rexed variety of the popular fancy breed and is very rarely seen. It was of very little value as a commercial fur.

The English Rex is the rexed variety of the English, and is also very rarely seen.

The Ermine Rex has always been one of the most popular Rexes and has been bred to a high degree of excellence. Blue-eyed stock were seen at one time, but at the present time all the Ermine Rexes are albino, i.e. red-eyed. The pelts were suitable for many forms of fur work, but never commanded such good prices as many of the other colours.

The Fawn Rex is a tan pattern Rex with a saddle of bright golden fawn gradually shading to a white belly. It is not often seen.

The Fox Rex, another tan pattern Rex, is produced in the four colours found in the normal fur Foxes. It is of course the rexed normal fur breed.

The Harlequin Rex is the counterpart of the Harlequin Rabbit and whilst not one of the most popular colours is being seen more often.

The Havana Rex is very popular. It is a self-coloured variety of a rich dark chocolate colour. The pelts were probably the most sought after by the fur trade, and the breed had the advantage that the majority of pelts could be used for the best quality of work. The pelts were used for all types of garments, and brown, being usually in fashion, was always in demand.

The Himalayan is a very striking Rex with its pure white body colour and sepia points; the standard also caters for chocolate and blue points, but at the present time breeders are concentrating on the sepia.

The Lilac Rex came both from rexing the normal fur Lilac, but also by crosses of Blue and Havana Rex, for the lilac colour is a dilute brown. Those animals produced by rexing the normal Lilac usually gave the best animals.

The Lynx Rex is a rexed variety of the Normal Lynx, a normal fur breed which originated in Germany but is not known in this country. Genetically it is a dilute brown Agouti. The top colour is orange-shot-silver, the intermediate colour being a

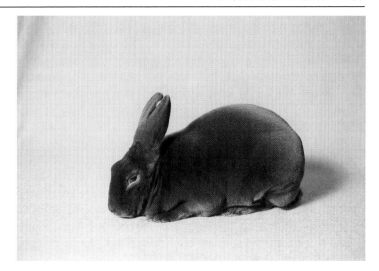

Fig. 2.33
Havana Rex

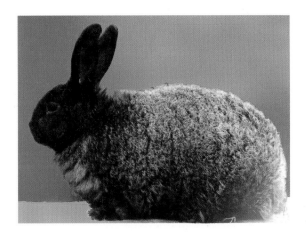

Fig. 2.34
Opossum Rex

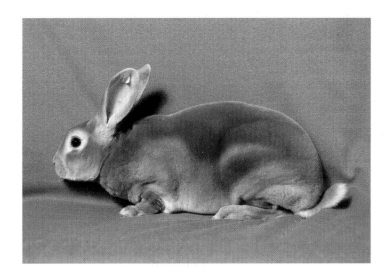

Fig. 2.35
Orange Rex

bright orange, with the undercolour white. The Lynx Rex is an Agouti and is not one of the popular colours.

The Marten Sable Rex is the rexed normal medium or light Marten Sable and is a tan pattern Rex with dark sepia-brown saddle shading gradually on the flanks, and with a white belly. It is somewhat less popular than the Siamese Sable Rex.

The Mini Rex is the newest addition to the Rex family, being first recognised in 1990. Apart from size it should be identical to the standard Rexes. The ideal weight should be 1.4 to 1.8 kg. Some countries have produced Mini Rexes of higher quality than are to be found today in the UK.

The Nutria Rex is a self-coloured Rex with rich golden-brown colour, but is now rarely seen, although in other countries it is considered to be one of the best of Rexes. Occasionally Nutria turn up in Havana Rex litters.

The Opal Rex is again rarely seen, although it was popular at one time. It is genetically a dilute Agouti and has a top colour of a pale shade of blue with a layer of golden tan between it and the slate-blue undercolour.

The Opossum Rex was produced in 1924 by T. Leaver of Kent, in an attempt to Rex the Chifox. Originally three black Chifox were used but later woollies from Argentes were introduced to obtain the silvering. The length of the undercoat of the Opossum Rex is about 25 mm and the guard hairs which project above the body coat are silvered, that is, devoid of pigment at the tips and curled. The coat is at right angles to the body, and thus presents a similar appearance from all directions. All colours were recognised. The character is recessive to normal Rex but the variety is now very rare. This is a pity for it is a unique and attractive breed.

The Orange Rex is a striking deep rich orange, carried well down the sides and shading to a white belly. The Orange Rex started as the rexed form of the New Zealand Red, and is genetically an Agouti although always classed as a tan pattern rabbit. It is a popular exhibition variety, but was rather too striking to have been popular with furriers.

The Orange Buff Rex is very rarely seen. It is a shaded variety with the saddle a deep rich clear orange shading into a beige or light clear biscuit colour over the remainder of the body. The breed was derived by selection from Orange Rex with orange-beige belly fur.

The Otter Rex is a relatively new colour variety and is indeed one of the very few importations of Rex since the early days in the 1920s and 1930s. The Otter Rex was first introduced from France in 1970. The original fur colour was a lustrous black

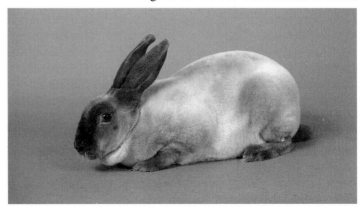

Fig. 2.36
Smoke Pearl Rex

with a slate-blue undercolour with the belly creamy white, being divided by a border of tan. Since its introduction the Otter Rex has been produced in blue, chocolate, and lilac as well as black.

The Satin Rex (see page 56) are Rexed versions of the Satin and can be either rough or smooth coated, They have never achieved the popularity of the other Rexes.

The Seal Rex is the Rex variety of the dark Siamese Sable, having a rich dark sepia (almost black) saddle with only slightly paler shadings on the remainder of the body. The Seal and Sable Rexes are often interbred to improve quality. The Seal Rex has one of the best pelts for the furrier and is certainly a popular exhibition Rex colour.

The Seal Marten Rex is the Rex variety of the dark Marten Sable, being a dark sepia shading to only slighter paler sepia on the lower flanks, chest and belly. This colour was separated from the Marten Sable Rex and given its own standard some years ago.

The Siamese Sable Rex is the rexed normal Siamese Sable of either the light or medium shades. The light shades were the least popular with furriers and the dark mediums the most popular. They are a shaded variety with a dark sepia-brown saddle shading gradually to a rich chestnut on the flanks.

The Silver Seal Rex became quite popular in the late 1940s, but their popularity died and they are very rarely, if ever, to be seen. The Silver Seal, the Rex variety of the Silver Grey failed to attain the smooth plush texture of other Rexes.

The Smoke Pearl Rex is a most attractive variety of the shaded group of Rexes. The Siamese Smoke Pearl Rex has a saddle of smoke-grey shading to pale grey on the flanks, chest and belly. It was produced from Sable Rex, being a Sable carrying the factor for dilution. Thus a Marten Sable Rex carrying dilution would give a Marten Smoke Pearl, and in fact this has been produced. The pelt of Smoke Pearl Rex is of such a delicate colour that it was used mainly for evening capes or trimmings.

The Tan Rex, a Rex variety of the normal Tan, has been produced but is not often seen.

The Tortoiseshell is a shaded-self rabbit with a rich bright orange top lightly dusted with brown ticking.

The Rhinelander (Fig. 2.37)

The first Rhinelander was imported from its country of origin, Germany, in 1965 but is still uncommon. It was created by a cross between rabbits with English and Harlequin patterns and is a tri-coloured breed.

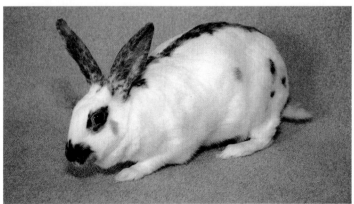

Fig. 2.37
Rhinelander

The Sables (Fig. 2.38)

There are two varieties of Sable – the Siamese and the Marten. In both varieties there are three colours, light, medium, and dark. The Siamese is a self-coloured rabbit, which carries the factors for light chinchillation, whilst the Marten Sable is a tan pattern rabbit (the tan, however, being replaced by white) also carrying the factors of light chinchillation. Both varieties are shaded. The Sables occurred at various times in litters of Chinchillas following the early importations. They were at first considered valueless and were discarded. Then they were kept and the name Maraaka was suggested for them, but was later not used. The Marten Sables most frequently occurred, and later Siamese Sables were produced in litters of Martens. The names by which they are now known were given to the two breeds as the Siamese resembled the Siamese cat, and the Marten, the wild Stone Marten, whilst the basic colour resembled the wild Sable.

The colouring of the Sables is a rich sepia saddle shading to a lighter sepia on the flanks and sides. The Marten flanks and rump should be well ticked with longer white hairs, and the belly white. The pelts of the light shades were not much sought after by the fur trade, the furrier much preferring the medium colour. The coats are of a high quality and the Sables are for this reason one of the most useful normal fur breeds. The weight is from 2.25 to 3.2 kg.

The Sallander (Fig. 2.39)

The Sallander originated in Holland, where it was first officially recognised in 1975. It is not well known in any other country. It derives from the Thuringer, and it is one of the most recent of breeds in England, its standard being recognised only in 1994. It is a thickset, well-rounded rabbit, weighing between 2.5 and 4.25 kg. The fur is dense and silky and the general colour is pearl, but the guard hairs cover the whole coat with a haze of pale charcoal. The animal is shaded but somewhat unusually, the darker shadings extend over the lower half of the body, the shadings therefore being the reverse of what is usually found. Apart from the colour it should be an identical rabbit to the Thuringer.

The Satin breeds (Fig. 2.40)

The distinctive feature of the Satin breeds is an exquisite satin-like texture and sheen which is produced by a peculiar modification of the hair, the scales being much flattened and the central hollow cells found in other fur types being either partly or completely absent. The mutation producing these structural modifications is completely recessive to the normal coat.

The mutation was first established in 1930 in America, but was only imported into the UK in 1947. Since then there have been several further importations. The original importations were of Ivory (albino) Satins and this still remains by far the most popular colour, although some other colours have been established. The coat is of a roll back nature and the fur length 25 to 32 mm. The adult weight is 2.7 to 3.6 kg. The Satin texture and sheen has been combined with the Rex coat to give Satin Rexes.

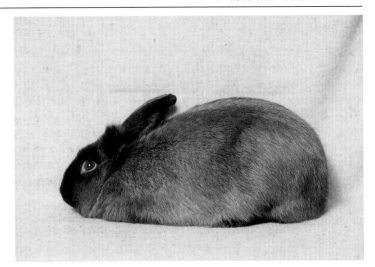

Fig. 2.38
Siamese Sable

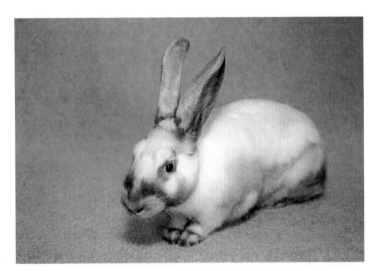

Fig. 2.39
Sallander

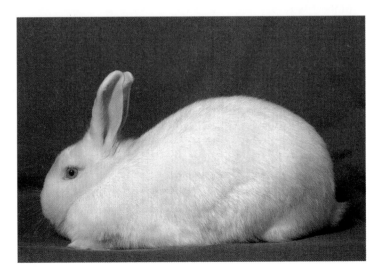

Fig. 2.40
Satin

The Siberian (Fig. 2.41)

The Siberian was produced in 1930, and is a modern normal fur breed and not to be confused with the Himalayan pointed Angora, once called the Siberian but now never seen. The breed was made for the purpose of producing uniform skins which would be easy to match. The self-coloured rabbits produced when breeding English formed a large part of the make-up of the Siberian which became quite popular during the 1939–45 war, but now is less so. The pelts were not a great deal sought after by the fur trade, for the colours were not entirely to their liking. The quality of the fur also required much improvement before they became of commercial value. The breed has, however, its fanciers. It is bred in black, blue, brown and lilac.

The Silver (Fig. 2.42)

The Silver is one of the earliest of exhibition breeds and today is one of the most popular of the early fancy breeds. It was usually said that the breed originated in Siam, but this was another of the myths that often surround the origin of breeds. The first mention of them is made by Gervase Markham in 1631 who speaks a good deal about a silvered rabbit, quite obviously a present-day Silver Grey. It is also singular that he gives the word 'richness' to their fur and talks about them as 'rich' rabbits, for an old name for the Silver Grey in France was 'riche rabbit'.

What happened to this stock of Silvers is unknown but Silver Greys appeared again in the 1860s amongst wild rabbits and in warrens in Lincolnshire, and were then known as Lincolnshire Sprigs, Millers, or Lincolnshire Silver Greys. The Silver Grey, the first of the colours, was shown initially in 1860, and rather later the Silver Fawn was introduced. These latter were known as either Silver Creams or Silver Fawns, and were not, contrary to fairly general belief, the same as the Argente-creme bred on the Continent at this time. The Silver Fawns were first produced in the UK by crossing a Silver Grey with a Fawn rabbit, and the original light fawn or cream colour has been deepened by selection to a deep bright orange. Following the introduction of the Silver Fawn came the Silver Brown, produced by crosses involving the Silver Grey and the Belgian Hare. The Silver Blue was not introduced until the 1980s.

The white ticking or silvering of the Silvers, which covers the entire body, is basically controlled by a mutation which is incompletely recessive, although there are a number of modifying factors which control the amount of ticking. The Silver Grey is a black rabbit with white ticking, the Fawn is a yellow with white ticking, the Brown is an Agouti with white ticking, and the Blue is a blue with white ticking. The silvering does not appear until after the first moult, i.e. four to six weeks of age, for the different varieties are completely black, Agouti Fawn or Blue when born. The silvering consists of the loss of pigment in the secondary guard hairs. To finish silvering some specimens take as long as six or seven months, although others complete the process much earlier.

Apart from being one of the most popular and attractive of exhibition rabbits, the Silvers are a most suitable breed for the older child. They are hardy and of the right size, and offer great interest to the child during the process of silvering. As adults they weigh about 2.7 kg.

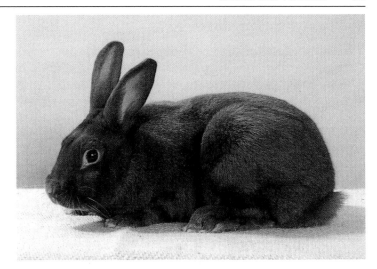

Fig. 2.41
Siberian
(Brown)

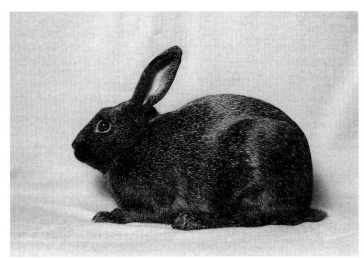

Fig. 2.42
Silver
(Grey)

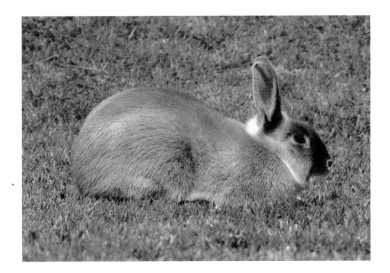

Fig. 2.43
Smoke Pearl
(Marten)

The Smoke Pearl (Fig. 2.43)

The first specimens of this breed were produced from Sables in the late 1920s in both the Marten and the Siamese patterns. They are in fact Sables carrying the factor for dilution. At first the breed was known as the Smoke Beige, but the name was changed to the present one in 1932 when the standard was first adopted by the British Fur Rabbit Society. The saddle is smoke in colour, shading to a pearly grey beige on the flanks, with the Marten type having the chest, flanks and rump ticked with longer white hairs, and a white belly. The weight is between 2.25 and 3.2 kg.

The Squirrel

The Squirrel was, as the Sable, from time to time produced in litters of Chinchillas. In the early days they were simply disposed of until an enterprising breeder in the mid 1920s considered they would be an attractive breed, much resembling the wild Siberian Squirrel, the furs of which were in demand by the fur trade. The breed was thus established and a provisional standard granted by the British Fur Rabbit Society in 1928. By the mid 1920s there were none being bred, but it was re-created in the 1980s, and the old standard re-instated. The Squirrel, being a blue Chinchilla, was produced again by crosses of Chinchilla and Argente Bleu. The colour is found in other breeds, e.g. Satin, and the weight is between 2.5 and 3.05 kg.

The Sussex (Fig. 2.44)

Originated in 1986 from a cross of Californian and Lilac, being used to improve the point colour of the Lilac Californian. The original Sussex descended from a brown tortoiseshell doe which appeared in a second generation litter. The Sussex Gold became standardised in 1991 as a normal fur breed, being a reddish tortoiseshell with brown or lilac shadings, and a preferred weight of 3.4 kg. It was followed by the Cream, being a rich pinkish cream, the top colour lightly ticked with lilac.

The Swiss Fox (Fig. 2.45)

Although originating in both Switzerland and Germany in the 1920s, for some reason it ceased to be bred in Germany but became popular in Switzerland from where it was introduced into the UK in the early 1980s, but is still not common. It is a medium-sized rabbit with a very short neck, weighing between 2.5 to 3 kg, with a coat that should be between 5 and 6 cm long. It occurs in White, Black, Blue and Havana (or Dark Brown). All colours are recognised. Most common are White, Black, Blue and Havana (or Dark Brown).

The Tan (Fig. 2.46)

The Tan rabbit was, like the Silver, first found in a warren containing wild stock into which some domestic rabbits had been introduced. The distinctive pattern of the Tan is due to a mutation from the wild Agouti. The basic pattern is a self-coloured back with a light-coloured belly and yellow flanks. Improvement consists in extending the yellow or tan colour over the entire belly, ears, nostrils, and feet and improving the

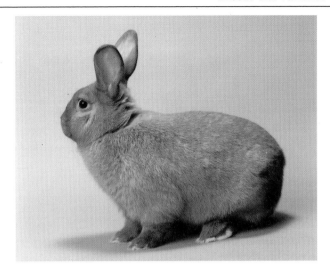

Fig. 2.44
Sussex
(Gold)

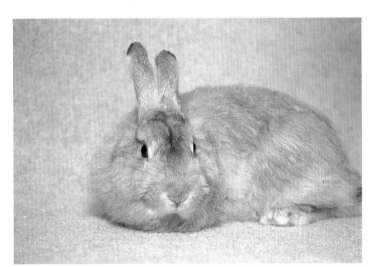

Fig. 2.45
Swiss Fox
(Fawn)

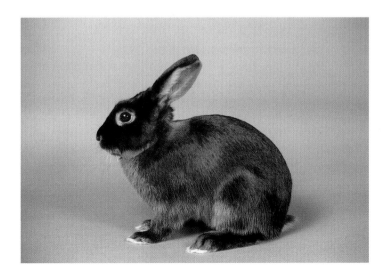

Fig. 2.46
Tan

colour of this tan. The adult weight is approximately 2 kg and the breed has four colour varieties, black, blue, chocolate and lilac.

The first Tans were found in the 1880s and were blacks. The dilution factor was introduced by using sooty fawn animals and thus blues were produced. The chocolates came next, being the recessives to blacks, and when the dilution factor was introduced into these chocolates, the lilacs were the last to be produced. Tans are one of the oldest breeds of rabbits and the National Specialist Club for the breed is over 100 years old.

The Thrianta (Fig. 2.47)

This is another Dutch Breed which was only recognised by the Dutch after the 1939–45 war, its standard being renewed in 1971. After importation into this country it was standardised in the early 1980s. The Thrianta originated by the crossing of fawn rabbits with Tans and is a brilliant orange-red in colour. It has attained little widespread popularity.

The Thuringer (Fig. 2.48)

The Thuringer originated in Germany from crosses between Himalayans (weighing approximately 2.5 kg) and Large Argentes (weighing approximately 4.5 kg) giving an adult weight for the Thuringer of the order of about 3.5 kg. In France where it is popular it is called Chamois de Thuringe to indicate the colour being very similar to the Chamois antelope found in the Alps, the same colour as shammy leather. Again the Thuringer has reverse shadings the general colour being yellow ochre or buff. The guard hairs are of a bluish black colour, which produce a haze of a pale charcoal colour. The markings consist of a general colour with shadings and belly colour. The belly colour and shadings are sooty (or charcoal) coloured, extending over the lower part of the body and fading towards the upper parts. The Thuringer was imported into this country and standardised in the late 1960s.

The Vienna Blue (Fig. 2.49)

Although there is sometimes debate concerning the origin of the Vienna Blue (and its other colour varieties) there is no doubt that it was first produced in Austria in the 1890s. The Vienna Blue was produced from crosses involving the Belgian Giant (almost certainly an early strain developed from the Patagonian) for size, and the Blue Lorraine Giant for colour. There is also little doubt that some Argente was introduced into the breed during its formation.

The Vienna Blue in Europe is certainly one of the most popular of all breeds and in some countries other colours of Vienna are recognised – White, Black, Grey, and Blue Grey. Of these colours, (and today only Blue is recognised in the UK) Blue, Black and Blue Grey have a weight of 3.5 to 5.5 kg whilst White and Grey have a weight of 3 to 5 kg.

The Vienna Blue has a superb coat and the blue is a superb colour. Already the Vienna Blue has had some considerable success in the exhibition world. At a recent show in Nurenberg there were 2230 Viennas exhibited out of a total of some 24 000, or nearly 10% of all exhibits

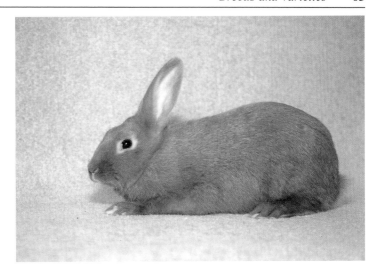

Fig. 2.47
Thrianta

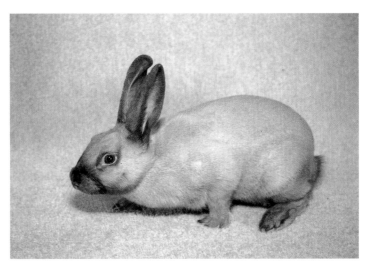

Fig. 2.48
Thuringer

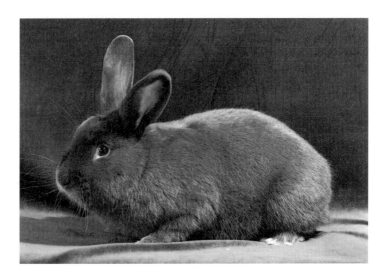

Fig. 2.49
Vienna Blue

Chapter 3

The Rabbit Fancy

The rabbit fancy in the UK (and indeed in most countries of the world) consists of large numbers of people, of both sexes and all ages, who are interested in breeding and exhibiting the different breeds of domestic rabbits. These people are known as rabbit fanciers.

A fancier is a person who has a passion to breed perfect specimens of a particular breed and sometimes more than one breed. The fancier builds up in his or her mind's eye a picture of the ideal animal, usually in the greatest detail, and this perfect animal he or she attempts, with all his or her skill and patience, to produce. The fancier quite apart from this passion, has a love and respect for the animals, and their welfare is a constant concern. There are some fanciers, in the truest sense, who do not exhibit at shows. Usually, however, the measure of success is judged by winning at such events.

The breeding of the perfect specimen, or as nearly perfect as possible, is the aim of the fancier. The winning of the supreme award at a major show is the confirmation that he or she has gone some way to achieving a dream. The importance of winning at shows varies a good deal from fancier to fancier. There are some who are bitterly disappointed if they do not win and in a few cases castigate the judges for what they consider their obvious (to them on this occasion!) lack of ability. The vast majority are however, philosophical about winning and know that there is always another show on another day, and more rabbits to be bred.

The true fancier does not keep such pleasure and fascination to him- or herself. He or she is always willing to help a fellow fancier or newcomer in any way he or she can. Possibly the distinction of a true fancier is that he or she is almost as pleased, when losing to someone to whom he or she has supplied the stock responsible for this, as when winning.

Although the domestication of the wild rabbit certainly began some two thousand years ago, exhibiting in this country dates only from about two hundred years ago, although the earliest society devoted solely to the exhibition of rabbits was founded in London in 1840 and was known as the Metropolitan Fancy Rabbit Club. At this time there were few breeds, and those very mixed and unstandardised. They differed greatly from their present-day counterparts. The English Lop (as it even then was called) was certainly the first breed to be exhibited although at the time the Silver Grey and the Angora had both been known for many years before. The two characteristics which were used in judging, but usually not at the same time, were ear length, measured in a straight line from tip to tip, and weight. The reason why the Lop at that time was the sole breed was that it contained both characteristics to the greatest degree.

The English or Butterfly Smut, as it was then called, was also present by the middle of the 19th century, but was not exhibited to any extent until a good deal later. In fact by about 1875 Belgian Hares, Himalayans, Dutch, Lops, Polish, Silver Greys and Siberians (at that time this name referred to an Angora with Himalayan markings and not the Siberian of today), all preceded the recognition and exhibition of English.

The fancy breeds were becoming well established during the latter part of the last century and the earliest National Specialist Clubs were being formed in the 1890s. It was not until after the 1914–18 war, however, that much development occurred in the fur breeds. During this latter period some of the present-day fur breed clubs came into existence, although it was during the 1939–45 war that the majority of existing fur breed clubs were formed.

RABBIT CLUBS

Almost every rabbit fancier will be a member of one or more rabbit clubs, some of which are local clubs, whilst others are breed or specialist clubs. The local rabbit club is one which has members interested in all the breeds of rabbits. The members usually live in a relatively small area. The local club will hold one or more shows each year, and in a few cases a local club may hold as many as nine or ten. At the peak period there were over 1000 local rabbit clubs in the British Isles affiliated to the British Rabbit Council (BRC), but currently there are about 150.

The local clubs are associations of interested breeders who meet fairly regularly and discuss rabbit topics. Sometimes there are lectures, social events, or visits to different places, but almost invariably there are shows. These shows may be Table or Box Shows where the exhibits are not placed in steel mesh pens but are brought to the judging table direct from the travelling boxes in which the owners have brought them. Alternatively they may be Open Pen Shows, in which the rabbits are individually penned in steel-mesh pens erected on wooden staging.

The specialist or breed club caters for, or looks after, the interests of its particular breed and each has the welfare of its own breed at heart. Some specialist clubs are recognised as being National Specialist Clubs, that is to say they are recognised by the BRC as the main Club for that breed in the country. There can be only one National Club for each breed and in 1994 there were 45 National Specialist Clubs. In general the standard for the breed is maintained by the National Specialist Club, which has members in all parts of the country. The National Specialist Club has an elected panel of judges, which usually has about 40 judges on it. There may however be as few as 25 or as many as 60. Each National Specialist Club will usually hold two main shows a year. These are the Adult Stock Show and the Young Stock Show.

Those breed clubs not achieving national status are Area Specialist Clubs. Their constitution and activities, with the exception of standards and the like, are very similar to the National Clubs, but of course they are (or should be) only active within a restricted area. This is usually a few counties, but may be the whole of Scotland, or Wales, or a third or so of England. At the present time there are 90 Area Breed Clubs affiliated to the BRC. Sometimes the Area Specialist Club is closely linked to the National Club and sometimes it is not. Usually, however no Area Club can become affiliated to the BRC unless the National Club approves of its existence.

Apart from local and breed clubs, there are other organisations whose members are interested in rabbits. There are, for example, over 80 affiliated agricultural societies at whose annual shows a rabbit section is included. There are school rabbit clubs, which are interested in rabbit keeping and exhibiting and it is a pity that more are not formed, for they can play an excellent part in education.

Similarly there are some public bodies which amongst their activities include rabbit shows, and also affiliated to the BRC are major Show Societies, National Rabbit Councils in other countries and the like.

THE BRITISH RABBIT COUNCIL

In each country in which there is a rabbit fancy, there is a central national organisation, which acts as a central governing body. This body has a number of different activities, including such things as licensing shows, laying down regulations for the conduct of shows, presenting a unified voice to government or other associations, and so on. On occasions there are in fact more than one body claiming to be the main body, but in fact this is rarely true.

In Great Britain the national or central governing body is the BRC. The great majority of clubs, societies and other organisations interested in domestic rabbits are affiliated to it. The BRC was established in 1934 by the amalgamation of the two largest central rabbit organisations at that time.

The objects of the BRC are:

- to protect, further and co-ordinate the interests of all British rabbit breeders;
- to assist and extend the exhibition of rabbits;
- to influence, advise and co-operate with central and local authorities, departments, educational and other committees and schools, in promoting the extension of the breeding of rabbits;
- to promote and encourage education and research of a scientific and/or practical nature for the welfare and benefit of the rabbit.

The BRC, apart from affiliated clubs and organisations, has some thousands of individual members. It issues a set of show rules, which regulate the exhibiting of rabbits and the organisation of shows in this country, and all good shows are held under these rules. In addition all shows are offered support in the form of Challenge Certificates and Diplomas, which are eagerly sought by members.

There are numerous activities in which the BRC engages to assist rabbit breeding. Not least is the provision of advice on every conceivable aspect, and the investigation of complaints and disputes, (though happily these are relatively rare). The ringing scheme, details of which are given in Chapter 5, provides a system whereby not only is each rabbit uniquely identified for its life but it can be returned quickly to its owner should it ever get lost. The ringing scheme has also a basic and important part in giving awards. Whilst the drafting and maintenance of most individual standards lies with the National Specialist Clubs, the issuing of all standards is the work of the BRC. Each member automatically receives a standard book and also, indeed, a yearbook. Many fanciers like to use a stud name or prefix. These are registered and maintained by the BRC. Each year, to well over 1400 shows, the BRC issues specials in the form of Challenge Certificates and Diplomas. These are awarded to the most successful exhibitors who apart from their pleasure in winning them, use them to claim further awards, such as Supreme Championships.

It is perhaps unnecessary to add that it is strongly advisable for all persons interested in the rabbit to join the BRC, as well as their local and breed club.

SHOWS

At one time, the Table or Box Shows of local clubs were not only great fun but the training ground for the newcomer, and indeed the novice judge. They were also a social occasion when members met for a convivial time, often of an evening. These have been largely superseded by the smaller pen shows of local clubs.

Moving up in levels there are the larger pen shows, the Area Specialist Club Shows, the Four Star Championship Shows, the National Specialist Club shows and then the major Championship Shows.

A system of star grading of shows exist, with different conditions attaching to different star graded shows.

● One Star shows have few conditions and are the basic level.
● Two Star shows require guaranteed prize money and there must be at least 15 straight breed classes.
● Three Star shows are confined to either National Specialist Clubs or are All Breed Championship Shows at which at least 30 Challenge Certificates are to be awarded, prize money is guaranteed, the judge or judges must be on either their National Specialist Club or the BRC Three Star panel.
● Four Star Shows have the same conditions as Three Star, but the grading is only awarded to those shows having the highest possible standard of organisation and venue.
● Five Star shows must be staged over two days, must have all the requirements of Four Star shows, and a full catalogue must be issued.

There are only two Five Star Shows, the London Championship Show held in October each year and the Bradford Championship Show held in January. Bradford, as it is commonly and affectionately called, has been held for the past 75 years and attracts several thousands of entries.

Table and One Star Shows are held more or less throughout the year, but the larger shows are mainly concentrated in June, July, and August for the young stock and summer shows, and October, November, and December for the adult stock and winter shows. The bulk of the specialist club young stock shows are held in July, whilst the majority of their adult stock shows are held in November or December.

Most of the shows are one-day events, whilst a few of the larger shows occupy two days. Table Shows are usually afternoon or evening affairs. All shows which are offered BRC support are advertised in the columns of the fancy press, in particular

Fur & Feather, a fortnightly magazine devoted largely to rabbit keeping and showing. There is, in this magazine, which is the official journal of the BRC, a show diary which contains full details of all shows being held in the following month.

The full set of prize cards at shows, which today are rarely given, consists of seven per class, i.e. 1st, 2nd, 3rd, reserve, very highly commended, highly commended, and commended. Almost invariably prize money is now confined to the first three winning exhibits in each class, or possibly the first four.

In addition to prize cards and prize money in each class, there are usually 'special' prizes on offer, which may be cash or special cards. Each National Specialist club, and many of the other specialist clubs, issue Certificates of Merit, or Diplomas or Club Certificates, for the best of their particular breed.

In the same way the BRC issues to shows applying for them, three kinds of 'specials'. The first are Challenge Certificates for the best of each breed or variety, and these CCs are awarded by the judge provided that he considers that the exhibits are up to Championship status. Challenge Certificates are graded in the same way as shows. Thus at a Five Star Show, the CCs are Five Star. Secondly, there is a Best of Breed Certificate, which is awarded to the best animal of a breed having several colour varieties, the CCs having being awarded to the best exhibits of different colours of that breed provided there are separate classes for the different colours.

The third type of special offered by the BRC is the Diploma. A Diploma is awarded by the judges at a show to the best exhibit in each of the sections for fancy breeds, normal fur breeds, Rex breeds, or to combinations of these sections. These Diplomas are awarded to either best exhibit in Show (if there is only one section), or to Best Fancy exhibit and the Best Fur exhibit (if there are two), or to Best Fancy exhibit, the Best Normal Fur exhibit and the Best Rex exhibit (if there are three).

In the case of the majority of Specialist clubs and the BRC, these special awards are only confirmed if the exhibitor winning them is a member of the club concerned or of the Council. After winning a certain number of CCs, a member of the BRC can claim another prize. Successful exhibitors will therefore almost invariably join their national specialist club and the Council, not only for the chance of winning these specials, but also for the other benefits which membership confers.

THE VALUE OF RABBIT SHOWS

All the present breeds of rabbits have evolved and been perfected to their present degree partly under the stimulation of the show table. Rabbit shows, apart from giving great pleasure and indeed in many cases excitement to many fanciers, have been a means whereby exhibitors can compare their animals and discuss the many problems which confront them, together with their solution. Shows have certainly led to the standardising of the different breeds and the ideal of each breed.

Perhaps no less important is the social side of showing. Very many friendships are built up at the pen side. Again, a great deal of useful information can be gained by visits to shows, for fanciers on the whole are anxious to encourage new rabbit breeders.

In each country in which domestic rabbits are bred (and these form the majority of countries in the world) there is both a rabbit industry, utilising the commercial or utilitarian characteristics of the rabbit, and an exhibition rabbit world, which is interested largely in producing beautiful animals. In some ways both sides have opposing views. At the present time it is only in the matter of mature fur that a possible similarity of interests occurs, for then both require a dense, well-coloured pelt. But there are very few fur breeders for commercial purposes at the present time.

It is sometimes argued that exhibitions of stock may place too much emphasis on 'beauty' points to the detriment of 'useful' points. The exhibition breeder, for example, is interested in producing a relatively few superlative animals. The commercial breeder is interested in producing a lot of animals suitable for meat or fur. Again, a few white hairs in a coloured coat are a serious disability to the fancier, but they will probably improve the natural fur, for they show that the pelt is natural and not dyed.

There are of course a very few breeders who sell exhibition stock for a living, or at least the major part of it, and more make a useful addition to their income by so doing, but these should not be classed as commercial breeders in the sense that the latter sell meat and dispose of the pelt as a very minor addition.

Provided that the clear distinctions between the exhibition and commercial sides of rabbit keeping are appreciated and the commercial points of a rabbit not confused with the exhibition points, then the two sides to rabbit keeping should not interfere with each other. Indeed, in many ways the exhibition breeder can assist the commercial breeder, and vice versa. The exhibition breeder has time, and usually the inclination, to experiment, whereas the commercial breeder is usually not prepared to do this.

THE PREPARATION OF SHOW STOCK

The British people have for a very long time held an enviable reputation for the breeding and showing of the highest quality of exhibition animals, and possibly nowhere is this seen to such an extent as in the rabbit fancy.

The aspiring breeder of exhibition stock must concentrate on developing the art of looking at and seeing his stock. Many fanciers never achieve this art! It is an interesting exercise to take the same animal and look at it under different light conditions and from different angles. It is surprising how many faults seem to immediately develop when the animal is looked at in good light, compared to its lack of faults when looked at in poor light!

Grooming

Good light is absolutely essential when examining and grooming animals for show. Another useful idea is to have a reasonably large mirror, so placed on the wall, that when the rabbit is being examined or groomed, its opposite side can be seen at the same time. This is particularly useful with the marked breeds but also helps with all others.

It is considered a grave offence for a rabbit to be exhibited in other than its natural state. That is to say, the removal of, say, white hairs or patches in a coloured animal, or the irregular cutting or colouring of the fur, is considered to be so serious that persons found guilty of attempting it are almost invariably prohibited from further showing. Thus the animal must be prepared in an entirely natural way. Its feeding must be so regulated that it is in perfect condition, and the lustre of its coat improved from inside, as it were. A really good animal may easily lose the premier honours unless it is in the best possible condition. Freedom from moult is also desirable, and the 'finish' of a rabbit will often be the only point which separates two animals on the judging table.

Probably the most constant method of preparation is by grooming with the hand. This allows the dust and dead hairs from the moult to be eliminated, and gives that little extra polish which is so desirable.

Some breeds must be taught to show themselves to the best advantage. Thus the Polish rabbit should 'sit up' to show itself off to the judge, the Belgian Hare should 'pose' well, and the Flemish Giant should sit to show the greatest length. All exhibition animals should be handled fairly frequently, to ensure that they are quiet on the judging table, but the only way in which the novice can learn to train his particular breed is by discussion with, and example, from an experienced fancier.

Apart from regular grooming with the hands (and the minutest amount of oil on either hand will assist), the other major point is in cleaning the exhibits, particularly the white breeds. These should always be kept in spotlessly clean hutches, for nothing is so difficult to remove as hutch stain, and nothing is so unsightly. For the shorter-furred varieties a piece of bread can be used for rubbing the dirty spots. French chalk or talc can also be used for cleaning up the white exhibits, as can a very little surgical spirit or a damp cloth, but care should be taken that all foreign matter is completely removed before the rabbit is exhibited.

Some grooming may be necessary when the exhibitor arrives at the show, but this is strictly controlled. It is therefore important that the travelling box in which the exhibit is taken to the show is of such a design and cleanliness, and is carried in such a way, that the rabbit reaches the show in the best possible condition.

When taking a rabbit to a show it is important to place adequate bedding in the box, and also a reasonable supply of suitable food. Food which is likely to stain the animal (such as carrots for white breeds) should not be used. During a fairly long journey, unless the ventilation of the travelling box is good, the rabbit may become travel soiled, and this will lessen its chances of success. Particular attention should therefore be paid to ensuring that the bedding is dry and the ventilation of the box good, otherwise all the care in taking the rabbit to the show may be of little avail.

EXHIBITING

The intending exhibitor will usually first exhibit at the smaller shows. At one time it was the custom for secretaries to send out schedules and entry forms, but this no longer often occurs. The surest way of finding which shows are to be held and when and where, is by looking in the columns of *Fur & Feather*.

His first step will be to find a copy of the schedule, which is a sheet giving details of the show and a list of the classes. In some cases, but now not often, an entry form is incorporated in the schedule, but if one is not sent to him then the exhibitor must make up his own.

The classes in a show are of two kinds, straight breed classes, and duplicate classes. Straight breed classes are classes for a particular breed or a colour variety, although the AOV (any other variety) classes may also be straight breed classes. The classes may also be limited by age or sex, for example Dutch adult, Dutch adult doe, Dutch under four months, etc. The exhibitor will select the appropriate straight breed class into which his rabbit can be entered. It can of course only be entered into one straight breed class at a show. He will next turn his attention to duplicate classes. There is a large variety of these and they include such classes as 'Breeders', in which animals of any variety or group may be entered if they have been bred by the exhibitor; 'Novice Exhibit', in which animals never having won a first prize at an open show may be entered; 'Challenge' classes for all varieties, and the like. The proportion of straight breed classes to duplicate classes at different shows varies a good deal, but it may be as low as three or so or as many as six or seven.

Having selected the classes in which he wishes to enter his exhibit, the exhibitor completes his entry form, including such details as his name and address, the straight breed class number, the breed, sex, and age of the exhibit (under five months, adult), the duplicate class numbers, the amount of entry fees enclosed, etc. This form is despatched in good time to the show secretary (the last date for the receipt of entries being given on the schedule), together with the appropriate entry fees, which usually amount to 20 or 25 pence per class at the smaller shows (which may sound very little, but the prize money is in proportion!). There is also at many shows a block entry fee system. This means that an exhibit can be entered into all classes at a show (which it is entitled to enter) for the single block entry fee.

On arrival at the show, the rabbit will be checked in, a small gummed label giving its pen number, will be attached to its ear or behind the ears, and it will be placed in a pen. When the time for judging arrives, the exhibits in each class are placed on a table before the judge by the stewards, who are asked, by the book steward assisting the judge, for the appropriate rabbits by pen numbers, and the judge, after examining each, places them in the order of their merit (Fig. 3.1).

All the details are put into the Judges Book, in which are listed all the exhibits (by pen number) in each class. The book steward will often record notes given to him by the judge, for he will need these for his report to *Fur & Feather*.

When the straight breed classes have been judged, it is the turn of the duplicate classes. In these classes, the judge will only require certain exhibits which have won in the straight breed classes. After each class is judged the slip from the judging book is sent to the show secretary, who, with his helpers, arranges that the prize cards are made out and placed on the pens of the winners. When the show is over the rabbit is returned, with or without prize cards, depending upon its success.

The judge has a further task to undertake, which he does on his return home. The task is to write a short report on the show and the winning exhibits for publication in the columns of *Fur & Feather*. Obviously people who could not attend the show are anxious to read the results, hence the need for the judge to send in the report in good time. There is often some confusion in the mind of the novice between the words 'exhibits' and 'entries'. As we have seen above, rabbits may enter several classes at the same show, that is first the straight class and then the duplicate classes. The number of exhibits relates to the number of animals at the show. The word entries relates to the total number of entries in all the classes. The number of entries therefore is usually several times larger than the number of exhibits.

There are two important general points that should be mentioned. First, although most judges have the same idea of what constitutes the best exhibits, it is only natural

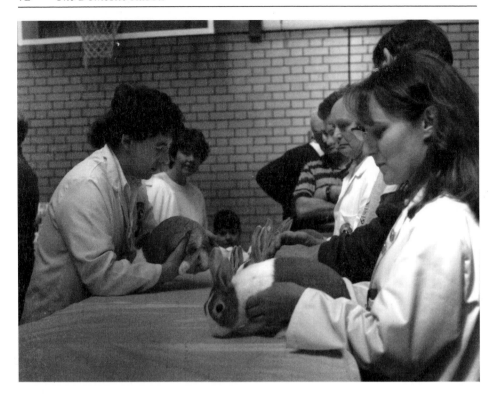

Fig. 3.1   A judge judging rabbits assisted by stewards on the other side of the table

that some judges give more weight to particular points than do others. For example, one judge will like a very fine silky coat in a Rex, whilst another will consider density of coat to be very important. Thus, by observing the slightly varying preferences of the judges, an exhibitor will be able to place his exhibits under those judges who will most prefer them.

Second, no fancier can be consistently successful unless he has a thorough knowledge of the breed which he exhibits, and also the points which are looked for by the judge. Nor will the greatest success come his way unless he takes care to ensure that his animals are in the best possible condition, and arrive at the judging table in this condition.

JUDGING

There are basically two systems of judging rabbits. The one preferred by all other countries in Europe, is the points system. That preferred and used solely in the UK is the comparison system. The Continental judging system is discussed below.

In the English system of judging by comparison, the judge has a number of rabbits on the table at the same time. He examines each animal and assesses its quality. Whilst the judge has a detailed understanding of the importance of each feature (for these are given that importance by the relative number of points in the standard allotted to each), he is also concerned with the balance of the different features. No matter how good a single feature is, unless it is to some extent in balance with the other features, it will be placed lower.

The judge then places the animals in order on the table, the best exhibit in his opinion being at the head with the others in descending order. He will frequently re-examine an animal which he has assessed before, to compare it with the one he is currently judging, and then place those two in relation to each other. If there are more than about seven animals in a class, he will first select a number and then return the others to their pens. More rabbits will be brought to the table and more will be returned until the class is complete.

Judging is a skilled task and carries much responsibility for the success of any show. Judging requires a great deal of experience, patience and integrity.

THE RABBIT FANCY ABROAD

In all countries where rabbit breeding is conducted, there are usually National Associations for both the exhibition and commercial sides of rabbit husbandry. The fancy national associations, older by far than the commercial associations, often have affiliated to them breed specialist societies which promote their particular breeds of rabbits, and clubs or groups of rabbits breeders in the same area. In addition, in Europe there is the European Association of Aviculture and Rabbit Breeding (EEAC), established in 1938, and concerned solely with exhibition organisations. It has membership from 14 member countries, and, with poultry and pigeons, rabbits are included as a section.

In most European countries, the USA, and many others, rabbit fancies exist and in each there is a central governing body. These are sometimes of great size and in one case numbers nearly 200 000 members. Their functions are very similar to the work of the BRC. In the same way, in the various countries, whilst the breeds are basically much the same, there are often variations of size and type, the breeders in the different countries having varying ideas as to the ideals of different breeds.

In general it is fair to say that, certainly in Europe, the shows are less frequent than in the UK, but usually very much larger. It is not unusual for the main shows to have upwards of 20 000 exhibits, and on occasions the major international shows have surpassed 30 000.

A second considerable variation between Great Britain and the rest of the world fancies is in the method of identification. In the UK rabbits are identified with a leg ringing system. Elsewhere each rabbit is identified with a tattooing system. The system varies slightly, but examples of typical notation systems are given in Table 3.1.

The most substantial difference, however, is in the system of judging. In the Continental system, the judge is issued with a card for each rabbit. There are separate cards for each different breed of rabbit. Each card contains details of the identity of the animal, its age, sex and weight, and a list of seven sections. The first three sections and the last are universal. These are:

(1) General appearance (Type)
(2) Weight
(3) Coat
(7) Presentation and condition.

The other three sections (4, 5 and 6) vary according to the breed. They are for specific breed characteristics. For example they might be:

(4) Colour
(5) Head, eyes and ears with the pattern
(6) The body pattern.

Each of these features is allotted a variable number of points, which are of course the points allotted to that breed in its Standard.

Table 3.1 Example of tattooing notation systems

France

	Left ear		Right ear
Month	Country of birth	Year of birth	Identity Certificate No.
2	F	3	AU 610
i.e. February	i.e. France	i.e. 1993	

Germany

	Left ear		Right ear	
Month	Year	No. in Register	Initial of State	Club No.
2	2	50	H	521
i.e. February	i.e. 1992		i.e. Hesse-Nassau	

Used by German Rabbit Breeders' Association

The judge, usually accompanied by a steward, goes to each pen in turn and assesses the quality of the animal in each of these seven sections. He allots the number of points which he considers the animal merits in each section. The points are then totalled and the winners are those animals with the highest number of points. The smallest amount of change in the points is one half. Thus it is inevitable that in a large show (and in the major shows on the Continent there may be several hundred animals in a single class!) there will be at least several animals with identical points. These are then, if necessary, separated by comparison.

The judges are meticulous in the assessing of quality and the allotment of points, and in exceptional circumstances only are allowed to assess more than eighty exhibits during any one day. Furthermore the exhibits are weighed before the judge sees them and hence the question of size is eliminated from their judgment, as the points for weight are allotted on a sliding scale.

In America there are two points of difference between the American and English Fancy, although the American system is also by comparison in the same way as in England. One difference lies in the identification of rabbits, which follows the European system of tattooing. The other difference lies in the number of exhibits which are placed in order. In the UK the judge has to find at best seven exhibits to which he is to allot places, and much more usual is the allotting of three or four places in each class. The number of animals the American judge has to list in order is a great deal larger and as many as 25 may be given a placing.

Chapter 4

Rabbits as Pets and Companions

Whereas the chief aim of the rabbit fancier is to produce as nearly as possible the perfect specimen of a particular breed, and the aim of the meat or wool producer is to produce quantities of meat or wool, the pleasure or reward of the pet or companion rabbit owner lies in the simple delight of the presence of the animal. Pet rabbit keeping has a long history, whilst the companion or house rabbit is a relatively new idea. The distinction between pets and house rabbits lies in that pets are almost invariably kept in hutches whilst companion rabbits are treated as companions and kept in the house. The name house rabbit is probably a better name for the rabbit kept in the house as a companion, for it is true in many ways that pets (and indeed rabbits kept by fanciers), are also in many cases companion rabbits.

Not all breeds are as suitable as others for either pets or house rabbits. For example, Angoras and the largest breeds, whilst being fascinating in other circumstances are less likely to be completely satisfactory for these purposes. It is essential that the prospective owner should see as many breeds as possible (going to a good rabbit show is an ideal way) before picking on one for him or herself. As with other forms of rabbit keeping, a breed which is really appealing to the rabbit keeper is important for success.

THE PET RABBIT

During the early Victorian era, when pet rabbit keeping developed rapidly, one of the important reasons why children were encouraged to keep rabbits was the belief that rabbit keeping, in particular, was of great benefit in helping to build the character of the child. That it taught self-discipline, kindness and consideration is undoubted, and this still applies today.

Since early Victorian days, the pet rabbit was certainly the most usual of boys' pets. For some reason, which is certainly not apparent today, girls did not then have many rabbits as pets. Today it is likely that there are at least equal numbers of boys and girls who have pet rabbits.

With the pet rabbit, there was, and still is today, often an element of breeding and many pet keepers sometimes find themselves with rather too many pets for their immediate facilities. Most people are also of the opinion that the pet owner usually has few rabbits. Whilst this is true with certainly the majority of pet rabbit owners, there are a surprising number of people who have numbers of animals. There are many cases where a person has 20 or 30 or even more animals, purely as pets. They have no interest in commerce of any sort and they do not exhibit. They are simply pet owners on a largish scale.

That pet rabbit keepers have enjoyed their hobby for a very long time is shown by the numbers of books published during the Victorian era which dealt with the subject fairly exhaustively. It is also indicated by the fact that George Stephenson, the inventor of the steam locomotive, kept pet rabbits throughout the greater part of his life (1781–1848) sometimes it is said in large numbers. It is reported that he had many friends who did the same and that at the height of his career rabbits, proved a great source of pleasure and relaxation to him and also to his friends.

Care and handling

The care and handling of the pet rabbit differs very little from that of the fancy rabbit. The hutches and equipment, whilst perhaps not being so elaborate, should be constructed on the same principles, and the feeding of the pets should conform to the same rules, although it is inevitable that the pets should get a greater proportion of 'treats' such as apples, baked bread and the like than the fanciers usually stock.

In most cases, there are some distinctions to be made between the companion and the pet rabbit. Whilst often there are more than one or two rabbits kept as pets this is not usually true of the companion rabbit, where it is most common to have one animal only, or at most two and the care and handling of companion or house rabbit differs somewhat.

THE COMPANION OR HOUSE RABBIT

It is only relatively recently that the idea of a rabbit being a companion and, except for certain times, living unconfined in a hutch has been widely recognised. Not only is it a recent innovation, but it is also probably the most rapidly increasing element in the rabbit world. The reasons for this lie in the nature of the rabbit.

Rabbits do not make a noise and do not get into neighbours' premises. In many establishments where dogs are not allowed, rabbits, unlike dogs, do not need to be taken for exercise. The rabbit soon becomes accustomed to any situation and the costs of obtaining and maintaining it are relatively low. Above all, however, is the docile but affectionate character of most rabbits. Rabbits come in all shapes, sizes and colours and it would be very difficult to be unable to find a breed or variety with which someone did not have an immediate rapport. Again the rabbit is extremely interesting to keep and watch. Rabbits are surprisingly easy to train and respond to handling and affection to a remarkable degree.

There are of course, as with all companion animals, some disadvantages that have to be overcome. Rabbits have strong back legs complete with claws! Unless properly handled and friendly to the handler, they can inflict nasty scratches. Also house rabbits need to be house trained; and their need to gnaw can cause problems unless this aspect is tackled. Whilst it is possible to leave rabbits on their own for a day or even two, (provided of course arrangements are made for their food and water), for longer periods someone has to be asked to attend to them.

There is also the question of the natural instincts of the rabbit. Adult bucks always mark their 'territories' by spraying urine and rubbing the scent glands on their chin against furniture. This is no problem with the pet rabbit housed in a hutch outdoor, but it is a problem in the house. The only way in which this can be prevented is by castration. If this is done at a relatively early age (say three to four months) these characteristics are eliminated. There are fewer problems with the doe, but many authorities, particularly in other countries, recommend the spaying of the doe which is a house rabbit. Both castration and spaying are also thought to improve the health of the rabbit and to ensure a longer life than would otherwise be the case. Both of these operations are fairly easy veterinary procedures and are usually attended by little risk. Whilst the above may sound forbidding, the problems can be relatively easy to overcome and a marvellous companion is thereby gained!

SELECTION OF RABBIT

The fullest consideration should be given to the selection of the companion rabbit and of course it should be obtained from a very reliable source. Some owners right from the start consider that there should be two rabbits together, for company. Whilst the belief that rabbits are 'lonely' if kept without one of their own kind is fairly prevalent, this is not so. However there is little doubt that two house rabbits together can be exceptionally amusing and interesting.

If the owner decides that two house rabbits are desirable (but it must be remembered that two rabbits take twice as much training as one!), then it is best to obtain litter mates, or at least animals of approximately the same age. If two rabbits are accustomed to each other then certainly there are fewer problems than might otherwise occur. If a new rabbit is to be introduced after the first rabbit has been in the house for a period then the first occupant may resent the newcomer and it will usually take a little time to accustom both of them to each other. This is again one reason why neutering is of benefit.

If a new rabbit is to be introduced then both animals should be confined separately when no one is present, to prevent any fighting. After some time they will become familiar to each other and establish friendly relations. Their hutches should be close together, so that when they are confined in them they can start to setle down.

TRAINING

Whilst there are a number of training processes (and rabbits can be taught many tricks which they greatly enjoy performing) the two most important for the house rabbit are toilet training and the prevention of damaging furniture and the like.

Rabbits are creatures of habit and prefer to soil in a particular place. The essence of toilet training therefore lies in ensuring that the place in which the rabbit soils remains available for him. A good system to use is to have a pen with a suitable mesh floor to put him in when he first arrives in the house. The pen is placed upon a solid tray filled with bedding, in a convenient corner of the room. The rabbit will select a corner of this pen which he will use. In this pen he remains for some days, and when he is let out, the pen is lifted off the tray, leaving the tray in place. He will tend to return to the tray when necessary and this instinct can be re-enforced with training. The pen is of course replaced on the tray whenever the rabbit is again confined. Sometimes it is found that the rabbit selects another place when he is let out. In this case, if it is convenient, the tray and pen should be placed in this corner. An alternative is to place a second tray in the second corner.

Instead of a pen placed upon the tray, a pen with an integral sliding tray underneath can be used, but this is not as good as the pen placed upon a tray. Whatever system is used some absorbent material is necessary to line the tray to absorb the urine. There are several types of suitable bedding. The cheapest and probably the most satisfactory is ordinary wood shavings, which can be purchased as bedding for animals.

Ideally the room in which the rabbit is confined, in the early stages of its training, should have a floor or floor covering which will not be damaged by the rabbit, either with its urine and faeces or by its scratching or gnawing. Whilst the faecal pellets will do no harm to most floor coverings, urine does so and should accidents occur a slightly acidic cleaner will correct the matter.

The prevention of damage to furniture is another matter. Undoubtedly a small block of wood placed in the pen, and available when the rabbit is out of the pen will greatly help. The rabbit will use it to gnaw upon, which is essential if his teeth are to be kept in proper order. A small piece of apple tree branch, about 4 or 5 cm or more in diameter and perhaps 20 cm long is ideal for this purpose but will need to be renewed from time to time. It is necessary to ensure that it is clean and free from chemicals. Another help to protect furniture is a very light spray of cat or fox repellant which can be purchased in aerosol form. For some reason rabbits are attracted to electric and other cables. Many cases of quite serious damage have been caused by their gnawing the covering of these until they bare the wires or in fact cut through the wires completely. It is essential that bare wires should be placed out of reach, or covered. All methods of animal training are much the same. A very few simple word commands, repeatedly given will relatively quickly produce a satisfactory result. The trainer should use each word consistently.

One last word may be said about outdoor runs. These are often advocated for the house rabbit (and indeed for pet rabbits). Provided the animals are protected from predators, are not allowed total freedom and particularly not permitted to continually run over the same area of land, all is well. However, rabbits continually being on the same piece of grass, for example, do tend to pick up harmful organisms.

Whilst brief instructions can be given as above, rabbits tend to be very individual in their natures, habits and likes as the owner will learn when he or she goes on with the fascinating business of keeping a house rabbit.

Chapter 5

Handling and Management

The management of an exhibition rabbitry or commercial rabbit farm consists of a large number of practices. To be successful, the rabbit breeder must attend to these details regularly. The experienced and successful breeder or farmer knows what to do, how to do it, and when to do it.

Successful management demands, above all, attention to detail. It is this attention to perhaps minor points which help turn an 'attendant' into a stockman. Management requires practice. The rules of good management may be laid down, and general instructions given as to what a breeder should do in certain eventualities, but after these rules and instructions have been learnt and digested by the breeder, he will require experience in putting them into operation. It is this experience, based on sound knowledge, which will teach him the essentials of his business.

Some breeders appear to have an inborn sense of management. It is usually difficult to analyse why or how a good stockman differs from one who is not successful, but generally, some of the difference lies in his ability to take trouble over the welfare of his stock and to recognise, almost instinctively, their needs.

Not all management practices are always suitable for all systems of rabbit keeping. For various reasons some item of management may be suitable for some conditions, whilst being quite unsuitable for others. This view is too often not appreciated, with the result that a good deal of bad advice is quite frequently offered to the rabbit breeder or to the rabbit farmer and indeed to the pet keeper. It is also true that some of the good practices in an exhibition stud are unsuited to the farm, and vice versa.

PURCHASING RABBITS

The majority of rabbit breeders are anxious to assist newcomers to rabbit keeping and to supply rabbits at reasonable prices. If the breeder who is to supply the stock is unknown to the purchaser it is often wise to purchase animals on approval although many breeders will not permit this. The novice should ask an expert to accompany him on his buying trip, or at least obtain the assistance of such an expert to examine his purchase on their arrival. This hopefully will help the novice to satisfy himself that the animal is worth the price to be paid and is exactly what he wants. If the rabbit is not satisfactory it should be returned immediately after feeding and resting, for unless it is returned within a day or two, the seller may be within his rights in refusing to have it back. Generally speaking, for obvious reasons, breeders will not sell stud bucks on approval.

There is an important distinction between buying a mated doe and a doe in kindle. If the purchaser buys a doe in kindle, then he can reasonably expect it to give birth to a litter, and in fact, a doe sold as such is really being sold on this guarantee. There is of course no guarantee that the litter will be satisfactory. If, however, a mated doe is purchased, the position is different. The breeder guarantees that the doe has been mated to one of his bucks. He does not guarantee that the doe has held to this mating, that is, that she will produce a litter.

There is no doubt that the best stock possible should be purchased. Very often 'cheap' bargains turn out to be very expensive. It is far better to purchase one or two really good animals than a larger number of poorer quality. It is usually advisable for the purchaser to visit the rabbitry from which a purchase is anticipated, before making his final decision. He can then observe how the breeder handles his stock, whether they are kept in a satisfactory manner, and so on. Such visits sometimes prevent what might otherwise have been an unfortunate purchase.

In the case of the rabbit farmer, it cannot be emphasised enough that the purchase of stock with which to commerce a rabbit farm is of the greatest importance; indeed it is true that the initial selection and purchase of animals is absolutely fundamental to success. Whilst the majority of suppliers can be relied upon to treat the newcomer with consideration, helpfulness and honesty, there are other establishments, some of them quite large and long-established where excellent salesmanship is only equalled by the poor quality of the stock.

Mention should here be made of the Accredited Breeders Scheme run by the British Commercial Rabbit Association. A skilled breeder who has a record of producing excellent stock can apply to be placed on the register. A detailed examination is made of the farm, the stock and the records kept and, provided that these meet a high standard, the farm is given accreditation. The object of the scheme is twofold. First, it is to ensure that new farmers have a known reliable breeder from whom to purchase stock, and second, it is an attempt to improve the average quality of stock throughout the industry. There is a third benefit. Arbitration is undertaken between the parties if that becomes necessary.

The inspection of the farms for applicants to the register is very detailed and covers such matters as management, hygiene, health, recording systems, performance of stock, quality of stock and the like. Any would-be commercial farmer would be strongly advised to visit such accredited breeders.

HANDLING

Although there are several ways of handling rabbits, there is no occasion on which a rabbit should not be handled gently but firmly. To allow a rabbit to feel insecure, and thus to cause it to struggle, will often result in damage both to the animal and the handler. If a rabbit continues to struggle it is often wise to put it down, allow it to recover its composure and then to pick it up again. The way in which a rabbit should be picked up will also depend upon its age and size.

The ears alone should never be used as the sole means of holding the rabbit. The most common method is to grasp the ears close to the head with one hand, whilst the other hand takes the full weight of the rabbit. In fact the hand holding the ears is really used for restraining and balancing the animal, the other hand taking the weight. In this method the palm of the hand 'cups' the back of the rabbit's head, and the thumb is placed at the base of the ears or the forehead (Fig. 5.1). This method is the best for animals over the age of four or five weeks. The rabbit appears to find it soothing if its forehead is gently stroked. A struggling rabbit held in this way can be stroked on the forehead by the ball of the thumb when it is very often calmed down.

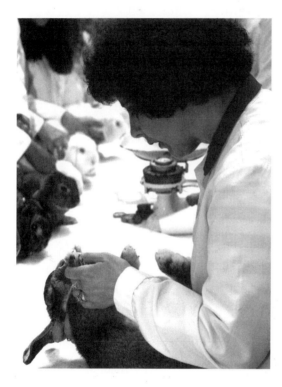

Fig. 5.1 Correct handling for examination. The weight of the rabbit is resting on the table

Although it is frequently suggested that the rabbit should be picked up by grasping the loose skin over the shoulders, this is generally not to be recommended. It is a fairly general method in Europe, but damage does occur, particularly when care is not taken to avoid digging the fingernails into the skin of the animal. If this system is used, the correct way is to use the flat of the fingers and not the tips. Far more damage can be done to the skin of the back by grasping it, than is ever done if the back of the head and the ears are used to balance the animal, with the weight being taken by the other hand or arm. If for some reason it is used, then again it should only be as a means of balancing the animal with the other hand placed underneath it.

For young rabbits up to about two or three months, a suitable method of handling is to grasp the animal across the loins, gently but firmly, with thumb in front of the hind legs on one side and the fingers opposite. This requires some practice, and is not suitable for larger rabbits, and particularly does in kindle. The fingers grasp the

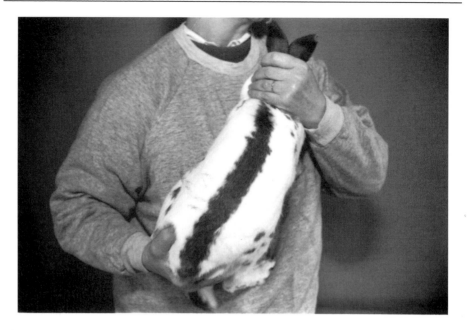

Fig. 5.2   Holding the rabbit to carry

muscles on one side of the spine whilst the thumb grasps the muscles on the other side. Care must be taken that the internal organs are not damaged. It is sometimes desirable to pick up a rabbit, particularly Lops, by placing the hand underneath the belly. Here again, the weight of the animal will partly be taken by placing the other hand over the rump.

The best way to carry an animal any distance is to hold it against the chest, with one hand taking the weight and the other hand cupping the back of the head and the base of the ears (Fig. 5.2). Alternatively, the forearm can be used, partly to support the animal and partly to hold it against the lower chest.

Rabbits should be removed or returned through small openings (for example a pen door at a show) in such a way that its claws cannot be caught in the side of the opening. Careless handling in such cases (for example, by dragging the animal through the opening head first) may easily cause damage. The rabbit should therefore always be put through such an opening hindquarters first.

If a rabbit has to be restrained when there is the possibility of struggling, for example when a wound has to be dressed, or when claws have to be clipped, it is advisable to wrap the animal securely in a cloth or sack. The rabbit must be wrapped up firmly, otherwise the procedure is worse than not doing it at all.

To examine the belly or breast, the rabbit should be held firmly over the rump, with the other hand holding the ears in the normal fashion close to the head, the thumb lying across the skull in front of the ears. It can then be turned over quite easily. In the same way, when sexing a large rabbit it is this method which is employed, but the animal can be laid on its back on a table, or on the lap of the attendant, or, if the handler is accustomed to stock, the animal can simply be balanced on the open hand whilst the fingers evert the sexual opening as described below (Fig. 5.3).

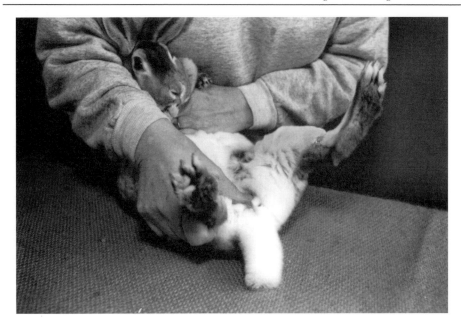

Fig. 5.3   Holding the rabbit on a table for sexing

DETERMINATION OF SEX

Apart from the sex organs, there is generally little difference between the appearance of the sexes, although the buck is usually the smaller of the two and often has a broader head. In the very young rabbit, the difference in the sex organs is so slight as to be difficult for the novice to determine. Undoubtedly the best way to learn the art of sexing is to have a lesson from an experienced breeder.

At weaning or later, the appearance of the buck's organ is circular, and the doe's organ is V-shaped. At this age it is easiest to sex by holding the head of the animal in one hand, balancing it (in the palm of the hand, this being held under the rump or for the less experienced preferably on the lap, the operator sitting down) with the middle finger holding down the tail. The index finger and thumb can then be used to evert the organ (Figs 5.4 and 5.5). At a still later age the penis of the buck can be easily obtruded, and the scrotal sac will also usually be visible.

Although it is usually not necessary, given good light and preferably a watchmaker's glass, the sex of animals one-day-old can be determined. It is easier to do it on the first or second day of life than a little later. This may be important when one sex is particularly desired and when the litters are being reduced in size. The baby rabbit should be held in the left hand with the head towards the wrist. It is necessary to hold the animal gently but firmly to stop it wriggling. The tail is held back with the index finger of the left hand and gentle pressure exerted with both thumbs on either side of the sexual organ, when the pinkish mucous membranes will be exposed. In the buck the organ, which will protrude slightly, appears as a rounded tip, whilst in the doe the organ appears slit-like and will slope slightly downwards towards the anus. In the buck a pair of reddish brown specks will be found near the vent, and the distance between the anus and the organ is slightly longer than that

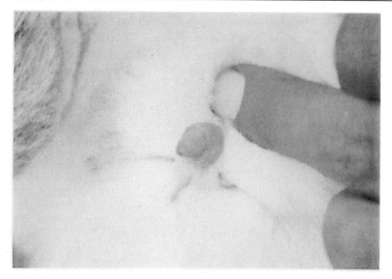

Fig. 5.4   Sexing the buck

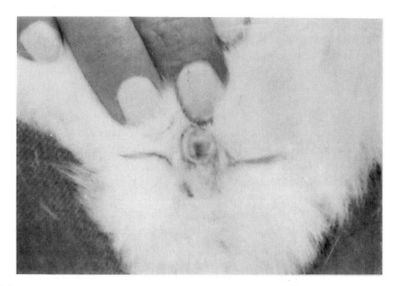

Fig. 5.5   Sexing the doe

found in the doe. The appearance of nipple spots is found at this age in either sex and therefore has no significance.

SELECTING A BREED

There is no breed which is best for any one purpose. In the case of Angora wool production there are indeed three breeds of Angora and in the case of the commercial rabbit farmer, when almost invariably the New Zealand White or the Californian (or derivatives from these breeds) are used. It is often recommended that the most suitable animals for meat production are cross-bred stock, but this is not so. It is only in some strains of stock (usually derived from the two breeds), where pure genetic lines are produced for the express purpose of crossing, that one could say cross-breeds were of use. The Rexes, of course, are undoubtedly the most suitable for prime pelt production, whilst for intermediate pelts, the Chinchilla and Chinchilla Giganta must be used.

Excluding, however, these rather specialised areas, the range of breeds is very wide, giving every colour, shape and size. Certainly there is always one breed to delight all comers. The interest to be derived from rabbit keeping is always increased when pure-bred stock is kept and, of course, the sale of surplus animals will always yield more attractive prices than can ever be obtained for cross-breeds.

There is a great deal to be said for the breeder keeping a breed to which he is personally attracted. There is little doubt that many breeders are more consistently successful with a particular breed to which they are most attracted, than they are with others.

The ideal way for newcomers to select a breed or breeds is to visit several shows after making a short list of the breeds which would seem to answer their purpose. There they will see specimens of the different breeds and can examine them and discuss their relative merits with their breeders. In this way they will finally decide on the best breed for their purpose, and then they should endeavour to continue with it for some time. Very early success may elude them and even experienced breeders must persevere with breeds new to them. Breeders who are continually changing the breeds which they keep rarely have consistent fortune with any.

PURCHASE OF STOCK

The novice rabbit breeder is often in some doubt as to whether to purchase young animals or a mated doe, or stock nearing breeding age. There is usually divided opinion on this matter. The purchase of young, newly weaned animals is rarely to be recommended to the novice, for it is most important that future breeding stock should be well reared. Young animals are more likely to suffer permanent injury from errors in management than are older rabbits.

The care of a mated doe, and one with a young litter, is perhaps rather more difficult than the management of nearly adult stock, and furthermore, it is often advisable to allow new animals to settle in to their new surroundings and management before breeding from them. Thus the purchase of stock approaching breeding age is usually the best buy for the novice breeder. He or she can usually buy does on the understanding that they can be returned to the seller for mating when they are ready.

It is always advisable to purchase a small number of animals and to increase their number slowly as experience is gained. It is doubtful whether the novice purchasing only one or two does at the start should also purchase a buck. He will not be used as frequently as would be desirable, and in general it would be better, under these circumstances, to use the services of the original breeder's bucks until such time as the novice has gained sufficient skill and knowledge, and has sufficient does to merit the acquisition of his or her own stud buck.

SENDING A DOE FOR MATING

At one time it was common practice for a well-known breeder to place bucks at stud. Many bucks having a good breeding and/or show record were advertised as being available; and does were sent (usually by rail in travelling boxes) to these bucks for service at a stud fee which of course varied according to the buck to be used. Today this practice is not so frequent as it was. Often the wisest course for anyone other than an experienced breeder is to discuss the matter with a good breeder and ask him or her to mate the doe to a suitable buck. The owner of a good stud is usually in the best position to know the qualities of his different bucks and can therefore pick the most suitable. Many rabbit fanciers are pleased to help novices in this way.

If the mating is to be a commercial transaction, the mating should be booked as early as possible, in order to ensure that the doe is mated at the right time for her owner's purpose. Before the doe is sent, complete agreement should be reached between the owners of the buck and the doe as to:

- the fee,
- whether a free second mating, or even a third, will be given if the doe fails to hold to the services,
- the length of time the stud buck owner can retain the doe for the mating.

With regard to the last point it should be noted that it is illegal for a stud buck owner to retain a doe sent him for mating for a period longer than the gestation period, i.e. 31 days, without the express permission of the owner. Thus, a time limit should be set, and if the doe is not mated within that period, she should be returned, or her owner contacted.

The owner of the doe should realise that the stud buck owner will usually try to be of assistance. Under no circumstances should a doe with the slightest signs of ill health be sent for mating, for this is grossly unfair to the buck's owner. Again, if the doe fails to kindle within a few days of the due date, the stud buck's owner should immediately be notified. It is unreasonable to expect a further free mating unless the doe is returned to him within a reasonable time.

VICIOUSNESS IN RABBITS

It occasionally happens that a rabbit becomes vicious and attacks all who attempt to handle it. Viciousness should not be confused with nervousness where an animal may attack a stranger, or a strongly developed maternal instinct, where a doe with a litter may attack a breeder who attempts to look into the nest. Although there are other factors, viciousness is usually the result of rough handling, which may also cause nervousness in rabbits.

Different breeds also vary greatly in this respect and while some are very docile, others are timid rather than docile, and yet others tend towards viciousness. It is in these latter breeds or, more correctly, strains of different breeds, that viciousness may develop. There is usually little that can be done with an animal that continues to be vicious, and unless the animal is required for some particular purpose it is best eliminated.

Some does are very temporarily vicious, either to the attendant or to their young towards the end of weaning, but this can usually be eliminated by putting her to the buck. Certain does may eat their young or scatter them at birth, and, although very rarely, others will attack and kill their young at a week or more old. Both cases rarely occur in a well managed stud. (It should perhaps be mentioned that rats may kill and eat parts of some young rabbits, the damage being wrongly attributed to the doe).

There are several causes of this abnormal maternal behaviour in the doe. There is little doubt that some of the cases are due to nutritional deficiencies or a lack of sufficient food. One very extensive series of cases was completely cured by improvement in the diet, deficiency in vitamin B having been diagnosed as the cause. Inadequate water, which should be left with stock at all times, is probably another cause. The doe, immediately following kindling, proceeds to eat the placenta or afterbirth, and may inadvertently eat parts of the young. The last cause, to which, however, undue prominence is usually given, is disturbance of some kind. If a doe is frightened, during her panic she may damage one or more of her young, and when this occurs she may start eating some when licking away the blood from any wounds so caused. There is a tendency for several features of abnormal maternal behaviour to occur at the same time. Coupled with the above, for example, there is often evidence of lack of maternal instinct in other directions. Often the nest is not properly furnished with fur, or the young are not born into the nest but scattered. With properly fed and managed does little trouble from this source should be experienced.

There is sometimes an interesting relationship between hutch size and viciousness. Small breeds (such as the Netherland Dwarf in particular) can become vicious if kept in too large a hutch. The trouble can be eliminated almost entirely by returning the animal to a hutch of the correct size.

THE CARE OF THE DOE IN KINDLE

After mating, the doe should be returned to the hutch which she will occupy when she litters, except of course when she is nursing young when she must be returned to her own hutch. The management of the doe during pregnancy will depend to some extent on whether she is also suckling a litter for at least part of the time, a situation very common in commercial meat production. In all cases there will be no change in management during the first part of pregnancy, although she should at no time be roughly handled. If she is suckling a litter for nearly all the period, (that is, she was mated very shortly after kindling), then her feeding will not change. She must be maintained on the highest possible level of nutrition.

On the other hand, if she was a dry doe at mating, then her feeding during pregnancy will change as discussed in Chapter 7, but until the third week she will be handled as any other adult. At the end of the third week, that is, about 10 days before she is due to kindle, the hutch should be thoroughly cleaned out and a good supply of bedding placed therein (unless, of course, the hutch or cage has a mesh floor), together with a nest box, unless one is left permanently in or on the outside of the hutch, or the system is not used. The design and use of nest boxes is discussed in Chapter 6.

It may sometimes happen that the doe will begin to make a nest early, and in this case the cleaning out should immediately take place. The doe will make her nest by carrying bedding material (and hay is best for this particular purpose) about in her mouth and forming a hollow mass from it. This she will line with fur plucked from her breast and belly. If the doe starts to make her nest outside the nest box, then it should be transferred therein and she will usually continue to make it there. Occasionally a doe is found that will refuse to make a nest in the box, or alternatively will make two or three. Some does do not line their nests satisfactorily. During cold weather the youngsters in these poorly lined nests are easily chilled, and some additional lining can be provided if some old nest linings, particularly those from does which have lost their litters early, are cleaned, sterilised and kept for further use.

The doe should not be unduly interfered with from this time onwards. She need not, indeed should not, be coddled. It is quite wrong to suppose that the least noise or disturbance will affect her. There are some does whose abnormal maternal behaviour is said to be caused by disturbance. If the disturbance is due to rats, dogs or cats, then occasionally this may be true. but otherwise reasonable disturbance, although to be avoided, usually does little harm.

BIRTH OF LITTER

When the baby rabbits are born the doe will usually place them in the nest, but if they are seen outside, they should immediately be placed in it. If any young appear to be dead after having been scattered, they should be gently warmed (a temperature of 37°C is ideal) possibly in an open oven, for it is remarkable how many recover in such circumstances.

The litter of young rabbits should be examined within 24 hours of birth. The attention of the doe can be distracted by offering some tit-bit whilst the nest box is removed, or she can be taken from the hutch whilst the litter is being examined, but usually if an external nest box is used this is not necessary. However, the young rabbits should not be frequently handled and many, particularly of the marked breeds, have been ruined by constant handling whilst in the nest. It should be the rule that the litter be examined periodically to see that they are progressing satisfactorily, but young rabbits should not be removed from the nest for display.

THE CARE OF THE DOE AND LITTER

On examination, the breeder must decide whether he will leave the entire litter with the doe (after eliminating any malformed or dead young), whether he will foster some onto another doe, or whether he will cull any. The size of the litter may vary between one and fifteen or even more, although between four and nine is more common, and the average will probably be about six or seven in most breeds, except in the case of commercial units, where it should be higher.

The number of young which the breeder will wish to leave on a doe will vary. Some who wish to have a few young of extreme size may leave only one or two on the doe, although this is really an unsatisfactory practice. If it is to be attempted, then the young should be removed after the milk flow has been stimulated, and then by one at a time.

In the case of meat rabbits, where the breeder has a good milking strain, the largest litter size will usually be the best. The maximum number of young to be left on the doe will again depend to some extent on the age of the doe, as well as the number of her previous litters. A young doe will not be able to rear as many young as will a doe with her third or fourth litter, and so one or two less should be left with her.

Usually the breeder of exhibition stock will leave five or six young with the doe, but the breeder interested in the general improvement of his or her stock as breeding animals will wish to improve their average capability in milk yield and other maternal characteristics and will therefore usually leave up to eight on each doe, except possibly for the doe with her first litter.

Fostering is valuable under certain circumstances but may have disadvantages (see Chapter 4). Foster does are often selected from the popular marked varieties, that is, Dutch or English, for apart from their general good qualities as foster does, it is possible to select the potential exhibition stock at a day or two old, and thus the badly marked young can be culled to make way for fostered young.

WEANING

There are three basic weaning systems. The first consists of a system in which the doe is required to produce three or four litters per year. The second is a system in which she is remated post partum, i.e. two to ten days after giving birth, when the young from the first litter are weaned usually at between 21 and 26 days. The mid system used in the commercial field for the production of six litters per year is the remating at some between 14 and 21 days, with weaning usually at 4 weeks.

Young rabbits should not leave the nest until they are about three weeks of age. At this time they will begin to eat some of the doe's food. If she is not feeding them well they tend to leave the nest earlier than 20 days or so, which will give an indication to the breeder that all is not well with his does or his management or feeding. Every endeavour should be made to provide the young rabbits with fresh and high quality food as soon as they leave the nest, to continue the high plane of nutrition which they have been having when suckling.

The hutch will, of course, have been cleaned out periodically from a few days after the doe kindled, and it is most important that for the first few weeks the youngsters should have clean and dry bedding, again, of course, except in wire cage systems.

The milk supply of the doe will to all intents and purposes be finished by the sixth week after kindling. Some breeders wean at six weeks, particularly in the summer, but this practice is not usually entirely satisfactory, except in the commercial unit where quite often young rabbits are weaned at four weeks of age. Some breeders go to the other extreme and leave the young with the doe for a long period, leaving them with the doe for up to 12 weeks. It is, however, except for particular reasons, unwise to leave young with the doe longer than at most nine weeks, for even at this age, or earlier, she may resent their presence.

There is no advantage to be gained by removing the young two at a time. It is sometimes suggested that this will help to dry up the doe's milk, but by the time any young are ready for weaning, the doe's milk supply will have almost if not entirely ceased. Indeed, such a practice will not enable the weaning to be done by removing the doe rather than the young. It is often found that if the young are left in the breeding hutch and the doe removed, probably direct to the buck for remating, and then to a fresh hutch, the young will not suffer any slight check which they might do on changing to new surroundings.

Occasionally a doe may be found to attack her progeny or to attempt to mate with them when they are five or six weeks old. The remedy is to mate the doe forthwith, when she will almost invariably become stocked. The trouble will then cease, although the young should be weaned ten days or so later.

GROWTH AND DEVELOPMENT

From the time the egg is fertilised until the resulting rabbit becomes really mature, and even later, it increases in weight and changes in conformation and the proportion of the various parts of its body. The increase in weight is growth. The change in conformation is development. Both are important to the rabbit breeder.

During the first half of pregnancy there is relatively little growth of the embryo, but during the second half the unborn rabbit grows very rapidly. Indeed, it is in the last ten days that 90% of the growth takes place. It is for this reason that the nutrition of the doe during the second half of pregnancy is so important. Although the unborn rabbit has priority over the needs of the doe in the way of nutrition, a doe which receives insufficient food will produce progeny much underweight. With a good doe, even under the best nutritional regime, the doe will have to call on her reserves to supply the milk for the young.

There are a number of factors which influence birth weight – that is, growth before birth (see Chapter 8) – but the most influential are controlled by the doe. Were this not so, a cross between a very large buck and a small doe would produce progeny of such size as to cause difficulty at birth, and this only very rarely occurs. After birth the typical growth rate of rabbits, if plotted on a graph of weight against age, shows a drawn-out S-shaped curve (Fig. 5.6).

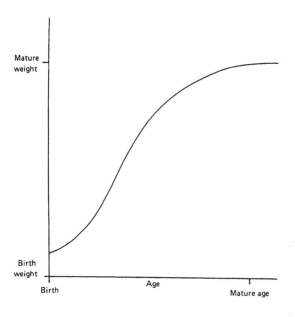

Fig. 5.6   A typical growth curve of the domestic rabbit. The actual weights for the various ages and the steepness of the curve will vary with the different breeds

The live-weight gain gradually increases to a peak and then levels off. With a knowledge of daily gain in weight and food consumption for that gain it is possible to calculate the age at which the most economic gain in terms of feeding stuff is obtained.

Factors affecting growth rate

A number of different factors affect growth rate. There is a basic pattern of growth determined by the inheritance of the animal. The larger breeds obviously grow at a faster rate than do the smaller breeds, but in some cases the rate of gain as a percentage of the adult weight is less. Superimposed upon the basic inherited growth rate are limitations due to the environment. The most important of these is the nutrition of the animal. Unless the food supply is sufficient, the rabbit cannot grow at its maximum rate. This can be very clearly seen in different sized litters. A doe suckling one young rabbit will not yield as much milk as she would if she were suckling several, but nevertheless the single rabbit will have much more than if it were in a litter of, say, five.

After weaning, the food supply also has a considerable influence on the rate of growth. It is not only the amount of food but also its composition which are important. A deficiency of one constituent will affect growth rate, sometimes very severely. Rabbits may be permanently stunted if their nutrition is poor. The earlier this occurs, and the longer the duration of poor feeding, the more severe is the stunting. Temporary stunting may also occur, but although the final growth weight may be achieved, the conformation of the animal so stunted may be changed.

Other factors affecting growth rate are disease, temperature, the season of year, and hutch size. This latter point is often overlooked. Overcrowding will almost invariably lead to a lowered growth rate, but again, an excessive hutch area will also reduce it.

Rates of growth

The different parts of the body, and indeed the different tissues of which it is composed, change in proportion as the animal develops (Fig. 5.7). For example, at birth, the head of the rabbit, compared with the rest of the body, is relatively very

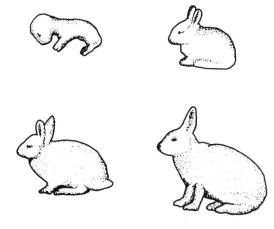

Fig. 5.7 Changes in conformation with age – rabbits at 10 days before birth, 3 weeks of age, 3 months of age, and fully mature. The size of each animal is reduced so that the eye to base-of-ear length of each is the same. (After J. Hammond)

large, weighing as much as one-fifth of the entire weight. When the animal is fully adult, the head will weigh as little as one-twelfth of the entire weight.

The changes in body proportions are brought about by the different parts growing at different rates. Some parts mature early and others late. In the same way, the different organs of the body develop at different times. The brain, lungs, heart and digestive system develop at an early stage, whilst the reproductive systems and the mammary glands, which are not required until a much later stage, develop later.

As well as the different regions and organs of the body, the different tissues develop at varying rates of growth. The order of growth is: brain tissue, bone tissue, muscle tissue and then fat. Thus if an animal is underdeveloped, its muscles and fat deposits will be much slighter than those in an animal well developed, although there will be less difference between the bones of the two, and even less between the brains.

An excellent example of the above laws can be seen in a rabbit of three or four months of age reared badly. Its head will be large in proportion to the rest of its body (compared with one of the same age, well reared) as also will be the intestines. The amount of bone will be in greater proportion to the muscle tissue than it would be if the animal had been well nourished, and there will be very little fat. The development of the sexual organs will be retarded.

To produce young stock with a high dressing-out percentage (that is, the weight of the dressed carcase as a percentage of the weight of the live animal), methods to increase the early development of bone, muscle and fat must be adopted, and must be brought into operation at an early age. Conversely, it is possible to increase the fineness of bone by slightly retarding the growth of the animal only when it is relatively young.

As the rabbit grows and develops, so the dressing-out percentage increases. At birth this percentage may be between 30 and 35%. At weaning it will have increased to 40 to 45%, whilst at slaughter the animal may dress out at 50 to 55%, and the very best animals even more. These percentages are about average for ordinary stock, but may be increased or decreased by the rapidity of growth. Thus young rabbits at weaning, which have been fed on a very high level of nutrition, may dress out at over 55%. A knowledge of these facts is most important to the breeder who wishes to obtain the heaviest carcase at the cheapest cost. By rearing stock slowly, the best advantage, purely in terms of feed, is lost.

There is sometimes a good deal of confusion regarding dressing-out percentages. This will obviously vary depending on whether the head is removed, and what organs (liver, heart, etc.) are left in. To have any validity, a dressing-out percentage must be measured immediately after processing, and before immersion in water, as is often the case. Immersion in water increases the weight of the carcase, sometimes considerably.

The appearance of yellow fat in the rabbit is controlled by a hereditary mechanism. In those rabbits which carry the factor for yellow fat, the yellow pigment, derived from the pigment in green foods, is not eliminated. Thus if the animal becomes fat and is then reduced in condition, the yellow pigment is concentrated. As the rabbit gets older the depth of yellow increases.

Although the quality, i.e. hardness, of fat depends to some extent on the foods given to the rabbit, fat deposited in a slowly growing animal will usually be of a softer quality, and therefore less desirable, than fat laid down during periods of rapid growth.

MOULT AND THE GROWTH OF FUR AND WOOL

The normal fur of the rabbit consists of two basic types of hair, the undercoat which is soft and varies in different breeds between about 12 to 32 mm and the guard hairs which are stronger and longer. In fact there are two types of guard hairs, the primary and the secondary. Each primary guard hair arises from one hair follicle whilst the secondary guard hairs arise in conjunction with a few undercoat or fur fibres from the same follicle. The fur fibres arise in groups from a single follicle. The length and form of the three types of hair are different, and the different proportions, forms, and lengths of the three types are responsible for the characteristic coat of the different breeds. The diameter of the undercoat hairs varies between 0.1 to 0.2 mm, whilst the guard hairs may be as much as 0.4 mm in diameter or even more.

These typical hairs have been modified in different breeds. For example, in the Rex the guard hairs have been shortened until they are about the same length or slightly less than the undercoat hairs, whilst in the Angora both types of hair are much increased in length.

All hairs consist of a medulla, a series of cells in the centre of the hair, a cortex, which surrounds the medulla, and the cuticle or scales, which overlap each other. In the undercoat hairs the scales cover the entire hair, but they are not present on the tips of the guard hairs which are swollen slightly to form a bulb. The normal undercoat hairs of the rabbit are slightly waved, but in the Angora the wool fibres forming the undercoat are crimped. In all cases the undercoat hairs are approximately uniform in diameter throughout their length, but guard hairs always have enlarged tips, and are not waved or crimped. There are several types of guard hairs which vary slightly in structure, but all types have the above general structure (Fig. 5.8).

The hairs arise singly or in multiples from a hair follicle, and growth from each half-hair follicle is more or less continuous. The first hairs to grow on the newborn rabbit are the guard hairs, but growth of the undercoat quickly follows and hair is

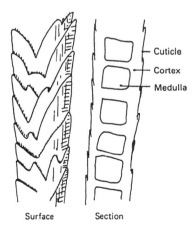

Surface   Section

Cuticle
Cortex
Medulla

Fig. 5.8   The structure of the hair

well developed after a few days. This first baby coat persists for between four and six weeks, and is much softer than the later coats of the same rabbit. The intermediate, or pre-adult, coat starts to replace the baby coat at five or six weeks of age, and is completed usually between 4.5 and 5.5 months although in the larger breeds it is often longer. On the completion of the growth of the intermediate coat, the pelt may be free of both loose hairs and new growth, that is to say, it is in 'tight' coat and free from moult. This occurs, for example, usually in the Chinchilla when the intermediate pelt was at one time in great demand for fur work. After completion of the intermediate coat, the growth of the adult coat begins.

Whilst the juvenile moults are dependent on age, the adult moulting pattern is more dependent on the season of the year. There are many factors which affect the growth and moulting of the hair, and depending on these, the adult coat may be completed at between six and eight months of age or even later. From this period onwards the rabbit will usually have two moults a year which are, however, variable and there are many exceptions.

Moult normally starts on the head and proceeds backwards and downwards. The areas of the flanks (in the region of the tail) and belly are thus the last places to be cleared of moult, and it is here that signs of moulting should be sought when the animal is being examined to determine whether it is in tight coat.

The moulting of the adult animal is really a continuous process, although the severity of loss of hair and growth of new hair varies considerably. The first moult is usually started in early spring, when the winter heavier coat is shed and the summer coat grown. This summer coat is less dense than the winter coat. It may not be until the autumn that the animal sheds an appreciable number of hairs and the moult is apparent. In some cases a very severe loss of hair and rapid growth of new hair may occur, when the appreciable moult period may be very short. In other cases the moulting period may be much longer.

Apart from what may be termed the normal moult, several other types of moult may occur. In the pregnant doe there is a loosening of the hair on the belly, thighs and chest, and she is thus able to pluck out fur easily to line her nest. The same loosening, which is due to the effects of hormones produced during pregnancy, occurs when the doe is pseudo-pregnant. There may be a double moult: that is to say, the rabbit may start and complete a moult immediately after a first moulting. This process may be further extended until the rabbit moults again immediately following the growth of new hair, and indeed several such moults may occur during the year.

Although the fineness of the hairs, and rapidity of their growth, and the length of moult period are determined basically by the inheritance of the rabbit (and this inheritance is by no means of a simple nature), these characteristics are much affected by environment, of which feeding and temperature are the two most important factors. A high level of nutrition will tend to produce a thicker fibre, but the increased density of the pelt (which is slightly increased by the thicker fibre) will not be so apparent, as the animal will be rather larger, and the actual density of the hairs thus slightly reduced. There is some relationship between size of animal and weight of hair grown, although this is not strictly correlated. Thus in the Angora, selection should be based on a weight of wool per unit weight of animal basis rather than on the basis of wool yield only.

The growth of an entire coat will impose some additional strain on the rabbit, and to assist it to overcome this strain, its nutrition should be good. The hair itself is composed very largely of protein, and rations designed to help in this way should therefore be adequately balanced. There are several abnormalities in growth and moult. In the Angora, areas of retarded wool growth may occur. These are usually small, the wool on the area remaining short. In certain cases of skin troubles, irregular falling away of the hair may also be caused.

MARKING AND IDENTIFICATION OF RABBITS

There are a number of ways in which rabbits may be marked, either permanently or temporarily, but only two systems of permanent marking merit consideration. They are ringing and tattooing. The only way in which animals for exhibition purposes should ever be marked is by ringing them with official rings, for otherwise they would be automatically disqualified.

Ringing

Rings, sold only by one central body, the British Rabbit Council, were introduced over 65 years ago and have since proved their great value. There are ten different sizes for the different breeds and they are shown in Table 5.1.

Table 5.1 Sizes, internal diameters and appropriate breeds of British Rabbit Council rings. It should be noted that very occasionally the ring size allocated to a breed may be altered, but the correct sizes are always available from the British Rabbit Council

Size	Internal diameter (mm)	Breeds
X	11.91	Netherland Dwarf
A	12.70	Polish
B	14.29	Argent Creme, Dutch, Himalayan, Mini Rex, Tan, Tri-colour Dutch
C	15.08	Argente Bleu, Argente Brun, Dwarf Lop
K	15.08	Miniature Lop
D	15.88	Cashmere Lop, Chinchilla, Deilenaar, English, all Foxes (except Swiss), Golden Glavcot, Havana, Isabella, Lilac, Perlfee, Sable, Siberian, Silver, Smoke Pearl, Squirrel, Thrianta
E	17.46	Angora, Argente, Champagne, Harlequin, New Zealand Red, Rex, Satin, Sussex, Swiss Fox
L	19.05	Alaska, Californian, Chinchilla Giganta, German Lop, Rhinelander, Sallander, Thuringer
G	20.64	Belgian Hare, Beveren, Blanc de Hotot, Pointed Beveren
H	22.23	Blanc de Bouscat, Blanc de Termonde, British Giant, English Lop, Flemish Giant, French Lop, Giant Papillon, Meissner Lop, New Zealand Black, New Zealand Blue, New Zealand White, Vienna Blue

When rings are purchased from the British Rabbit Council, the number of the rings (and no two rings have the same number in any year) are recorded against the name and address of the purchaser. When a ringed animal is sold or in any other way acquired by another person, then the ring number is transferred to that person in the records. In this way the ownership of any rabbit which is lost can instantly be found. The rings are also used as a check at shows, to ensure that the correct rabbit is sent back to the owner and to ensure that the rabbit to which a special is awarded is correctly awarded.

Rabbits should be ringed by placing the ring over the hock joint on one or other of the hind legs of the animal. Some breeders use one leg for bucks and the other for does, but there is no regulation concerning this point. The animal should be ringed at between 8 and 10 weeks of age except in the case of smaller breeds where earlier ringing is desirable. After this age there is some difficulty in getting the ring over the hock joint. After the rabbit is ringed it bears a permanent identification for life. Although the hock joint grows to a size which makes the removal of the ring from the live rabbit (without destroying the ring) almost impossible, the ring, if of the correct size for the breed, does not cause the rabbit any discomfort. Although it is a requirement that all exhibition stock must be ringed, many breeders ring the majority of their stock, for they find it a most suitable method for keeping records.

It is desirable that the ring should be checked from time to time, to ensure that the rabbit is comfortable with it. Sometimes hay or such like will get caught up in the ring which may constrict the leg and cause swelling. Sometimes a ring is put upon a rabbit which grows larger than is required for the breed and again the ring may constrict the leg. It is an excellent idea to check the ring, giving it a turn or two each time the rabbit is handled. The UK is the last country in the world, apart from Australia, New Zealand and Japan, in which ringing is used. In other countries tattooing is the method of permanent identification adopted.

Tattooing

Tattooing, although having some disadvantages, and not being entirely satisfactory for show animals, is a useful method of permanently marking rabbits. Usually a tattoo punch is used, although a mounted needle in which the number is pricked out can be employed, the latter method, however, being rather laborious. The inside of the ear is first cleaned with a degreasing fluid such as spirit, to remove any grease. The tattoo mark is then made, and specially prepared ink is liberally applied and massaged well into the tiny holes made by the punch or needle. Black ink is normally used, although red usually shows up better on dark coloured animals. It is sometimes suggested that tattooing is cruel but this is not so. If there is much tattooing to be done a tattooing box, in which the rabbit is placed, with its ear projecting, is used.

Other methods of marking

Other methods of marking, which are not normally employed (although in the commercial field they are becoming used more frequently) are numbered tags, similar to poultry wing tags, which are clipped through the ear, numbered studs which are similarly clipped through the ear, and for very young animals, ear notching. These systems are quite unsuitable for exhibition animals.

For marking very young animals temporarily, for example when two groups have to be amalgamated under a foster doe but when each must be identified, the use of a stain is satisfactory. There are several which can be used, but the two most satisfactory are acriflavine, and a solution of picric acid in 50% alcohol. This latter should be used with care and brushed on lightly. Different animals can of course be marked on different parts of the body, and the dyes will remain until the moulting out of the nest coat. If there are animals in only two groups, then one is marked and the other not.

RECORDS AND RECORDING SYSTEMS

The basis of improvement of any domestic animal depends on selection of future breeding stock. This selection must be based upon accurate knowledge, and, as the human memory is extremely fallible, accurate records are essential. With certain notable exceptions, recording is not greatly practised by rabbit breeders, although the necessity for it is now being more widely recognised. Quite apart from the ability to select stock on their performance, records allow breeders to assess their management. Recording will quickly show when and where their management fails, and only with satisfactory records can they trace the introduction, and therefore make easier the elimination of a particular fault.

Without accurate records, losses from disease will almost invariably be underestimated. With a stud limited in size, some stock have to be eliminated. Recorded animals can be eliminated easily on the basis of their profitability or otherwise. Accurate recording requires accurate observation. It is hardly surprising therefore that many breeders who introduce recording systems become more closely aware of their stock, and thus increase their knowledge.

Changes may occur in various characteristics of a strain over a period of years at a rate that is so slow as to make the breeders unaware of the changes unless they keep records with which they can compare these characteristics year by year. Thus in many cases early warning of undesirable trends means that they become known in time to prevent their full development. It can be seen then, that records are essential, and it is surprising therefore that so few are usually kept. The main reasons are that they can, if not properly arranged, be time-consuming, and unless they are correctly analysed, may be of little use. It is most important to remember that records are a means to an end, not an end in themselves.

An animal may be forced, for a short period, to produce at a very high level, but thereafter may be more or less valueless. It is necessary to obtain records over as long a period as possible to obtain a true picture. The longer the period over which records of individual animals and a stud are kept, the more valuable they become. Short-term records may be useful for some purposes, but may be valueless or even misleading for others.

Records fall naturally into three classes. There are those which are concerned with the financial aspect of the rabbitry, and little need be said about these, for such records are usually well understood, or, in the case of the exhibition breeder, ignored. It is advisable, however, to keep a financial record which allows the various items of expenditure to be analysed. Considerable saving can often be achieved when the respective costs of different items are clearly identified.

Apart from financial records, the two other classes of records are concerned with the management and the selection of future breeding stock. They are of course fairly closely related, and in many cases overlap. Very often management records can be extracted from individual stock records. For example, the overall figure for infertility in the rabbitry, which may well be related to certain management practices and feeding, will be obtained by an analysis of the breeding records of the stud bucks and does. Mortality records on the other hand will assist management by outlining trends in disease, or show where undue numbers of animals are dying. Whilst it is perhaps more important that the commercial breeder keeps accurate mortality records it is no bad thing for the exhibition breeder to do the same. It is very important to include all deaths. A review of the mortality record over the year produces a surprising figure in the majority of cases.

The recording needs of the fancier and the commercial farmer are different, for the commercial man requires above all an accurate assessment of growth gain per kilo of food used, and a record of what might be termed the commercially important characteristics of his animals. The items to be recorded in any rabbitry will depend upon the time which the breeder is prepared to spend on this aspect of management, and also on the purposes for which the rabbitry is maintained.

Hutch care

For day-to-day management in the exhibition rabbitry a hutch card (Fig. 5.9) can be very useful. On this card, which must be properly fixed to each hutch (a sheet-metal holder to give a solid backing for writing is useful), details of matings are entered, and thus a check of any card will give dates of kindling or weaning. These cards, as with all records, should be completed when any event to be recorded occurs.The hutch card is replaced in the commercial field by several records or registers.

HUTCH No:			SIRE:	
NAME:			DAM:	
RING NO:				
DATE BORN:				
DATE MATED	BUCK	RESULTS	NOTES	

Fig. 5.9   The simplest of hutch cards, placed, preferably, in a metal holder on the outside of the hutch. Details are entered as they occur. The number kindled and weaned are usually entered in the results column. This record card needs to be amplified for the commercial breeder

MATING AND LITTER REGISTERS

In general, the breeding efficiency of the stock is important in all types of rabbitries, and thus the results of each mating, the number of young in all litters, and, in the case of the commercial breeder or the exhibition breeder who is concerned with the growth of stock, the milk yield of the does (measured by the weight of the litter at 21 days), the growth rates and, partly, the resistance to disease will be recorded.

A simple system which would cover these points consists of a mating register (Fig. 5.10) and a litter register (Fig. 5.11). These two records will form the basis of the entire system, and from them a number of important facts can be elicited.

Mating No.	Date	Buck No.	Doe No.	Result		Notes
				Date	Litter No.	

Fig. 5.10 The mating register. All matings are entered in the register. If no litter is produced after a mating, then the details (e.g. missed, pseudo-pregnant, etc.) are entered in the notes column

Litter No.	Sire No.	Dam No.	Birth			Weaned		Weights		Disposal	Notes
			Date	Bucks	Does	Bucks	Does	21 days	Weaning		

Fig. 5.11 The litter register. Used to record details of all litters born. In the case of the exhibition breeder, except where weight is of importance, the columns for weight are often taken out. In the case of the commercial breeder where early growth is important, weights at 21 days and weaning should be included. These details are used (with the does' record cards) for analysis purposes for selecting future breeding stock

In a commercial rabbitry, where large numbers of rabbits will be dealt with, it is hardly likely that records for individual animals will be maintained, although an analysis of the litter records for both sire and dam will give satisfactory data for the selection of breeding stock.

In the Angora rabbitry, however, a full record giving such details as ring number, stud number, date of birth, sex, parentage, and wool yield at each clipping, may be required. Individual growth rates for special animals in the rabbitry may be required by the breeder, although only certain animals are usually recorded in this way, for the work can be laborious.

In a commercial rabbitry for meat production the dressing-out percentage of at least selected animals, or the gradings received from the processor, will often be of value both in deciding which families or strains give the better carcases and are therefore incorporated. These same details will also give a picture as to whether management is of the right standard. A low dressing-out percentage (for any particular age) will mean that the animals are not being managed and fed to the best advantage. If the coat quality is of some importance, the records may well be designed to show the quality of all coats, and whether the moult period was long or short. On this point, both the fur breeder and the fancier have the same requirement.

The recording of what might be termed 'fancy points' presents rather more difficulty than does the recording of such characteristics as weight, growth, litter size, etc. Although there are several systems for evaluating the quality of exhibition animals, each breeder's system, and the points which he or she will allocate to any particular characteristic, will vary. But none will deny that a knowledge of how an animal is bred, or of its efficiency as a breeding animal, even if its main purpose is for exhibition – or the breeding of animals for exhibition – is of great value.

It is obvious, then, that any characteristic can be recorded, as well as any detail of management. When the breeder has decided on the basic qualities that he or she wishes to record, he or she will then devise a system. Any system must be so designed that it helps to ensure accuracy. The only thing worse than not keeping records is to keep records which are inaccurate. These are quite definitely a danger.

The system must be flexible and should be capable of modification. It should contain sufficient detail to allow the breeder to compile all the data which he will need, but it should not require the duplicate entry of any item except, of course, when figures are transferred to analysis sheets. The system should not be costly, either in time or money, although cost is a relative term and the improvement of stock, management, and profit is the prime consideration. The system must be capable of easy analysis, for in general records themselves need analysis before their full use can be obtained. Good records should be physically and materially well kept. Slips of paper, although sometimes useful, are easily lost, a stout book is not.

Whilst all the above principles refer equally to exhibitors and commercial stock, different types of records are usually kept by both. For example, for commercial farmers, particularly those who hope to sell breeding stock or are going to rear their own future breeding stock, it is essential for them to keep those records which will allow them to select the best animals for this purpose.The only way they can do this is by judging the qualities of the parents of stock. Thus in addition to the mating and litter records mentioned above they must record the performance of each litter, or at least those from animals or strains they believe are likely to produce good stock. They certainly need to know total food consumption and total weight of litter at time of slaughter, albeit that some of the young are to be retained. Thus an excellent system is the use of a card for each litter (Figs. 5.12 and 5.13) and the doe record (Fig. 5.14).

Whilst for the meat producer who is not so concerned with the improvement of breeding stock (some farmers purchase all their replacements), then the most simple record that should be kept is the total of food consumed and liveweight sold.

It is obviously necessary when one is dealing with a large number of animals to have some system which projects all the tasks – against cage numbers – which have

Date Born	No. Alive	No. dead	No. fostered	Litter No.	
				Doe No.	
		Total weight at		Litter parity	
		Kg	g	Buck No.	
At 10 days				Notes	
At 21 days					
At weaning					
At disposal					

Fig. 5.12 The single litter record card. Used by the commercial breeder to record number alive and liveweights and food consumption of all litters which may contain potential breeding stock. On the reverse (see Fig. 5.13) details of food consumption are recorded. Usually the amount put into feed hoppers is recorded daily, and the totals of each week added at appropriate times

Food consumption in kg   Cage Numbers

Doe No.							Litter No.									
Weeks	1	2	3	4	5	6	7	8	9	10	11	12	13	14	15	16
Enter on right totals of food put into hoppers																
Brought Forward	/															
Totals																

Fig. 5.13 Reverse side of the single litter card (see Fig. 5.12). Amount of food (in kg) is put into columns and totalled at end of week. Up to weaning the totals will include that given to the doe and young. Note that each cage into which the litter may be transferred is put onto the card, the solid one being crossed out

Doe Number   Cage Number

Mating No.	Date	Buck No.	Litter			Fostered		Weaned			Note Number
			Date Born	No. Alive	No. Dead	+	-	No.	Weight		
									kg	g	
1											
2											
3											
4											
5											
6											
7											
Dam No:			Sire No:								
Discarded date:			Reason								

Fig. 5.14 The commercial doe record. Records details of *all* visits to the buck and the results. The reverse is often used for notes relating to particular matings, nest building, etc. Young fostered to the doe (+) and from the doe (–) should be entered. The card, with single litter records if kept, is used to analyse the performance of the doe

to be completed, the whole in the form of a diary. For example, having checked the day for a mating and having completed that mating, the day for the provision of the nest box might be entered, and so on.

MORTALITY

The subject of mortality is of much importance. Except for recording numbers dead at birth, and decreasing litter size which indicates deaths, mortalities should always be recorded separaretly and on the days when any occur. A simple mortality register is given in Fig. 5.15, which gives columns for the different important age groups. A final column exists in which the number of any note written concerning that particular day's or week's deaths can be inserted. At periods, depending upon the size of the establishment, these columns are totalled. If this record is to be of the best value, all deaths must be included. A review of this record at the end of the year will usually produce figures which are surprising to the rabbit breeder.

DATE	NEST BOX	11-21 DAYS	21 DAYS TO WEANING	WEANING TO SLAUGHTER	GROWERS	ADULTS	NOTE No.

Fig. 5.15   The mortality record. Each day, any deaths discovered are totalled for each age category and entered. Some mortality records have more detailed analysis of ages, but there is usually of no added benefit

Sometimes a breeder will use a diary or day book to record any items of interest in the rabbitry and will include details of losses or accidents. A true picture of these losses cannot be seen or assessed unless the details are extracted and presented in a much reduced form, such as monthly totals. The mortality record is a better way of recording these details.

Periodically, once the breeder has accumulated records, it will be necessary to analyse them to obtain the general information which is required. It is impossible to stress sufficiently that series of figures by themselves are of little value. They need analysis, collation and use. If, for example, it were seen that the fertility of the stock was decreasing, the purpose of the records would not be achieved unless the reasons were sought out and eliminated.

In the analysis of records, the prime purpose is to reduce a mass of figures to a few details of information in a usable form. One way of doing this is, of course, to plot the figures on a graph and thus obtain a 'picture'. This is an ideal method for growth rates, or for monthly totals of losses.

The bucks will have been used for a number of matings throughout the year, and the details of these must be reduced to understandable figures. If the number of all matings, the number of all resulting litters, and the number of all young produced by each buck are totalled and the average litter size calculated, a good deal of information is obtained. For each buck there is a set of four figures only. In the same way the number or percentage of fertile matings compared with infertile matings of each doe (and of the different bucks), the average weight of her young at 21 days (the best index of her milk yield), their average weight at weaning, the number of young in the litter, and so on, will be calculated from the different registers.

In the case of the buck, a buck performance analysis card is of value (Fig. 5.16). The figures are obtained and listed from the mating register and doe cards, and then totalled. In the same way the details of the doe are calculated by totalling and averaging the columns on her record card (Fig. 5.14) supplemented, if these are kept, with the single litter cards of her young. The important parameters for the selection of both bucks and does are accurately produced from these analyses.

Date	Doe No.	Doe		Palpation		Kindled		Nest Box	
		Mated	Refused	Doe in Kindle	Doe Empty	Yes	No	Alive	Dead

Fig. 5.16   Buck performance analysis. Used in comparison of bucks. All the information is taken from the mating register and totalled over a period to give average results. In more advanced analysis, comparisons of other bucks used with the same does and over the same periods are made

All comparisons from these analyses must be made on the basis of the same characteristics recorded under the same conditions, i.e. food regime, period of the year and similar housing, etc. It is also important, for example, not to compare young bucks with fully mature bucks, or only the first few litters of one doe with the subsequent litters of another. Food consumption between weaning and 8 weeks of age cannot be compared with food consumption between weaning and 12 weeks of age, and so on.

It may appear from the above that the time required for even a simple recording system would be great. This is not so. As an indication it may be stated that to fully record a stud of some 20 does with 4 bucks, kept meticulously in an exhibition stud, occupied less than one hour per week, although the time spent in the analysis of the records at the end of the year was excluded from this figure.

In this age of the computer some institutes, government departments, commercial firms or enterprising farmers have produced computer software which allows nearly all the records to be entered and analysed, and which then produces a daily work rota of work to be done against cage numbers. There are a number of such software programs available in different countries. These do, of course, reduce the labour of keeping the records themselves, but the most important feature of computer programs is that they most easily and very quickly allow for the important part of record keeping – the analyses of the records.

CULLING

The criteria on which the principles of the selection of stock must be based are dealt with elsewhere (see Chapter 9). There are, however, a number of reasons for eliminating animals from the rabbitry. Culling in this sense should be a more or less continuous part of the management.

Production stock, that is, does being used for the production of meat and fur or laboratory animals, which are not producing well, should automatically be eliminated. Any animals which do not thrive well should be culled, but it is worthwhile attempting to find out whether or not some management or feeding practice might be at the root of the trouble.

Abnormalities such as deformed limbs, and abnormal conformation such as 'chopped-off rump' (where the rump is cut away sharply), should not be tolerated, nor should, for example, malocclusion of the teeth. There are, of course, a number of breed faults in each breed, and animals showing these to a well-developed extent should also be culled.

Age is often given as a reason for eliminating animals from a rabbitry. Age alone, however, is not a sufficient reason. Does will inevitably have smaller litters as they grow older, but in some cases it may be worthwhile to continue to use an old doe which produces excellent quality young. In the same way age alone should never be a reason for discarding a buck which has proved itself to be a good getter of stock. Sound management, however, demands severe culling, and the rabbit breeder is fortunate in having quick breeding and fecund stock which allow this. A veterinarian will carry out this service for the one-rabbit keeper.

ROUTINE EXAMINATIONS

Closely allied with culling is the need for routine examinations of the stock. The good stockperson will be quick to notice any signs of ill health in his or her animals, but opportunity should be taken of thoroughly examining the animals before each mating, or preferably at more frequent intervals. Each breeder should develop some system or order for these examinations. Lack of a system almost invariably means that important points will be missed. A well-thought-out system of observation will also enable the breeder to accomplish the work more quickly. A suitable system is as follows: the weight of the animal is noted and the relation of this to size will give an indication of its condition. With a rabbit in very poor condition the projections on the side and top of the spine can be felt, whilst with one in less poor condition the projections on the top of the spine only can be easily distinguished. The condition of the coat will give further information regarding health. A harsh, dry, staring coat indicates poor health, whilst a patchy coat may indicate moult (perfectly normal) or parasitic infection or damage due to fighting. The condition of the belly fur should not be ignored. A hand run over the body will give indication of the presence of cysts, whilst if the legs are stretched out any deformities may be noted. The nostrils and eyes, and the ears, followed by the teeth (the lips being drawn back), can next be examined. Details of any wet patches or 'drooling' from the mouth should be noted. Discharges from the eyes, nose, mouth, ears, sexual organs and anus must not be overlooked. It is important to look deeply into the ears, for the first signs of trouble can only be found in this way. The mammary glands should be noted in the doe, and the sexual organs everted as though sexing. Sound examination must be based on a thorough system and on practice, and the only way for a breeder to become proficient in this art is to practise it.

CASTRATION

Castration, although sometimes advised, has little application in the rabbitry. Although many breeders claim the contrary, all experimental evidence shows that castrated animals require rather longer to attain the same weight as their litter mates which are not castrated, the castrated animals require more food to achieve that weight, and the carcases are no better. In some cases it may be that when Angora bucks are kept for woolling some of the fighting may be prevented, although this is not always certain.

Surgical castration consists of the removal of the testicles of the buck as soon as they have descended from the abdominal cavity which may be as early as two months, but is usually between three and four months. The rabbit must be held firmly by an attendant, whilst the operator stretches the skin of the scrotal sac over a testicle and makes a clean incision with a sterilised knife. The testicle being released, is drawn through the incision, and the cord is severed by scraping through it. The second testicle is removed in the same way. The cut must be made at the lowest point of the scrotum to ensure good drainage. The wound should be swabbed with a mild antiseptic, and the animal placed quietly by itself in a clean hutch. The animal should be fasted for the previous 24 hours before the operation. Some skill is required for this operation, and the novice is recommended to try on a dead rabbit or to watch a demonstration before practising himself.

WARRENS AND COLONIES

The original method of rabbit keeping, which extends back over many centuries, was the warren. Usually, although not always, the warren was entirely fenced and the foodstuffs were brought in by an attendant, the stock being otherwise semi-wild. The mortality due to the build up of disease, was great and the system is never to be recommended. In recent years, this system has been modified to some extent and runs similar to the way poultry runs are used for keeping stock, but again the system is not really successful. Occasionally the system is used purely as a breeding unit and a number of does run with some bucks for 25 days or so, after which they are removed to a breeding hutch. Sometimes the young are returned to the colony or compound until three-months-old when they are grouped in further colonies according to age and sex. A modification for the running on of meat stock is the use of wire-floored colony pens, and this is much to be preferred to the old type compound.

SUN IN THE RABBITRY

As any breeder can observe, sun will completely fade the coat of a coloured rabbit quite quickly, and discolour a white one. On the other hand, sunlight is of undoubted benefit to breeding stock and growing young. Thus the breeder will have to compromise, and usually the rabbit keeper, particularly of exhibition animals, will exclude the direct rays of the sun whilst admitting plenty of fresh air and light.

WEIGHING RABBITS

Weight is of much importance to all rabbit breeders. It gives an excellent indication of the stock's progress and of impending troubles. For the commercial producer, growth is linked fairly closely with profit. For the exhibition breeder, weight is important for either the stock must not exceed a certain weight, or they are required to be as heavy as possible. It is therefore surprising to find that scales of some description are not amongst the most common items of equipment. Under BRC Show Rules a pair of scales must be available at every show, and an exhibitor may sometimes save a fruitless journey for his or her exhibit by weighing it if perhaps it is close to the permissible limit.

The weight of the same rabbit may vary a good deal throughout the day and from day to day. When routine weighings are used, it is important therefore to weigh always at the same time each day, when more consistent results can be obtained. A spring balance with a suitable box, into which rabbits can be placed easily, is usually satisfactory, as is also the spring balance with a pan on top, provided that the pan is quite secure and the scales not liable to fall over. The ideal weighing machine is the normal old fashioned weighing scales with a suitable platform, and give the most uniform results. With any type of scales it is desirable to check the accuracy from time to time with an exact known weight.

DETERMINING AGE

There are various indications which the experienced breeder may use as a guide to the age of any rabbit. These indications are, however, varied by different circumstances, and can therefore be misleading, unless all the circumstances are taken into consideration. The claws of the rabbit do not project beyond the fur until the animal is nearing maturity. They continue to grow and become more curled as age advances. If the rabbits are kept on a solid floor the claws will wear and will thus be shorter than if the animal had been kept on, say, a wire-mesh floor.

A slight indication is given by the feel of the ears, although this simply allows animals of the year to be distinguished by their rather softer feel from animals of two or three years of age in which the ears feel slightly tougher. The general development of the rabbit does not give such a reliable guide unless the breeder is very experienced, for it is affected greatly by external factors. The normal age to which rabbits live varies between 5 and 8 years, although some of over 10 or even 12 years have been known.

REGULARITY OF ROUTINE

Perhaps the most important aspect of rabbit management refers to regularity. Rabbits are very much creatures of habit, and a regular routine is of great importance in achieving good results. Not only do the animals benefit from this regularity of care and management, but the breeder is enabled to conduct his operations with the least waste of time, and with the least possibility of error.

MANAGEMENT OF ANGORAS

Angoras are a specialised breed with coats which may measure as much as 15 cm or more. They require rather specialised management. One aim of management is to prevent the wool from matting or becoming stained, and thus stock are never bedded on the usual bedding materials but are kept on mesh floors, and hay for feeding is not fed loose but in some sort of hay rack.

The coats of exhibition Angoras are allowed to grow to their full length, and frequent grooming with brush and bellows is necessary. For stock for woolling, however, which are clipped every 12 weeks, such grooming is not necessary. The highest prices are obtained from wool which is plucked from the animal rather than clipped.

KILLING

There will be occasions when the rabbit breeder will need to kill stock. For those who are unable to kill stock, the assistance of a local butcher or another rabbit breeder can probably be obtained. In general, however the rabbit keeper should be able to kill rabbits quickly and humanely.

There are two methods which are normally adopted, but for small-scale commercial purposes the method in which the neck is dislocated is the only one to be recommended. This method consists of holding the rabbit securely by the back legs with one hand, whilst the head is grasped with the other. The fingers of the hand will pass under the chin, and the thumb will lie on top of the head behind the ears. With the hind legs being held securely, the chin is pressed up whilst the base of the head is forced down, the whole operation being done quickly but with insufficient force to pull the head off the animal, and this may occur fairly easily with a small rabbit. A slight sudden give will indicate the dislocation of the neck. This method (Fig. 5.17) requires a little practice, and by far the best way of learning is to have a demonstration by a competent person.

The second method is by a blow with either a stick or the side of the hand. The stick should be about 35 cm long and fairly heavy. The animal is held with head downwards in one hand or sat on a table with the ears held forward (Fig. 5.18), when a blow can be given to the base of the skull with either the hand or the stick. Care

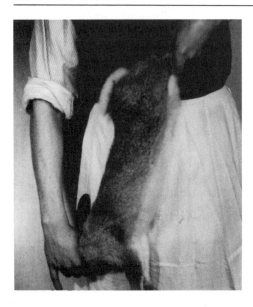

Fig. 5.17   Killing by dislocation of the neck

should be taken that the blow does not hit the shoulders, otherwise the carcase may be discoloured, and the killing ineffective. This method is usually thought to be the easiest, but once proficiency has been attained with the dislocation method no trouble should ever be experienced, except possibly with an extra large and old rabbit.

When the rabbit is held with the head hanging down the ears will usually be held fairly tensely when the animal is alive, but will be quite loose when the animal is dead. Immediately after killing there is some reflex kicking but this soon ceases. If the rabbit is being killed for table purposes, then it should not be fed for 24 hours prior to killing.

Rabbit processing or packing stations exist to process young animals from rabbit farmers. The most usual and satisfactory method of killing in these establishments is

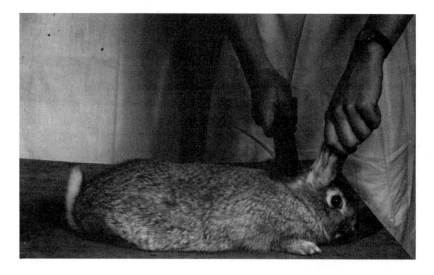

Fig. 5.18   Killing by blow with a heavy stick

by an electric stunner followed by decapitation, or by bleeding, both producing a whiter meat.

There are also some humane killers available which are effective and easy to operate.

PREPARATION OF CARCASES ON A SMALL SCALE

Rabbits for meat should always be killed after a period of up to 24 hours or so without food, although water should always be available both for humane reasons and also to assist in preventing weight loss. After killing, the animals can be pelted (skinned) immediately, or they can be left for a short period to allow the flesh and fat to firm a little. It is not advisable to allow the carcase to get cold before skinning as this will make the operation more difficult.

If the use of the pelt as a high-grade fur is contemplated, care must be taken in the pelting process. This has a decided effect on the subsequent value of the skin. Every effort should be made to keep the fur quite clean, and to ensure that the cuts are made in the right places in order that the fur will be of the correct shape when dried, and without torn and ragged edges.

The rabbit for pelting is suspended by its back legs either on hangers (see Fig. 6.18) or on nails pushed between the tendon and the bone of each leg. A knife cut is made through the skin, but not into the flesh, from the inside of the hock joint to the vent, and the skin eased off the leg with the fingers. The skin is then cut away at the hock joint, and when the other leg has been similarly treated, the skin is loosened over the hindquarters and the tail bone cut through, or alternatively the skin cut through high up on the tail. The skin is then pulled down over the body sleeve fashion, the front legs being skinned in the same way. It may be necessary to loosen the skin from the body. When the ears are reached, the skin can be cut off the body, or the base of the ears cut through, and the skin taken off the head. The method will depend on whether the carcase is to be sold with head on or off.

After removal of the skin, and not before, the veins in the neck should be cut to allow the release of blood, which will make the carcase appreciably lighter in colour. The skins should be hung up and not thrown in a heap, for this will lead to deterioration.

The so-called 'Ostend' method of dressing rabbit carcases was the only one acceptable to the butcher's trade up to the early 1950s. It still continues at the present time in some of the Continental trade. The method consists of opening the belly with a cut just in front of the vent for about 10 to 12 cm, and removing the offal. Care has to be taken when making this cut to ensure that the intestines are not cut. The pelvic bone is cut through or left intact, depending on the wishes of the buyer, but in either case it is essential to ensure the removal of the part of the intestine which runs through the pelvic bone. The kidneys and liver are left in the carcase, but the gall bladder, the small greenish sac attached to a lobe of the liver which contains a bitter fluid, is carefully removed to prevent contamination. The feet are removed from the front legs which are then inserted into slots cut into the ribs. The back feet are cut off below the hock and the legs inserted into each other, thus pressing out the thighs to give a better appearance.

The carcase, having been dressed, is normally placed in iced water for a period of up to four hours, when it is cut, pre-packed and, if necessary, frozen at –20°C. For local consumption the cooling in iced water and freezing may be omitted, but blood and other stains must be removed. Customarily in processing and packaging for the retail trade packs of various sizes and types are produced.

Although the commercial rabbit farmer produces only young rabbits for sale, the hobbyist or fur enthusiast can produce the ideal size of carcase for the domestic consumer, of approximately 1.5 to 2 kg in weight. Thus the medium-sized normal fur breeds yield, when in prime coat, an ideal carcase which is also one from an animal not more than about six months of age. The Rex breeds will give a carcase rather larger.

Carcase faults which detract from the appearance and therefore price are blood or other stains, finger marks, yellow fat, bruising, cuts in the flesh, dark flesh resulting from poor bleeding, etc.

Dressing losses

The weight lost between liveweight and carcase weight is known as the dressing loss, and is usually given as a percentage, i.e. the dressing-out percentage. This is the carcase weight as a percentage of the liveweight. The dressing-out percentage has an important influence on profit and loss, and is affected by several factors. For mature animals the dressing-out percentage is about 60%, and for younger animals it may be reduced to 50% or even less. An animal which has been reared on a low level of nutrition will, before it reaches maturity, have a lower dressing-out percentage than one reared on a high level of nutrition. A very fat adult animal will dress out at a higher percentage than will a lean adult. The dressing-out percentage will of course be affected by the removal or otherwise of the head and organs. When an animal is cut and packaged, the head is not included but the liver usually is.

HANDLING OF FURS

After the pelt has been removed from the rabbit it is hung up until it can be dealt with, although this should be as soon as possible, to prevent damage. It can then either be put on a wire or wooden stretcher or it can be cut down the belly line and nailed out.

If the pelt is not cut open and nailed out it is dried on a stretcher (see Fig. 6.19) and when dried it is known as a cased skin. This method is suitable for handling the poorer grade skins, for it is very quick. It is not satisfactory, however, for the highest quality of pelt which is to be used for fur work. These must be nailed out on a pelt board.

The pelt is cut down the belly line and placed fur downwards on the board, and a nail (and furriers' nails 30 to 40 mm long are ideal) inserted at the root of the tail (which is cut off). The pelt is then pulled slightly to prevent wrinkling and a nail inserted at the nape of the neck. Further nails are then inserted alternately on each end and side. If one end or side is nailed first, then it is unlikely that the pelt will be correctly nailed out. The nails should finally be about 25 to 30 mm apart. No matter how good the original pelt, it will lose some of its value if it is incorrectly stretched during nailing.

After the pelt has been nailed out, all fat and flesh should be removed with a blunt knife. If fat is not removed it will 'burn' the pelt. The fat should be scraped off. Under no circumstances should any pieces be pulled, for the skin is composed of diagonal layers and the pulling of what appears only the surface film may tear the skin in half.

When the pelt has been cleaned it should be hung up to dry. It should never be dried by artificial heat or exposed to the direct rays of the sun. The best method is to hang the pelt boards in an airy shed. The pelts may take anything from two or three days to two weeks in bad weather to dry. When quite dry they are removed and stored until dressing. Air-dried pelts, provided that they are protected from the ravages of moths, will store in boxes for long periods. Indeed they store better when air-dried than when dressed. It is important that they should always be stored leather to leather and fur to fur, for the slightest amount of grease on the fur will cause damage. They should always be stored flat; folding or rolling will usually lead to cracking.

SELECTION OF ANIMALS FOR PELTING

The value of the skin will depend, amongst other factors, on its freedom from moult. The fur from a moulty skin will always tend to 'slip', that is, to drop out, consequently it is important that prime furs should be taken when there is no moult. Unfortunately the rabbit may not be in 'tight' coat (i.e. completely free from moult) for very long, and opportunities should not therefore be missed.

Absence of moult can be detected by examining the skin of the animal. If the fur is blown apart then, in coloured breeds, the skin will appear bluish in those areas where the rabbit is moulting. These same patches will, when the animal is skinned, show on the skin side as blue patches. The colour is due to the pigment of the new hair showing through. Moult in white furred breeds is more difficult to detect, but the presence of dead hair is a good indication, as also is shorter hair which is growing. The belly fur is often cut away before the furrier makes up the pelts, and therefore a few moult marks on the belly are not so important. However, moult marks on the back must be avoided, or the value of the pelt may be reduced by as much as half.

Rabbit furs, even from animals of the same breed or same strain, vary a good deal in colour, density and texture. Thus the commercial buyer needs to match a bundle of pelts to make any article of clothing, otherwise the article will appear patchy. It is for this reason that dyeing is used to such an extent in the fur trade. Matching of pelts is a highly skilled operation, but nevertheless matched pelts bring enhanced prices.

The number of rabbit pelts required for the making up of different articles varies between 40 for a full-length coat, 28 for a hip-length coat, 14 for a large cape or stole and 8 for a small cape. Thus if a breeder is able to match up sufficient pelts to make a bundle for any of these, his profit will be increased.

DRESSING AIR-DRIED PELTS

Dressing is the means whereby an air-dried pelt is turned into a supple, thin-leathered pelt, by tanning the raw skin into leather. The dried skins are first cleaned and then soaked in a fluid which softens them. They are then fleshed, that is to say, the thin membranes overlying the true leather are removed. During this operation circular or flat knives are used and any nails left in the pelts may cause serious damage. The fleshing is one of the most important operations, for upon it will depend the thinness of the final leather, a matter of some importance to the furrier. After the fleshing the pelts are pickled to tan the leather, and the excess fluid is then removed by using a centrifuge. The skins are then manipulated to produce the softness required in the finished leather, and finally cleaned by revolving in large drums with sawdust, which is itself then removed. It will thus be seen that the whole process involves considerable skill and knowledge, and the use of expensive equipment. It is only with these that a good dressing can be achieved, and it will be seen why home dressing of pelts is not usually to be recommended.

Chapter 6
Housing and Equipment

'We now come to what appears the simplest of all matters, and which yet, if it be not well contrived, will have a most influential effect in causing failure. From a tea-chest to a worn-out port-manteau or a leaky tub, anything has been thought good enough to keep a rabbit in. "Everybody," says Cobbett, "knows how to knock up a rabbit hutch". If the rabbits themselves could only speak they would tell us that many a body sets about it in a bungling manner, and proves himself profoundly ignorant of the fundamental principles of rabbit architecture.'

These words, written by Delamere more than 140 years ago, are as true today as when they were written, except in the case of the most modern intensive rabbit farms. Elsewhere, the average quality of rabbit housing has undoubtedly improved, although the designs are in general the same, but there are still many very unsatisfactory hutches. They are unsatisfactory because they cause loss of time and money to the owners and discomfort to the occupants.

The variety of hutches is enormous, and the final design will depend largely on the requirements of the owner. It is therefore desirable to deal with the general principles of housing in order that the breeder can work out designs most suitable for his or her purposes and pocket.

The development of the intensive commercial rabbit industry – as it has done in so many other ways – has changed many features of housing and equipment for the commercial breeder. The farmer is concerned to reduce labour to the absolute minimum; the fancier, whose great interest is his or her stock, is not so concerned. Indeed the fancier usually considers any time spent with the animal a pleasure. At one time it was thought that completely open-mesh pens would be of great help in reducing the incidence of disease, but this has not proved so. Certain disease conditions are controlled to an extent by mesh, others are aggravated by the use of this material. Nevertheless the labour saving aspect has meant that mesh cages are now almost universal in commercial farming.

Again, many rabbit farmers, who are concerned with a carefully controlled environment, with temperature and humidity levels kept within quite close bands, usually have to invest considerable sums of money. The fancier does not need to do this and, because in many cases a colder atmosphere is better for the stock, would be foolish to do so. This is not to say, however, that ventilation is not important to the fancier. It is very important but, because of the usually small scale and the often open air conditions, expensive ventilation systems are not required.

Thus there is a divergence of systems between the exhibitor and the professional rabbit farmer, and this fact should be remembered when considering what follows. The first part of this chapter deals with some general principles, and housing and equipment for the non-professional and rabbit keeper on a small scale. A second part considers commercial aspects.

THE RABBITRY AND RABBIT HOUSE

The rabbitry may consist of a few odd hutches or a well-designed building or group of buildings in which have been built a number of hutches. The layout must be carefully planned, for the ease of management, and the attractiveness of the unit depends largely upon correct grouping and spacing of hutches. If a new building is contemplated, then full consideration should be given to details of further expansion before the rabbitry is built. Very often the rabbitry will be enlarged and unless this expansion is foreseen and provided for, a bad layout will usually result. It should be remembered that work in a badly designed rabbitry may easily take twice, or even thee times, as long as the same work in one which is well designed. And the work is less pleasurable.

For the smaller breeder there is also the question of the appearance of the rabbitry. Under the present law, embodied in the Allotments Act of 1950 and the Environmental Protection Act 1990, no landlord may prohibit rabbit keeping unless, amongst other things, it constitutes a nuisance. It may well do this if the appearance presents an ugly view to neighbours. Also under the Environmental Protection Act a nuisance can be caused if the buildings and hutches are not constructed satisfactorily.

There are several advantages and disadvantages of indoor rabbitries, i.e. hutches enclosed within a building:

- stock and attendants will be completely protected from the weather;
- coats will not be faded by strong sunlight;
- winter breeding is cert inly easier and more successful;
- losses of young during winter probably a little less.

Also in recent times, with the advent of the two viral diseases of the rabbit, it is safer to keep rabbits protected from flying insects.

Against these are the disadvantages that young animals should have some sunlight (when they are not to be exhibited as youngsters), stock usually have slightly denser coats when kept outside, the moult period may be slightly longer inside a building, and the initial cost of the building could be relatively high. Furthermore there may be problems arising from poor ventilation, which never occur when rabbits are housed outside.

For these reasons the most desirable system for the exhibition breeder (except for a well-ventilated shed or house) is often to be found in the stack of hutches with a shelter or at least an extended roof, or perhaps facilities for enclosing the hutches in some way (Fig. 6.1).

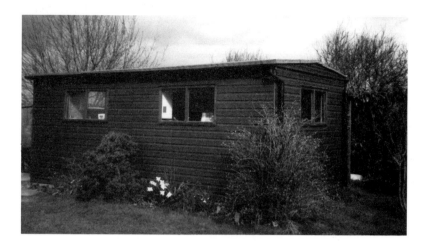

Fig. 6.1   An ideal building for the rabbit exhibitor

Some arrangements must be made in the rabbitry for the storage of food, bedding and equipment. In all cases the food and bedding store should be vermin-proof, and large bins of either metal or wood are ideal for some of the food. At the present time, when probably most food is purchased in factory bags, this is not of such importance. It is also important to have a suitable bench or table on which to handle stock when small rabbits are concerned. A well-designed table-trolley is useful in the commercial establishment.

A very common arrangement in many rabbitries is that in which rows of hutches face each other. This saves much time, especially if the width of the passageway between is sufficient for the easy passage of a trolley or small cart (Fig. 6.2). The doors of the rabbitry must also be large enough to admit the largest barrow which is to be used, and if the floor level of the rabbitry is above that of the ground outside, then a ramp should be made to the rabbitry floor.

Probably most rabbitries are insufficiently lighted. The ideal system is the use of hopper type windows, which assist in the control of ventilation, situated between the level of the top of the hutches and the eaves. In large-span buildings, additional roof lighting is often desirable, and the installation of electric light is usually found to be essential in commercial establishments when a 16-hour day (or something similar) is required. Windows should preferably face north or east so that strong light does not fade the coats of the stock, and when roof lighting is installed it may be necessary to have some form of blind to prevent the direct rays reaching the stock.

The actual location of the hutches within a building is important. Mention has already been made that passages between stacks of hutches should be sufficiently wide. Stacks should not be placed tight against a wall, an air space of at least 25 cm being desirable between the rear of the hutches and the wall. This allows free

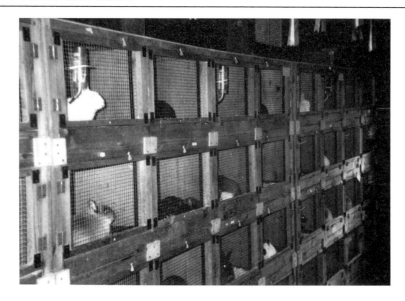

Fig. 6.2 The interior of the building shown in Fig. 6.1. Note that the hutches are stacked four deep. This is because the breeds the exhibitor keeps are the smallest and are completely happy with the hutch height. The housing shown is for the Polish breed

ventilation of the building and assists in the prevention of dampness.

The floor of the rabbitry should be solid, impervious to rats and mice, and easily cleaned. It should also be non-absorbent, non-slippery, durable and dry. A concrete floor is probably the best type if properly laid, that is, a minimum of a 5 cm thick layer of good concrete over 10 to 15 cm of well rammed coarse aggregate. The top layer of concrete can with advantage be reinforced with a 12.7 mm mesh galvanised wire netting, which assists in preventing vermin from entering the rabbitry (Fig. 6.3).

Earth floors and floors made from bricks absorb urine and are very difficult to clean and keep hygienic. The ease with which a good floor can be kept clean will

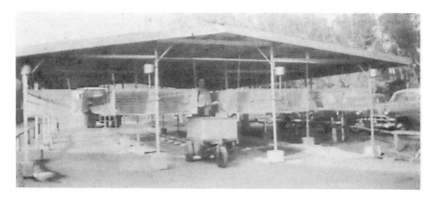

Fig. 6.3 An American rabbitry built over a concrete floor. Note suspension of cages giving a completely clear floor and the water breaker tanks mounted near the upright supports

quickly repay the initial extra cost. It is advantageous to have the floor sloping slightly to a gutter to facilitate washing.

The rabbitry roof should be of a material that provides some insulation against both cold and heat. A corrugated iron roof, unless it is laid over insulating material such as glass fibre mat, is bad for this reason. Corrugated asbestos cement sheet is probably the most satisfactory material, but a wooden roof covered with a heavy quality roofing felt is as good, though more expensive.

It is unusual, except in a larger commercial undertaking starting from a 'green field' site, for buildings to be specially constructed for a rabbitry. In general, existing buildings are more often adapted. Shelters and sheds are, however, another matter, although, of course, a controlled environment is not possible. They are much less costly and easier to erect. The shelter may consist of an extension of the roof of the top hutch in a stack, or it may be independent. For roofs extending more than about 60 cm, additional supports must be erected, and 60 cm does not really provide adequate shelter, particularly for the attendant. Good protection is afforded by a shelter extending 1.25 m from the hutch front.

Attention to the comfort of the attendant is definitely important, for unless work can be carried out in reasonable comfort it may be skimped, particularly during the winter months, when attention to detail is so important.

An ideal shelter may be made by extending the roof some 1.25 m from the hutch (Fig. 6.4). This roof must be supported by a framework consisting of 60 × 60 mm timber resting on a heavier beam running parallel to the hutches. The heavy beam is supported by uprights at 2.5 to 3 m intervals. Ideally these uprights are rested upon concrete footings. The roof must be anchored securely to the framework to prevent it being blown off by high winds. The use of corrugated asbestos cement sheet gives added weight to the roof, and thus assists in preventing it being blown away. Sometimes a light framework is fixed between the uprights, and wire netting attached to the framework, thus forming an enclosed rabbitry at low cost. In those areas where myxomatosis and VHD amongst wild rabbits is common, there is much to be said for preventing the entry of mosquitoes into the rabbitry and mosquito-proof material can be used as well. Even a shelter of this nature can be made more or less mosquito proof.

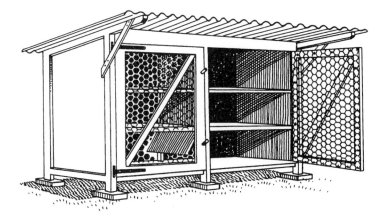

Fig. 6.4 A six-hutch stack with extended roof. Note centre partitions are hinged at top to allow two hutches to be made into one

Sacking stretched over the wire netting also gives added protection. It is common in America for the uprights of the shelter to be used for the support of hutches, a system which both reduces the cost, and allows complete clearance under the hutches.

VENTILATION AND LIGHTING IN THE RABBITRY

The control of temperature, relative humidity and ventilation in a controlled environment commercial house is most important. Indeed it is one of the most fundamental necessities for success in that form of housing. Good ventilation is so important, but in many cases also so expensive that in many areas the commercial 'open air' farm system, in which natural ventilation is more easily achieved, has many devotees and the system is probably gaining over the totally controlled environment house.

Whilst the proper ventilation of the non-commercial rabbitry is as important as in the commercial field, it would be unusual for the same amounts of money to be spent upon it as is done in the commercial field. Therefore general details are given here which apply to all conditions, with further points relating to the fully controlled commercial house being discussed later in this chapter.

Ventilation

Ventilation is essential for the removal of noxious gases, pollutants, moisture, dust and heat. In badly ventilated conditions, the moisture content of the air, with the polluting materials, increases as does the temperature. These conditions are particularly harmful to animals, but are very suitable conditions for disease organisms. Both this increase in disease producing organisms, and the various stresses exerted on the animals by the bad ventilation interact to produce mounting problems. In winter, the amount of moisture that the air can hold is reduced and thus the relative humidity increases and adds to the difficulties. Ammonia is produced by bacterial action on material in the urine of the animals. The increased concentration of ammonia in badly ventilated conditions causes damage to the rabbits which are then more easily infected with disease organisms.

During the course of the day rabbits give off a surprising amount of heat and moisture which add to the problems. Similarly, badly maintained watering systems which leak are harmful. The accumulation of manure and urine in the rabbit house is often overlooked as a source of increased requirements for ventilation. The adequate removal of this at appropriate intervals is most important.

Whilst insufficient ventilation is bad, too much may be even worse, particularly in the colder weather. The need then for control of ventilation is clear. Signs of inadequate ventilation are: a smell of ammonia, condensation, too high a temperature or relative humidity compared with the outside air, and a marked difference in the temperatures recorded by a maximum–minimum thermometer. This latter indication shows that the insulation of the building is poor.

Relative humidity

The ideal relative humidity (the amount of moisture vapour in the air as a percentage of the total amount the air could hold at the same temperature) of an indoor rabbitry is under 75% at a temperature of about 16°C. It is of course impossible to maintain such relative humidity, or the ideal temperature for the breeding of exhibition stock of about 10 to 13°C, unless there is special control, and it would be rare, outside a laboratory, for such control to be incorporated in a rabbitry. Thus the next best alternative is to ensure that the relative humidity should not be higher than that of the outside air by more than about 5%, and the temperature should not differ from that outside by more than about 5°C. Usually it is preferable to have both temperature and humidity lower inside the rabbitry than outside, except in cold weather.

Inlets and outlets for ventilation

Ventilation must, however, be under control for, depending on the outside conditions, a varying amount of inlet and outlet space will be desirable. As warm air rises, the inlets of the ventilation system should be low and the outlets high. If the inlets are too high, the cold air entering the rabbitry prevents the escape of the foul air and condensation occurs. It is essential that the air inlets should be of a suitable size to adequately ventilate the rabbitry in the hottest conditions. It is also essential that apart from being adequate in size the inlets are suitably placed. In all cases the outlets in unpowered ventilation systems should be of a greater size than the inlets. The actual sizes of the inlets and outlets are difficult to calculate, but for the very worst conditions of heat and humidity something like 45 cm^2 per kg liveweight of animals in the shed or house is necessary. In the very coldest conditions a good deal less than this (17 cm^2) is required, and should be catered for by having openings that can be restricted to 15 cm^2. In unpowered ventilation systems the outlets should be at the highest points in the rabbitry (Table 6.1).

Table 6.1   Maximum air speed and ventilation rates

Approximate temperature (°C)	Maximum air speed (m/sec)	Maximum ventilation rate (m^3 per kg liveweight per hour)	Maximum unpowered inlet (cm^2 per kg liveweight)
3–6	0.1	0.65	17.0
7–10	0.12	0.9	20.0
11–14	0.2	2.0	27.0
15–18	0.3	3.9	34.0
19–22	0.4	6.15	42.5
23–26	0.6	10.0	45.5

The avoidance of draughts is important. Draughts are occasioned by too high an air velocity. The maximum air velocity which may, under any circumstances, flow over an animal should not exceed 0.6 m per sec in the hottest conditions. The ideal is about 0.1 m a sec. There are various devices for measuring air speed, but the simplest by far is to use a lighted candle. With an air speed of less than 0.1 m a sec there is no deflection of the flame. If the flame is bent over to slightly less than 45° from upright, the speed of the air movement is about 0.6 m a sec. Other speeds are proportional. The important point to remember when using the candle-flame method is to ensure that the wick is not shielded by the candle, that is to say, all wax should be cut away leaving the wick protruding from a cone point.

Inlets may consist of porous bricks, grills, piping let into walls, and windows. The outlets may be ridge openings (either fixed or preferably adjustable), louvre boxes, ventilation cowls, or high windows. There should be periodical inspection of both inlets and outlets to ensure that they do not become blocked.

Temperature

In some rabbitries, at certain times of the year the temperature may become so high as to affect the stock. Apart from ensuring that the ventilation is adequate, and using a form of construction (e.g. a double roof) that will insulate the rabbitry from the sun's rays, the only method of lowering the temperature is by sprinkling water on the walls, floor and roof of the buildings and/or hutches. In a badly ventilated rabbitry this procedure would, however, only make matters worse, but under good ventilation conditions the temperature may be reduced by as much as 5°C.

ESSENTIALS OF GOOD HOUSING

Although there is an infinite number of types of hutch, the principles underlying the construction of the best types are the same. There are certain essential points which must be considered if housing is to be suitable. The shed or rabbit house should be included in this consideration as well as the hutches themselves. Essential conditions for the hutch are that it must be:

- sufficiently large and of the right dimensions for the purpose for which it is intended;
- comfortable and escape-proof;
- sanitary and capable of being easily cleaned (Figs 6.5–6.7);
- convenient for the easy handling of stock and the servicing of their requirements;
- well constructed of sound materials, but as cheap as possible;
- structurally strong and sound and well made;
- so constructed that the animal can hurt neither itself nor the hutch;
- so constructed that fresh clean air can, but draughts cannot, enter;
- so designed that there is good visibility of the animals at all times.

There is obviously no best type of hutch, but it is always desirable to so construct hutches that they can be easily modified for different purposes. For example, a large breeding hutch should be capable of division to make two hutches for running on youngsters. It is sometimes practicable to remove the divisions between breeding hutches to make larger colony hutches, and so on.

TYPES OF HUTCHES

No one hutch will be suitable for all purposes, and the types of hutch required will depend on the system operated by the breeder and his reason for keeping rabbits. For meat production, breeding hutches and growing on colony pens will usually be required. For pelt production, although the young rabbits can be run on together for

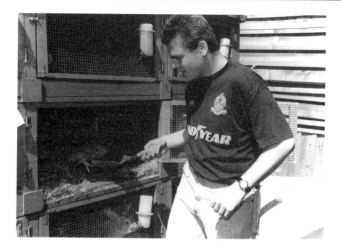

Fig. 6.5 Cleaning out an outdoor hutch kept for adult Rex bucks

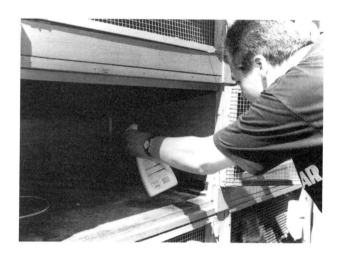

Fig. 6.6 Spraying the interior of the hutch with disinfectant

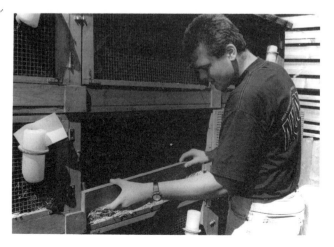

Fig. 6.7 Replacing the litter board after cleaning out

a short period in colony pens, they will eventually need separation into single hutches, and the same system, possibly running the young in pairs rather than in colonies, will be used by the exhibition breeder.

When hutch accommodation is limited it is preferable to have hutches which by partitioning can be adapted to suit either breeding stock or individual animals. Stacks of hutches can be divided with removable partitions, partitions hinged to the roof, or with removable double hay racks which fit the entire depth of the hutch. Different breeders will insist on solid partitions, whilst others will wish to have partitions, even if separated by a gap, which will permit the animals to see each other.

The number of hutches for young and single adult animals produced from each breeding hutch will again depend largely on the requirements of the breeder, but often the number of these hutches is underestimated. For the exhibition breeder a minimum of four hutches for single animals or pairs of young is desirable for every breeding hutch, and for adult pelt production, more would be required. For the meat producer the number of hutches of different types depends upon the remating cycles.

Hutch and pen sizes

The different breeds of domestic rabbit vary in weight from just over 1 to 7 kg or more. The size, or rather the outstretched length of different breeds also varies, and in some cases the outstretched length of a breed is greater than that of a much heavier breed. For these reasons the sizes of hutch must also vary according to size and breed. There is also an argument that the smaller younger animal may require a greater size proportionally than the heavier older animal. Too small a floor space results in overcrowding, which quite apart from the welfare point of view, is a predisposing condition to a number of troubles including disease and poor growth.

A simple generalised standard for hutch size is to allow 1000 cm^2 of clear floor space for every 0.5 kg of weight of adult. This standard is rather too severe on the smallest breeds, but perhaps a little overgenerous on the largest. Thus the average size of breeding hutch to be aimed at is about 75 × 60 cm for the smallest breeds, 100 × 60 cm for medium-sized breeds, and 125 × 60 cm and upwards for the largest breeds.

Due allowance must be made for any utensils which may take up floor space. For example, an internal nest box will certainly take up to about 1350 cm^2, and a hopper attached to the door a further amount. The height of the hutch must be adequate. Low roofs are very unsatisfactory, both from the point of view of ease of handling, and because they certainly affect ear carriage. The minimum height of hutch for the small breeds should be 40 cm although 45 cm is much better, and 50 cm desirable in the case of the largest breeds. This height again refers to uninterrupted space. A 45 cm high hutch with 10 cm of bedding on the floor (not a good idea!) is not satisfactory.

It is desirable to allow as much space as possible for young, growing rabbits, except in commercial meat production, where as little as 900 cm^2 is used per young fattener, although this level is too small when animals reach six or seven weeks of age. In fact, within reason, the only limitations which should be imposed should be one of necessity and ease of management. In small hutches 1800 cm^2 per young rabbit should be regarded as the minimum. In larger colony pens, although this amount is desirable, it could be reduced slightly. The larger the colony pen, the (slightly) less the amount of floor space required by each youngster. Again, the amount of floor space required will depend upon the size. For almost fully grown stock the above figure would be a definite minimum.

Colony pens may be of any size, although it is never desirable to have more than about 30 young together, as accidents sometimes occur through panic. It follows, therefore, that the maximum size of colony pens will usually be about 6 m². This does not of course refer to the warren type of colony, which may cover a large area, and is in general not a satisfactory system of keeping rabbits except possibly in developing hot countries for meat production.

Mating or buck hutches for stud bucks should be rather larger than hutches for single adult animals, and it is an advantage to have them rather narrower from front to rear than the customary 60 cm to allow for easier handling. In all cases the hutch door should open the full width of the hutch so that the buck or doe can be rapidly caught and separated if fighting starts. In single tier hutches it should be possible to lift the roof easily. Here it might be mentioned that it is sometimes the practice to have mating hutches which are reserved solely for mating purposes to which both buck and doe are brought, rather than single buck hutches to which the does are brought. This is not a satisfactory procedure, for the buck will often waste time by examining it when first brought to a strange hutch. There is also the ever present danger of disease being spread in this way.

Flooring

The floor of the hutch is most important, for on its construction will depend much of the ease of management. The floor may be solid, part solid and part perforated, or completely perforated (self-cleaning), through which the faeces and urine drop.

The solid floor has been largely superseded in America, and entirely superseded in this country in commercial undertakings by the perforated floor. In the non-commercial rabbitry, however, by far the most common type in this country is the solid floor. The reasons are that it may be slightly cheaper, bedding can be used with it, there is possibly less trouble from sore hocks, although this is by no means certain, and draughts are eliminated. The solid floor is certainly preferred by the exhibition breeder and the pet rabbit owner.

There is a good deal to be said in favour of both types, particularly when both are well designed and constructed but the mesh floor assists to some extent in disease prevention, and it certainly saves labour in cleaning out. The wire-mesh floor has become the universal standard in intensive commercial meat production throughout Europe. Probably the tendency in the future, particularly with the development of metal hutches, will be in favour of the perforated floor.

The semi-solid floor which consists of part-boarded section and part mesh, has little to recommend it, for it has the disadvantages of both other types, without their particular merits. The only point in its favour is that it certainly does keep bedding dry, but under good management this would be accomplished on solid floors.

Unless the perforated type of floor is properly constructed, it is unsatisfactory. In the past many of the cases of unsatisfactory mesh floors have been due to their construction with the wrong material. The only suitable material for these floors is welded wire mesh (sometimes woven mesh is used but is not satisfactory) of not less than 1.5 mm diameter. The wire mesh must be galvanised (after welding) to prevent rusting. Mesh made of previously galvanized wire is not satisfactory.

Self-cleaning perforated floors must be mounted over a tray or a sloping sheet of metal or plastic or over pits. The faeces drop through the floor and are easily collected for removal. In the case of a sheet, this directs the faeces to a central channel for collection. It is usually necessary to clean the sheet down when cleaning out. More sophisticated pen systems have moving belts which transport the faeces to a collecting point.

Solid floors can be constructed of wood or exterior quality ply. The latter has the advantage that the floor can be made from a single sheet, and there are therefore no cracks through which moisture can drip into the hutch below. Even with tongue-and-groove boarding this sometimes occurs.

When fitting floors it is sound practice to seal them on the floor supports with the use of one of the plastic sealing compounds, and to secure them to the battens with countersunk screws and screw cups.

Some laboratories overcome any difficulties arising from solid or perforated floors by using pans or trays which fit the entire floor and which are removed complete with the bedding for cleaning. Another system is to stand a perforated floored hutch, with a large mesh, on a tray filled with bedding, simply lifting the hutch on to a new tray and to remove the old one for cleaning. It is doubtful whether either of these two systems would find much favour with the rabbit fancier, although a modification of the first idea is discussed later under 'Hygiene' trays or units, page 137.

A type of flooring quite common on the Continent in the small farm non-intensive type of farming, is the slatted floor. This consists of slats 25 to 50 mm wide and 12 to 18 mm thick, placed at 12 mm spacings. These floors, although suitable for Angoras, have little to recommend them for other breeds.

Hutch doors

The efficiency of the hutch doors will have a marked effect on the management of the rabbitry. A slight delay in opening each door will amount to a very considerable period throughout the year in a large rabbitry. Doors which can be opened by the rabbit are a great nuisance.

If feeding and watering can be done without opening the doors, so much the better. The operation of the door will not then be of such importance. The door will usually be hinged at the side and swing outwards except in the case of wire-mesh cages when it is invariably hinged on the top. It should open in such a way that it does not interfere with the movements of the attendant, and it is desirable that all doors should swing the same way – away from the normal line of travel of the attendant.

In some cases, it is an advantage for the door to cover three hutches in a stack at once, although some breeders prefer one door for the two top hutches and a single door for the bottom, which assists in preventing the escape of the occupants of the bottom hutch. If, however, there is a good litter board on the bottom hutch (and there should normally be one for each hutch) then this problem is very slight, and a door to cover the three hutches is satisfactory.

There are a number of designs for doors which swing inwards, or which slide along the front of the hutch, or which are hinged at the base and swing outwards.

These types of doors are usually suitable for special purposes only, and apart from the type which tilts into the hutch and lies close to and parallel to the roof, these designs are not entirely satisfactory for the general breeder.

An excellent system is a combination of litter boards and doors, the three doors being fastened together with an upright bar (Fig. 6.8). The bar keeps the litter boards in each hutch closed, and usually the litter boards are also independently hooked to the hutch frame. The litter boards are hinged as well as the doors, and the advantage of this method is that the wire netting of the door frame is in the same plane as the face of the litter board. This ensures that there are no projecting edges for the stock to gnaw.

All doors should be uniform and should be strongly constructed with suitable

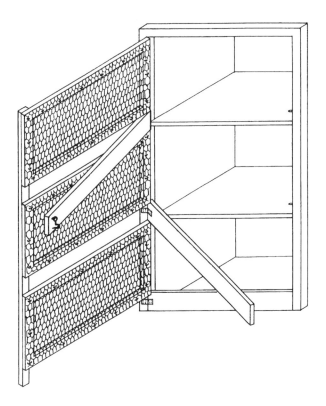

Fig. 6.8   Combination litter boards and doors. Note that the wire mesh covers the entire inside surface of the door frames and is also in the same plane as the litter boards thus preventing the stock from gnawing these

braces to prevent sagging. Adequate clearance should be left between the door and the frame to prevent jamming if the door swells slightly in damp weather. Door hinges are important. 'Unusual' hinges found in many rabbitries, such as leather straps, twisted nails, wooden buttons, etc., are great time-wasters. A good T or strap hinge is undoubtedly the most satisfactory, for it also assists in preventing the door from sagging.

The above discussion on doors refers, of course, to the typical three-tier type of stack hutch made of wooden framing. There are a number of variations for single-tier metal hutches, one of the best being that type of door which wholly or partly covers the top and not the sides, and opens upwards and backwards. A pulley system with weights can be used whereby the door or 'lid' of the hutch can be lifted and then remains in any position.

Another system which is adopted on one of the largest Angora farms in Denmark is the use of a movable frame rather than a door. This frame fits over the openings of six hutches. The frames are moved along the stack of hutches as work progresses, and the owner considers the system to be the most advantageous as it eliminates troubles due to hinges, doors swinging into the passages, and so on. There has not appeared to be a problem with the spread of disease.

DETAILS OF HUTCHES

Good materials and good workmanship are always desirable, and in the long run a great economy. Extra time taken in good construction will be fully repaid during the years of use. All exposed edges of wooden-frame hutches should be covered with metal strip, and as far as possible asbestos cement board sheeting, if used for walls, or wire mesh to cover the door, should be fixed to the inside of the wooden framing. Ledges and difficult corners should be eliminated.

Litter boards, about 13 cm high, placed at floor level across the opening of the hutch, prevent the young and the bedding from falling out of the hutch when the door is opened. They can be fixed to the framework of the hutch with hinges or with metal guides.

Roofs of hutches should extend at least 15 cm to the rear of the hutches and, preferably, guttering should be fixed to prevent water dripping down the backs of these. The roof must slope sufficiently to carry off all water and must of course be completely weatherproof.

Door fasteners often cause a good deal of trouble. They should be of such a type that they are easily opened by the attendant but not by dogs or the stock themselves. If possible, a type which closes when the door is swung to should be used.

MORANT HUTCHES

The Morant system was first introduced by Major G. F. Morant in 1884, the idea at that time being that these outdoor movable hutches in which the rabbits could graze should be used for commercial rabbit keeping. Each Morant was a large movable hutch, or ark, with the floor partly or wholly covered with a fairly large mesh of usually about 40 mm. The hutches varied in size from about 90 × 125 cm upwards, large poultry arks being adaptable to the purpose (Figs 6.9 and 6.10).

The system had some disadvantages in that a good deal of land was required because the animals could not be frequently grazed over the same land. Fairly light soil was necessary and the field had to be fairly flat. Morant hutches were often laid on rails during the winter and used as colony hutches when a solid floor was placed in them. Increasing labour costs stopped this system when wire-mesh pen meat farming developed, although occasionally in one form or another Morant hutches are still used.

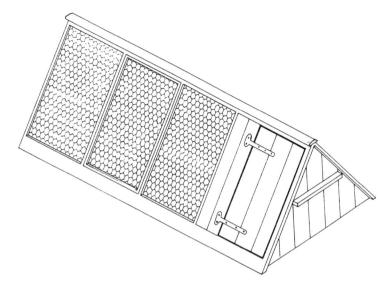

Fig. 6.9   A large type of Morant hutch or ark

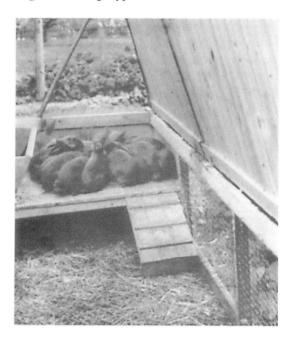

Fig. 6.10   The interior of a Morant hutch showing the raised solid floor portion

COLONY PENS

The colony system entails keeping groups (up to about 30) of young rabbits, in large pens. It is an excellent system provided it is carried out correctly but is mainly used for meat rabbits up to the age of at most 4 months. It is sometimes suggested that such systems are more humane than any other, and allows the animals to enjoy a more 'natural' existence, but this is open to doubt. In the past, large colony pens consisting of enclosed areas similar to poultry runs have been used, but the most satisfactory colonies are undoubtedly those on wire mesh. A solid floor may be divided up by partitions of wire mesh about 1 m high, to form solid-floored colonies.

Colony pens should not be too large. The construction of a metal type of pen is based on an angle-iron framework with a strong mesh. It may be necessary to support the mesh floor and for this purpose angle-iron may be used, with the mesh supported upon the apex of the angle. It is essential to ensure that the floor is rigid and can fully take all the weight which is likely to be placed upon it. Very often, cases of failure in such floors are found to be due to inadequate support.

THE COSTS OF HOUSING

Many rabbit keepers, particularly those who contemplate a small rabbitry, endeavour to make their hutches at the lowest possible costs. That poorly made, 'cheap' hutches are usually in the long run very much more expensive in terms of maintenance, renewal, extra time involved in management and the comfort of the animals, than well made, 'expensive' hutches, is rarely considered.

In any enterprise the cost of housing must be balanced against subsequent cost of management, and cost of depreciation. A cheap hutch made from scrap boxes from a greengrocer could be constructed for a few pence, but there is little doubt that its life would be comparatively short, and the time wasted by operating it through one year would be great. It can easily take two or three times as long to manage a badly constructed rabbitry as it would do if the same rabbitry were well made.

From a number of surveys of commercial rabbit farms, it becomes apparent that a figure of seven hours per doe per year would be a fair estimate of the time required for all operations, and even greater efficiency could possibly be obtained. It is necessarily quite impossible to give more than generalised statements on this question, but it would be fair to say that, provided the cages were well made and well designed for labour-saving operation, a very high figure for initial outlay would not be uneconomic, particularly when it is considered that the life of the hutch could be some 15 years or more.

It is possible to build or have built sets of metal hutches with self-cleaning facilities for an amount which is literally only one or two hours of paid labour. Many commercial farms do in fact manufacture all their own cages. There is also the further point that with well designed equipment, some reduction in the incidence of disease would be achieved. With the saving of only one or two young rabbits a year (a conservative estimate), the increased cost of the hutch would be repaid.

The subject of housing costs – indeed, the wider subject of all costs in the rabbit industry – has been scarcely considered in this country. It is obvious that a great deal of investigation and attention to this important subject is necessary in the future.

It should not be assumed from the above that it is recommended that the most expensive housing should be purchased or made. It is only that attention should be drawn to the very prevalent fallacy that the most economical housing is that which can be made for the lowest cost. When planning a rabbitry, after the designs have been worked out they should be costed, and the only satisfactory way in which this can be done is to draw up a bill of materials (allowing in most cases about 7% for wastage) and cost each item and then the labour of building. Quotations could be obtained from hutch builders, which will provide a standard, and in the long run experienced workmanship may be best.

STACKING OF HUTCHES

The majority of non-commercial hutches in this country are stacked in three tiers (Fig. 6.11). The reason is generally that space in rabbitries is at a premium, and the cost of tiered hutches is rather less per unit than is the cost of hutches in a single tier. However, in almost all large commercial undertakings, the single-tier system forms the basis of the majority of rabbitries, and generally speaking the floors of these single-tiered hutches are of mesh, allowing the faeces to drop on to the ground below. It is argued that single-tier housing requires less labour, but this is only true when feeding and watering can be accomplished without opening hutch doors. When solid floors are used, the single-tier system has probably not a great deal to recommend it.

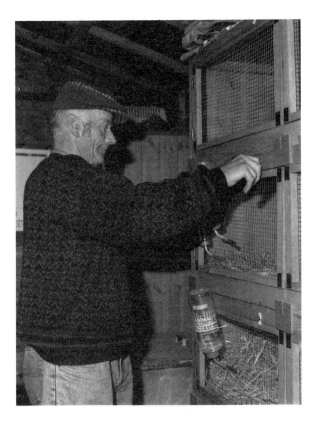

Fig. 6.11 Portion of the *Fur & Feather* rabbitry. These hutches are designed for small to medium sized breeds of rabbits. (As they get older they are transferred to larger hutches.)

The floor of the bottom hutch of any stack should not be less than 20 cm from the ground, and 30 cm is preferable. With hutches 45 cm high, this will mean that the floor of the top hutch is about 1.3 m from the ground, which is not too high for easy management.

MATERIALS FOR HUTCH CONSTRUCTION

In this country the majority of hutches (except for those for the commercial rabbit industry) are manufactured from wood, although more and more attention is now being given to metal hutches, and laboratories have used these for many years. Wood is now relatively expensive, and after a wooden hutch has suffered some wear it often becomes increasingly difficult to clean it easily and well. Exposed edges must be protected, for some rabbits will do considerable damage by gnawing. Unless wood is carefully treated it has a tendency to absorb urine, and consequently will tend to smell rather more than hutches made of other materials. Nevertheless, the majority of hutches are made of wood and it is unlikely that the majority of fanciers' hutches will be replaced by metal hutches. Wood is also, of course, much easier to use than is metal.

Manufactured boards

There is a wide variety of manufactured boards, including Sterlingboard, plywood, 'Weyrock' and the like. These are suitable for the rabbit breeder.

Metal sheet

Metal sheeting, particularly in the form of corrugated iron, has often been used for hutches and shelters, but in general it has little to recommend it. It tends to be excessively hot in summer and excessively cold in winter, and, in humid conditions, condensation is high.

The same objections do not apply entirely to aluminium sheets, which have few disadvantages except that of cost. It is probable that this material will be increasingly used, particularly for all-metal hutches. Aluminium or alloy sheeting is also much used in other countries for the construction of equipment such as food hoppers and the like, where 1.5 or 1 mm sheet is ideal.

Wire mesh

Wire mesh or grid is essential in every hutch. It is used to cover doors on wooden hutches, and for hayracks. Poor quality wire netting is a very bad investment. Badly galvanised netting will soon deteriorate, as also will too light a gauge netting. Before purchase the netting should be examined for faults, particularly cracking of the galvanising and sharp splinters. Both sides of the mesh should be examined, one side is usually worse than the other and of course the smoothest side should always be used towards the animals.

The thickness of the wire is denoted by a gauge number; the higher the number, the thinner the wire. The thinnest wire which should be used in the rabbitry is 1.5 mm. A good quality, well galvanised woven wire has many uses, and is sometimes used for floors, but the ideal for this purpose is welded wire, which is being increasingly used.

Concrete

Concrete hutches have been used on the Continent, on some occasions prefabricated units being marketed. Concrete is not, however, really suitable for housing of rabbits, although it makes an excellent floor for the rabbitry and foundations or blocks for supporting uprights of shelters. In the same way, although bricks and breeze blocks are sometimes used, they are not satisfactory.

Roofing

Roofing felts and bituminous roof coverings are excellent when they are in places that do not come into contact with stock, for example, as a covering over wooden shelters. They are not suitable for hutch construction.\

EQUIPMENT

Certain equipment is essential in the rabbitry, but in addition there are other items which, if properly constructed and used, make management easier. There is frequently a good deal of prejudice against labour-saving devices; often they are contemptuously labelled 'gadgets' and ignored. This is sometimes due to previous experience with badly designed equipment and sometimes because of ignorance.

Each item of equipment should save time, should improve management, ease of operation and the comfort or welfare of the animals. When a new item is being considered, it should be given a fair trial to see whether it meets these conditions. All items should be strongly made, and should be capable of being easily cleaned. Above all they should not be a danger to stock. Splinters, protruding nails, sharp edges of metal, all will cause damage.

Feeding equipment

Feeding equipment should be sufficiently large to enable all the occupants of the hutch to feed at the same time, and it is advantageous for feeding and watering equipment to be so arranged that feeding and watering can be accomplished without opening the hutch door.

Pots and troughs

Pots and troughs of glazed earthenware, with an inturned lip to prevent animals scratching out food have always been popular, although now being widely replaced by food hoppers. Enamel pots, galvanised iron and plastic pots are all useful but do not have the weight of the earthenware type and are more likely to be thrown about or tipped up by the animals and usually wear badly. The idea of fixing the pot to a board on which the rabbit has to stand when eating, thus preventing the pot from being thrown about, has some disadvantages, and consequently a pot fitted into the wire of the door is the best type. Pots or troughs should not exceed about 75 mm in depth and should be only sufficiently wide for the animal to reach the bottom. It is important to remember that there must be sufficient trough space to allow all animals to feed at the same time.

Automatic food hoppers

Automatic food hoppers save much time and labour. They are easily fixed to the door so that the trough projects into the hutch with the opening for filling remaining outside. The lip of the trough should not be fitted more than about 110 mm above the floor of the hutch. In some cases it is as well to divide the hopper up into several sections in order to allow for several different foods being fed at the same time. Hoppers are of course only suitable for concentrated foods such as pellets or cereal.

An excellent type of hopper of circular design, which must, however, be placed entirely within the pen, has also been developed. It is particularly suitable for colony pens, and can be bolted to a wire-mesh floor to prevent tipping up. A narrow mouth and sloping divisions prevent the young rabbits from sitting on the mouth of the hopper and soiling the contents.

Racks

Hay and greenstuff racks prevent these feeding stuffs from being contaminated by the stock. The usual type is a simple piece of wire mesh fixed to a corner of the hutch. This type is unsatisfactory, and the best designs incorporate the following features:

- filling should be possible from outside the hutch;
- the angle at which the hay is held should not be too flat (i.e. too much parallel to the floor) as the rabbits will then pull the hay down, which may result in seeds, dust, etc., falling into their eyes;
- there should be some form of trough to catch the leaf from the hay (which is the most valuable part);
- the construction should be such that the young rabbits cannot injure themselves by getting caught in the mesh.

A rack made by fixing a panel of wood at an angle to the door outside the hutch is satisfactory, although it does obstruct light. The rabbits pull the material through the mesh of the door.

Undoubtedly the most satisfactory type is the rack made as a unit and placed between two hutches, thus forming a partition and serving as a rack for both hutches (Fig. 6.12). A major advantage of this type is that it can be used to split up a range of hutches into various sized units. The most suitable mesh for the hay rack is welded wire of 25 × 50 mm, the longest side of the mesh being vertical.

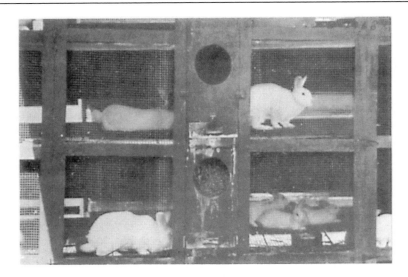

Fig. 6.12 Wood and woven wire mesh hutch stack. The central unit has hay racks serving two hutches and a combined concentrate feed draw. These units can be removed to double the size of a pen

Watering systems

Watering systems and utensils can be of very varied designs. There is the simple pot at one extreme, and at the other the fully automatic system which, if it is well made and installed, requires attention only rarely, and that attention being confined to flushing out the system once monthly. All systems or utensils should be easy to clean, so fitted that they cannot be spilt, and the water cannot be contaminated by the stock or with bedding, easily removed or filled from outside the hutch, and so placed that stock of all ages can drink easily.

The glazed earthenware pot when fixed half-way through the door (Fig. 6.13) is suitable, but liable to contamination. A semi-automatic system consists of a glass bottle from which comes a 6 mm diameter glass or metal tube through which the water passes when the animal sucks at it. There are several metal tubes with single

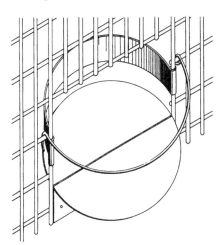

Fig. 6.13 Holder for feed or water pot. The pot rests on the base which consists of two halves bolted together on either side of the mesh. The wire hook keeps the pot in place although allowing it to be removed easily. The unit is only suitable on hutches with good mesh on the doors or in wire mesh pens. Instead of the base bolted on the wire mesh, the pot can be rested on the floor of the hutch

balls in them to prevent dripping, from which the rabbits soon learn to drink (Fig. 6.14). If the glass tube is home-made, it is important that the edges are smoothed by placing the end in a flame. The bottle can be easily attached to the hutch door with metal-expanding wire or straps.

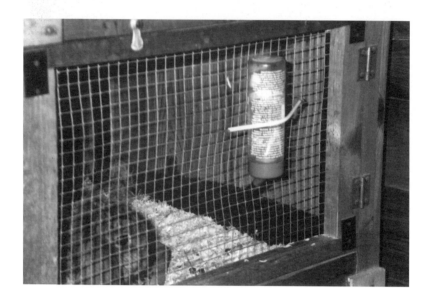

Fig. 6.14   Water bottle on hutch front, held in place by expanding wire clip

The objections to the latter systems are that in freezing weather the bottles are often broken, leaving the rabbits without water, and they are laborious to fill. Also, unless protected from sunlight, algae tend to grow on the inside. Plastic bottles overcome the first problem.

The automatic systems of watering all consist of piping running through, underneath, or against a line of hutches, into which are fitted cups, valves, or a combination of the two (Fig. 6.15). The cost of installing these systems is high, and sometimes trouble is experienced through jamming up of valves or inlets. Freezing troubles can be overcome by running a suitable electric cable (usually lead-covered hot-bed cable) through the pipes, the electricity being controlled by a thermostat. Low voltage cable is necessary.

Open channels running alongside hutches are not suitable as they easily become contaminated and blocked, and assist in the spread of disease.

Many breeders prefer to use open pots, and there is some evidence that certain types of valves do not allow the stock to drink sufficiently. Where large numbers of pots have to be cleaned and filled, a simple type of gun attached to a lightweight hose can be very useful. A double trigger action produces either a high-speed jet of water suitable for swilling out the pot, or a large volume at low pressure for filling.

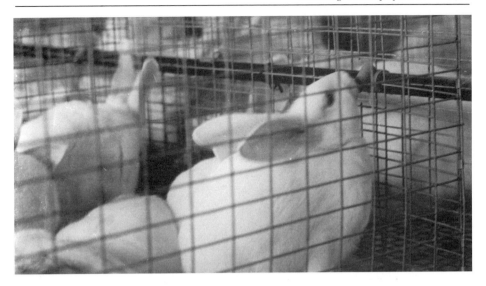

Fig. 6.15   Rabbit drinking from automatic water valve

Nest boxes

Nest boxes are one of the most useful and essential items of equipment. They are now almost universally used in commercial farming. They eliminate the usual (but unsatisfactory) practice of having a partition in the hutch, and allow the doe to make her nest in an enclosed box instead of on the floor of the hutch. If the nest is made on the floor, the young very often leave it too early, thus becoming liable to chilling, and to picking up contaminated food, or food which is unsuitable for them. Unless there is some barrier the doe herself may pull youngsters which are suckling from the nest with harmful results. A nest box also simplifies the examination of the litter, for it can be lifted out of the hutch and the youngsters examined at leisure. It also gives extra protection to the baby rabbits, and the top gives the doe a place where she can escape the worrying of the young rabbits just before weaning.

A good nest box should be designed to:

- a suitable size in which the doe can kindle and nurse her young;
- be capable of ensuring that the temperature can be easily maintained at about 30°C within the nest, but the young must be able to huddle together in the early days, and in warmer conditions after some days must be able to disperse a little to keep cooler;
- ensure that the nest and young can be easily observed and handled;
- allow easy cleaning and disinfecting and the urine to escape;
- ensure that the young cannot easily get out of the nest (or be dragged out by the doe), but if they are can easily get back;
- prevent the doe and the young being hurt.

There is a great variety of nest boxes made. Some have lids (preferably hinged) so that they can be easily opened, which are placed on the hutch floor and these are commonly used by fanciers. Further types of nest boxes are discussed later in the chapter.

The type shown in Fig. 6.16 is made of 12 to 15 mm thick wood. Satisfactory nest boxes for medium-sized breeds are 20 cm wide, 25 cm high and 38 cm long, and these sizes can be modified slightly for the largest or smallest breeds. The top of the box should be hinged to allow it to be fully opened for examination of the nest and for cleaning.

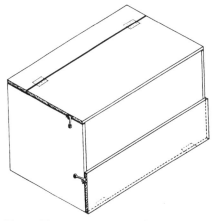

Fig. 6.16   Ideal type of wooden nest box. Note both top and front are hinged for easy cleaning

Travelling boxes

Travelling boxes should be light, strong, and of the correct size for the comfort of the rabbit. The box must not be so small as to cramp the rabbit but neither should it be too large so that the animal feels insecure and is thrown about in it. The ideal size of the box is not only relative to weight but also to size. For example a suitable size for a Belgian Hare must be larger than for say a Californian which is of approximately equivalent weight. Suitable sizes for different breeds are given in Table 6.2.

Table 6.2   Travelling box sizes

Breed	Length (cm)	Width (cm)	Height (cm)
Argentes Bleu and Creme, Dutch, Dwarf Lop, Himalayan, Mini Lop, Netherland Dwarf, Polish, Silver, Tan	35	20	30
Argente Champagne, Chinchilla, Deilenaar, English, Golden Glavcot, Harlequin, Havana, Isabella, Lilac, Medium Lops (i.e. Cashmere), Perlfee, Rhinelander, Sable, Siberian, Silver Fox, Smoke Pearl, Squirrel, Sussex	38	23	35
Alaska, Belgian Hare, Blanc de Hotot, Californian, New Zealand Red, Rex, Sallander, Satin, Swiss Fox, Thrianta, Thuringer	45	25	35
Angora, Belgian Hare, Beveren, Black, Blanc de Bouscat, Blue, Blue Vienna, British Giant, Chinchilla Giganta, Flemish, Giant Papillon, Large Lops (i.e. English and German), New Zealand White	45	30	35

Ventilation must be good, but the box must not be draughty. It is best to keep separate boxes for does and bucks. A buck sent to a show in a box which has previously been used for does may not arrive in the best condition.

The commercial rabbit industry often uses one-journey travelling boxes. Typically a strong fibre board purpose-made box of approximately 37 × 39 × 22 cm with a number of holes punched round just under the lid, is satisfactory. Whilst these were originally made for short journeys, hand held, they can be used repeatedly for accompanied travel. They are usually available from veterinary surgeries and the larger pet shops. For air journeys certain specifications are laid down which must be adhered to. These generally consist of a light wooden frame with wire mesh on the sides and top. Travelling boxes should have a quantity of clean straw as bedding. This is more satisfactory than wood shavings or sawdust. Some commercial bedding is also satisfactory. Angoras and Cashmere Lops should stand on a wire tray placed at the bottom of the box. Bedding should not be used in the box. This will prevent their coats becoming soiled during the journey. Upon arrival at the show the exhibitor will remove any shavings or sawdust from the show pen and place a similar type of tray at the bottom. A suitable frame for an Angora measures 43 × 43cm.

The weight of the travelling box should be as low as possible consistent with strength. Weight has some effect on the costs of transport.

The standard exhibition travelling box should be raised on two slats or metal rails nailed to the bottom, which prevents the box touching wet floors. A chain should be fixed to the lid to prevent the hinges from being strained when the box is opened. Whilst a metal tray fitted inside the box prevents the floor from becoming soiled and assists cleaning out, it is not usually so fitted. Adequate ventilation is supplied by holes in the end of the box or by ridge ventilation, but draughts are prevented by baffle boards installed inside the box.

The fastening of the box is important and it should be reliable but easy to undo, for a great deal of vexation can be caused to stewards at shows by difficult catches. Some form of carrying handle gives an additional safeguard. It is attached to both ends of the box and not only to the lid. A strong leather strap is excellent.

Hygiene trays or units (Fig. 6.17)

These make useful accessories in hutches. A unit consists of a metal tray over which is fitted a metal grid. If placed in the corner of the hutch used by the rabbits the majority of faeces and urine will be collected and can easily be removed. Cleaning

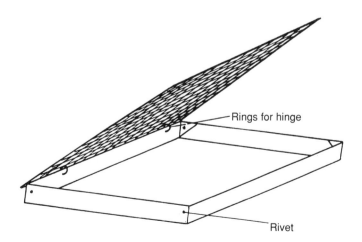

Fig. 6.17 Hygiene unit

of the entire hutch can therefore be less frequent, and rotting of wooden floors by urine can largely be prevented. Any metal may be used, although aluminium alloy is probably the most suitable. The tray should measure at least 30 cm square by 4 cm deep, and the grid should be made from welded wire grid of 19 mm mesh of at least 2 mm wire. The grid is attached to one side of the tray by wire rings or clips, and should overlap the other three sides. The tray can be improved by extending two sides of the tray to a height of 12 or 15 cm, these increased sides being placed against the hutch back and side.

Cleaning equipment

This is essential in all rabbitries. A scraper may consist of an ordinary hoe (those with straight sides are best) with the blade straightened to slightly more than a right angle with the handle. A 45 cm handle is quite long enough. Some breeders prefer a narrow scraper, but 20 cm wide is probably the most useful. A second type of scraper consists of heavy gauge metal sheet 18 cm wide and 15 cm high with one long edge bent over to form a tube for the handle. One or two stiff brushes, one with a short handle, for hutches, and one for the rabbitry floor, are desirable. A wheelbarrow or manure trolley is necessary for the larger rabbitry, but in no circumstances should this barrow be used for food or clean bedding.

A rabbitry table

This is essential for the handling of stock. Any table which is firm and large enough is suitable. The table should also be of the right height for easy handling, and a movable table has advantages. An old tea-trolley may be easily adapted although these are often too light and 'wobbly'. The table top should be covered with sacking to prevent the rabbits from slipping. A false top covered each side is better still, one side being used for bucks and the other for does. Both sides should be clearly marked. A mature buck will usually be much quieter on a top that has not recently carried does.

Holders for skinning rabbits

Whilst far less necessary than in previous times, holders for skinning rabbits can save considerable time when there are a number of rabbits to be handled (Fig. 6.18). A slotted iron bar, about 40 mm wide, bent to slightly more than a right angle, with the slot 6 or 7 cm long and 2.5 cm wide at the mouth and tapering to a point, makes a highly suitable holder. The holders are fixed in pairs about 20 cm apart, the slotted piece coming away from the wall. Any sized rabbit can be hung from these holders, for each leg is pushed into a slot above the hock joint, the swelling of which prevents the leg from slipping through. A variation of this design for those breeders who prefer a swinging type of holder is easy to make, rather in the shape of an inverted clothes hanger, with slots in either end. If a large number of rabbits are to be pelted, a number of these holders should be used to hold the animals for bleeding and cooling after pelting.

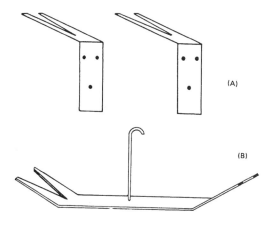

Fig. 6.18 Holders for skinning rabbits. Type A is fixed to a beam or wall, each holder of the pair being 20 cm apart. Type B is tied to a beam by the hook and thus is enabled to swing

Pelt boards and stretchers

These are essential for all breeders who sell or use the skins they produce, whether they are sold for hatting fur or as prime fur skins. Pelt boards are best for the furrier skins, but for hatting fur skins, which are usually sleeved, pelt stretchers are preferable for ease and quickness. Pelt boards are made of fairly soft wood and should be 0.6 m wide and 0.75 m long. It is always better to have the boards too large than too small. If 40 mm battens are screwed to both sides of the boards at the top and bottom, then both sides of the board can be used for a pelt, as the pins or nails used for nailing out the pelts will be shorter than this.

Pelts should, however, only be nailed on both sides when the board can be hung freely. When it is hung against a wall, only one side can be used. For nailing out pelts, 40 mm pins should be used. Heavy gauge furrier's pins are excellent.

Pelt stretchers are made either of wood or wire, the latter being preferable. A 1.5 m length of steel spring wire of 3.5 mm is used. The centre of the length of wire is wound for several turns round a 50 mm diameter pipe, the ends of the length being left about 30 or 35 cm apart. A variation of this type consists of a stretcher having shoulders. Wooden adjustable stretchers (Fig. 6.19) are also easy to make.

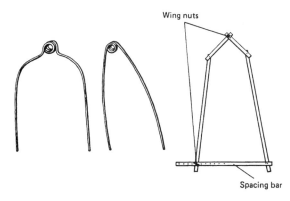

Wing nuts

Spacing bar

Fig. 6.19 Pelt stretchers. The wooden type on the right is adjustable

BEDDING

All solid floors must be covered with suitable bedding. The main essentials of good bedding are:

● that it should have good absorbency;
● it should not be dusty or stain the animals;
● it should if possible assist to eliminate odours;
● it should not be harmful to plants when the manure is used for the garden or field.

A variety of bedding materials is available including sawdust, straw, hay (the poorest quality), wood chips and shavings, leaves, peat moss, and even soil. Usually that bedding material which is cheapest is selected by the rabbit breeder, although in most cases sawdust is usually the most suitable, at least as a base. The best sawdust should not be dusty or damp, nor should it have too strong a smell. The same characteristics apply to wood shavings, which possibly now form the bulk of the bedding used by rabbit breeders. Sawdust and wood shavings have the advantages of absorbing moisture well, being good deodorisers, being generally unpalatable to stock so that they will not eat the bedding, and finally, do not stain the rabbits' coats. Peat moss, whilst having most of the same advantages, has the grave disadvantage that there is a tendency to stain coats, particularly with white breeds. A problem with straw, which is well liked by many breeders, is the disadvantage that stock may eat it and, if it has been contaminated, may pick up infections in this way. The same objections apply to hay. Hay also does not have such good absorbing powers as any of the others and is moreover much more costly. Dried leaves are often used, but it is doubtful whether they have much to recommend them. They break up easily and their absorbing powers are not high. Although dried soil and cinders have been used, there is little to recommend them. There is little doubt that the most satisfactory bedding system is sawdust or wood shavings for absorbency, overlaid with straw.

There is a widespread fallacy that sawdust may be injurious if used in the garden. Sawdust is, however, a valuable addition to the soil, although in a fresh condition it may cause a slight but temporary shortage of available nitrogen. This is, however, soon replaced.

After hutches are cleaned out, a sprinkling of lime before the fresh bedding is put into the hutch will assist in keeping the hutch sweet. The depth of the bedding, and the frequency of changing, will depend on the type of stock, the type of bedding, the type of ration, and the weather conditions. Thus no guide can be given, except to say that the bedding should not be allowed to become damp; as soon as this occurs, it should be changed.

Bedding which the pregnant doe will use to make her nest should be carefully chosen. The nest box should first be lined with at least 12 mm or so of sawdust, on top of which should be placed some bedding. Hay, best chopped into 15 or 20 cm lengths, is probably the most suitable material. An additional amount of the hay should be left in the hutch, from which the doe will prepare her nest. Angoras should not be bedded on hay and straw as this can become entangled with their wool. Angoras that are kept as pets can be bedded on barley straw, but their wool should be clipped every three months. Exhibition Angoras should be kept in hutches containing wire show trays, with newspaper placed beneath the tray.

MANURE

The amount of manure produced in any stud will depend upon a number of factors such as breed, rations fed, amount of bedding used and so on. Obviously a bulky ration will produce more manure than a concentrated ration. The weight of rabbit manure varies between about 450 to 640 kg per m³, and a large breed doe with young would produce throughout the year some 0.34 m³ of manure, that is to say, between 150 and 200 kg. It is necessary that adequate storage or disposal arrangements should be made.

Rabbit manure, again contrary to widespread belief, is one of the most valuable manures of all livestock, as can be seen from its analysis. On a dry matter basis the manure contains approximately 2.7% nitrogen, 1.5% phosphoric acid, and 1% potash. The amount of fresh manure required to produce 45 kg of dry manure is, however, only about 64 kg compared with some 110 kg of horse manure, and as much as 220 kg of manure is most valuable.

In some countries the clear manure, that is, manure from self-cleaning hutches, or separate from the bedding, is dried, ground and sold as a concentrated fertiliser. When dry, the manure has little smell and is easily handled.

Many gardeners like to use a liquid manure, and an excellent type may be made by soaking rabbit manure in a barrel of water. The faecal pellets (about 3 kg per barrel) should be enclosed in a coarse sack and suspended in the barrel for a few days. An occasional stirring will be of benefit, and the contents of the sack after this time should be returned to the manure heap, the liquid manure now being ready for use.

Fresh manure can be applied immediately to the soil, when no loss of the more soluble constituents occurs. If, however, the manure contains a good deal of bedding, then it will probably be more beneficial to allow it to rot before application. A layer of soil some 50 mm thick over a heap will efficiently prevent the breeding of flies and prevent any smell.

Although rabbit manure should be freely applied to the garden and to crops for the stock, some breeders, particularly those with small gardens and in urban areas, may find difficulty in arranging adequate disposal. Under no circumstances should manure be burnt, for quite apart from the waste, the resulting smoke will almost certainly be a nuisance to the breeder and neighbours and problems may easily arise from such breaches of the Environmental Protection Act 1990. The most suitable solution to such a problem is an arrangement with a local nursery gardener or allotment holder (one can always get details from the Local Authority Allotments Officer) who will usually be extremely pleased to make regular collections.

Some people do not like to use hutch cleanings containing sawdust and wood shavings because it is often said that this material encourages soil pests. This is completely untrue. The only immediate disadvantage in the use of raw shavings or sawdust is that there is a slight loss of nitrogen (although this is made up later). There is no disadvantage if the material is used as a mulch, and it is excellent for this purpose, conserving moisture, controlling weeds, improving soil texture and so on. If, however, about 4% by weight of sulphate of ammonia is used at the same time as the hutch cleanings, the immediate loss of nitrogen is overcome completely. Another way of overcoming the small problem is to use the manure for pea or bean crops, which provide their own nitrogen supply. If the hutch cleanings are composted, then the result is an excellent product for the garden.

Earthworms

In many countries a system of using earthworms under single-tier hutches to convert the manure into humus has been established for a number of years with good results.

This system has been developed almost worldwide. Alternatively, raw manure is collected from the rabbit house and placed on worm beds which are kept moist by sprinklers and produce an excellent and saleable manure product.

In the indoor system the worms are enclosed in wooden or metal-sided bins placed beneath the hutches over the soil. There must be no floors to the bins in order to allow the worms to retreat into the soil when conditions are unfavourable, and to allow free drainage. Normally the sides of the bins are about 30 cm high. The normal species of worm used is *Eisenia foetida*, known commonly in this country as the Brandling, although in America, domesticated types are sold in cultures to rabbit breeders. Provided the bins and the worm population are sufficiently large, no odours develop, and neither do flies breed in the manure. The worm-transformed manure is removed every six months or so.

It can be seen that the system is considerably labour-saving, but unfortunately until about 10 years ago there was little interest in the use of worms to transform manures from many different farm animals into usable material. At the present time the development of such concepts are being increased by interest from such organisations as the Rothamsted Research Station.

THE COMMERCIAL RABBIT FARM

The above completes a survey of the housing and equipment used in the small rabbitry and largely by the exhibition breeder, much of which may also apply to the intensive rabbit farmer. There are, however, many differences in the commercial rabbit industry where a number of the items of equipment, as well as the cages themselves, differ, due largely to the need for the maximum reduction in labour.

There are two schools of thought concerning the ideal environment under which commercial rabbits are bred. The first insists that a carefully controlled environment, where the temperature, ventilation, and humidity are kept within fairly rigid limits, is essential. The other adopts the view that a considerable degree of fresh air is far more important and that both the extra costs of feed required if the temperature is allowed to fall with that of the outside air, and a corresponding possible reduction in performance, are balanced by the improved health, the reduced cost of maintaining a heating and ventilating system, and the reduced cost of the capital buildings necessary for the controlled environment.

TUNNEL HOUSE

A further development in recent years is the tunnel house which was developed in an attempt to have low cost housing. It consists essentially of a metal framework over which plastic film is fixed. Various types of insulation can be built in and it is usual to have openings along the lower sides which can be closed when appropriate. Fairly standard sizes are 3.6 m wide, 2.5 m to the ridge, with the tunnel being built in 2.5 m modules.

The advantages are:

● it is inexpensive;
● it has good natural ventilation;

- it is capable of being moved from site to site;
- environment control costs are eliminated;
- size can be easily increased at any time, without disturbing the occupants.

The disadvantages are:

- it probably requires a higher level of management;
- it is more difficult to achieve the highest possible production;
- food costs in winter are increased slightly;
- there are problems with freezing of water systems in bad weather;
- it is more difficult to keep out vermin;
- it is not so permanent.

Whichever of the three systems is eventually proved to be the best, there is no doubt that the best possible insulation of any type of rabbit house is very desirable, not only indeed to keep the temperature up in winter, but also to keep it down in summer, and to prevent condensation which can be a severe problem. The ideal temperature in the controlled environment house lies between 15 to 18°C (although this is rarely maintained in cold weather). Ventilation is necessary in the controlled environment house to keep temperature and humidity at the desirable levels, to change the air and to remove the gases and moisture produced by the animals and arising from the faeces and urine.

The first calculation that has to be made in the matter of ventilation is the maximum weight of livestock likely to be housed at any time in the building, for it is weight of livestock rather than anything else which controls the ventilation rate. The ventilation system can be powered or unpowered and can be of a negative pressure, that is to say, powered fan withdrawal of air, or positive pressure with the use of fans to bring in air and then allow the air to be released through unpowered outlets. The negative pressure usually appears to be the most satisfactory.

The maximum speed of air throughout the building will vary with the temperature, as will of course the requirements for the amount of air being passed through the building. Table 6.1 gives some norms for the maximums that should be permitted at any time in a controlled environment.

There is no doubt at all that draughts have a very bad effect on all stock, and every effort must be made to eliminate them. The direction of the flow of air, which can be established by the use of smoke generators of various sorts, should be controlled in such a way that the air flow is not directed onto the animals. Furthermore, the direction of flow must allow the removal of the warm air. Unless correctly directed, the incoming air may trap the exhausted air. Sufficient has been said to indicate that skilled advice should be obtained if there appears to be any problem.

Commercial houses at the present time are often modified from buildings which have previously been used for other purposes. Naturally a purpose-built building has much to commend it but is usually a good deal more expensive than the cost of modifying an existing building. It is usually necessary to pay much attention to the matter of insulation. Without this, the cost of controlled environments is likely to be prohibitive (Fig. 6.20).

There are a few planning points which should be considered whether the house is to be constructed or modified from an existing building.

- The width should allow the correct multiples of pens with adequate passageways in between, with no pen closer than 20 cm to a wall and clear passageways (between external nest boxes) of a minimum of 1 m.
- The total length should be a multiple of the length of a block of pens, if pens are so manufactured, or of a pen.
- Height to eaves should give an ideal total density of liveweight of between 3 to 5 kg per m³ (always providing the ventilation is to be satisfactory).
- Walls should be as smooth as possible. Ledges should be kept to a minimum. If windows exist they should be fine netted to prevent entry of flies and vermin.
- Doors must fit well and doorways be sufficiently large to take the widest trailer likely to be used.
- Floors are very important. Concrete, sloping to good gutters are certainly the best type. Earth floors below pens are satisfactory provided good concrete passageways are built in.

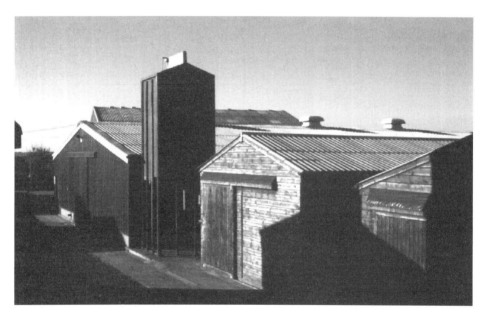

Fig. 6.20   A group of commercial buildings (all insulated). *From left to right*: fattening shed holding 3500 rabbits, bulk feed bin gravity feeding through the building wall, and two breeding sheds each holding 100 does. (Courtesy of Tony Barber)

THE MANUFACTURE OF PENS OR CAGES

Pens or cages are almost invariably manufactured from wire mesh, the most satisfactory way being to use panels clipped together. The gauge of the wire from which the mesh is manufactured is important. For the floors a minimum of 1.5 mm is essential but it is much better to have 2 mm or even 2.5 mm. It is always necessary to check that the wire is galvanised after welding and is free from sharp points and splinters. When the mesh is not square, the shortest length wires (i.e. those closest together) should be underneath to assist in the prevention of sagging.

Meshes for floors vary in size. Many rabbit farmers consider a mesh of 19 mm square to be the best size for floors. Others favour 15 mm square, whilst others consider a 50 × 13 mm mesh satisfactory. A 13 × 13 mm mesh is too small for satisfactory results and larger sizes than 19 mm square allows the legs of smaller rabbits to be trapped. One important consideration with welded mesh floors is that they must be rigid to prevent sagging and 'bouncing' which helps create sore hocks.

At the American Rabbit Research Station, perforated steel sheet floors with 15 mm square holes at 21 mm centres were designed in the hope that the larger surface would prevent sore hocks. This type of flooring was not as satisfactory as 15 mm welded mesh, due to the fact that there was considerably more labour required to keep the floors clean, and the surface retained the moisture during the foggy and rainy seasons, which increased the prevalence of sore hocks. Thus the 19 mm welded mesh was the recommended type.

Meshes used for walls and tops of cages can be of a larger size than those for floors, and also of a lighter gauge. The maximum size of mesh is usually considered to be 25 × 50 mm. The wire mesh should be heavily and well galvanised. As a result of constant use, cleaning, and attack by urine chemicals, galvanising becomes damaged. Some highly successful establishments have their cages regalvanised but this is only worthwhile when the cages are of the best possible quality in the first place.

Cages can be purchased ready-made or manufactured by the rabbit farmer himself. They can be made from roll wire or from bought panels. In both cases, clip pliers or ferrule pliers must be used to fasten the mesh or the panels together – a common mistake is to put too few ferrules or clips in place. A useful tool is also a type of plier with sharp points which open outwards which is used to open and remove the rings or clips and ferrules.

The top of the cage must be so fixed that it will operate as a door through which animals can be removed. Various openings may also have to be cut in the mesh to allow feed hoppers and external nest boxes to be fitted. Whenever openings are cut into the mesh, care must be taken to ensure that all the ends of the cut wire are cleaned away to prevent the rabbit being snagged while lifted out of the cage.

Cages vary in size but tend to be 90 × 60 × 40 cm high which are slightly smaller than the dimensions recommended in the MAFF Code of Practice for rabbits. There are many cages a good deal smaller than these figures, particularly on the Continent but eventually the sizes recommended in the Code of Practice will be required.

The actual *minimum* sizes recommended in the Ministry of Agriculture Code of Recommendation for the Welfare of Rabbits (issued in 1987) are as follows:

Doe and litter to 5 weeks of age	0.56 m² total area
Doe and litter to 8 weeks of age	0.74 m² total area
Rabbits 5 to 12 weeks of age	0.07 m² per rabbit
Rabbits 12 weeks and over, other than those used for breeding (multiple occupation cages)	0.18 m² per rabbit
Adult does and bucks used for breeding	0.56 m² per rabbit
The minimum height should be 45 cm.	

Cage configuration

There are various configurations of cages (Fig. 6.21). The first and most usual is the 'flat deck system' in which all cages are on one level. The so-called 'Californian'

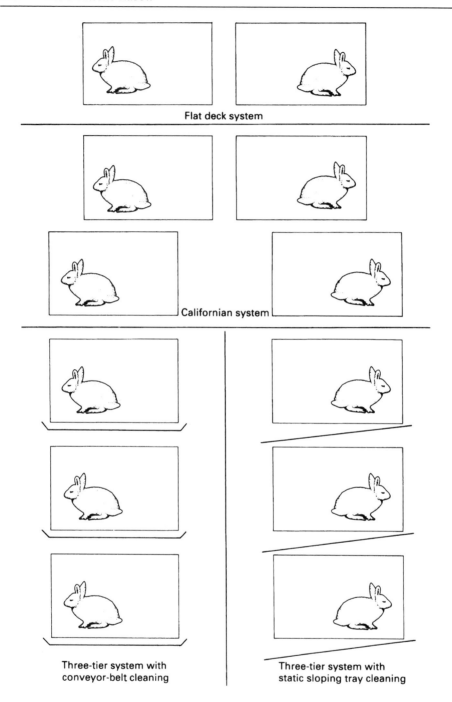

Flat deck system

Californian system

Three-tier system with
conveyor-belt cleaning

Three-tier system with
static sloping tray cleaning

Fig. 6.21   Various types of typical arrangements of mesh pens

system has two levels, with the rear cage set above but behind the front cage. Two-
or three-tiered systems are of three types. The first has solid floors as previously
described. The second has sloping trays which allow easier removal of faeces. These
two types are of use only to the smallest farmer. The third type which has manure belt

conveyors are used in fully automated systems.

The most common system is the flat deck system. All the cages are on the same level and can therefore be maintained at the ideal height for servicing. Manure disposal is simpler than with other systems except perhaps the fully automatic housing, but this is expensive. Installation of flat deck cages is also the most simple. The disadvantage of the flat deck system is that the number of cage units in any one house is less than with other systems, and hence the capital housing costs per cage are higher. The housing density that can be achieved with three-tier automatic systems is considerably greater; however, the individual cage costs are also higher, there is an enhanced labour cost per unit and the ventilation requirements become more complex. Throughout Europe in the intensive systems of rabbit farming the most usual form used is the flat deck system.

Cage supports

The cages must be supported, and the method of support has an influence on the ease of working. Cages should not be supported on small walls erected for this purpose, for this prevents good ventilation and encourages the build-up of gases from the faeces. Furthermore, the droppings accumulate on the tops of these walls with consequent risk of disease.

Cages should therefore be supported by suspension from above or, alternatively, round steel supports can be used. Whichever system is adopted it is important that the cages should be firm and that the fixings, whether they be wires or steel tubes, do not interrupt the efficient working of the rabbit house.

Watering

Watering is achieved by automatic watering systems, of which there are several. No success would attend any commercial undertaking which did not use such a system. The usual system is a low pressure one, with piping – usually plastic and a very minimum of 8 mm internal diameter – to all cages, with drinking nipples tapped into the piping. The best nipple drinkers that can be found should be used. Poor (usually cheap) nipple drinkers can cause untold trouble, the amount of water that can be lost from faulty nipples is remarkably high, and this excess water can itself be the source of problems. Blocked nipples cause reduced performance from the animals, quite apart from welfare considerations. The piping usually runs from a low pressure storage tank connected to the mains with a ballcock. This storage tank should not be too small and must be sited at the appropriate height above the level of the nipples. This height, and hence the water pressure, at which the tank must be situated to give the appropriate pressure, usually varies between 75 cm and 2.75 m. These heights give water pressures at the nipples of 0.5 to 1.75 kg. When the tank is being installed, it is best not to fix it in position until the whole system has been connected up, for it may have to be raised or lowered. Water coming into the tank should be filtered and the tank covered to prevent dirt getting into the water. If the pipe runs are long, then covered vent pipes should be incorporated, although in such circumstances it is better to have intermediate breaker tanks.

The animals learn very quickly how to use these drinkers. The nipples may be fixed to the cages or fixed separately and project into the cages at the right level. This latter arrangement allows pens to be moved without disturbing the watering system. The height of the nipples is important. Whilst the best height for adults is 20 to 25 cm that for very young animals is 12 to 15 cm. If the nipples are too low then adults have difficulty in drinking and often cause the nipples to leak by pushing against them. The best compromise is to have them at a height of 15 cm. Nipples should be easily reached by the stockperson to ensure that leaking nipples can be corrected. Rapidly depressing the operating pin will often cure a leaking nipple.

Some nipples are manufactured to work at 45°, others vertically and some horizontally. It is important to follow the manufacturer's instructions in this, and also in the matter of the proper height of the low pressure tank in relation to the level of the nipples.

Freezing up does not occur in controlled environment houses, but it may be a problem in other systems. There are two solutions. First, a low voltage cable may be fed through the water pipe which will satisfactorily keep the temperature above freezing. Second, the water may be pumped continuously through the water system and the water in the tank kept heated by a small immersion heater. The first method is usually a more satisfactory solution than the second, except in cases where the rabbit house gives a fair amount of protection.

Feed hoppers

The only suitable type of feed hopper for cages is the J type, manufactured of steel sheet and then galvanised. The hopper is fitted to the outside of the cage with the trough projecting into the cage. The typical hopper is 15 to 20 cm wide and the capacity should always be sufficiently large. It is unusual that a 4 kg hopper would be too big. It must be securely fixed to the cage front to prevent the animals from dislodging it, but at the same time it must be fairly easily removable to allow for regular cleaning. This is particularly necessary if, as sometimes happens, it is sprayed by the bucks or becomes wet from a leaking water nipple.

Some designs of feed hoppers, known as self-cleaning hoppers, have a mesh incorporated at the bottom in order that dust from the food, produced as well by the rabbits scratching at the pellets, may be eliminated. These self-cleaning hoppers should have a hinged flap underneath the mesh which then allows the stockperson to see how much food is being wasted in dust. The scratching of the food and the habit which some young rabbits have of sitting on the hopper can be eliminated by having dividers running from the back to the front of the trough and upwards.

The important features are the correct height of the lip and the correct width of the opening of the trough. The hopper must be mounted so that young can feed easily, the width of the hopper should be sufficient to allow feeding but too small for young to climb in, and the base should bring the food forward to be easily available. For colony pens large circular hoppers are very satisfactory (Fig. 6.22).

Nest boxes

The use of nest boxes for the fancier was commented upon earlier in the chapter and reference should be made to the comments made there. In the case of the meat rabbit

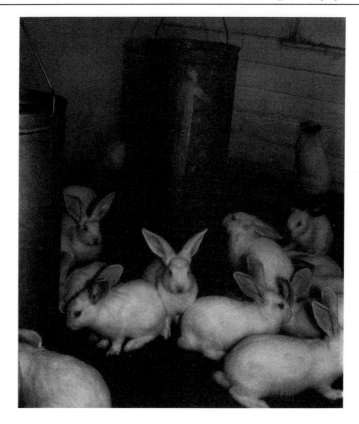

Fig. 6.22 Young meat animals in a wire-mesh-floored colony pen with extra-large circular feed hoppers

in wire mesh cages the nest box is essential. The nest box is required to attempt to keep the temperature in the centre of the nest to approximately a constant 30°C (which is the best temperature for young), to prevent the young from leaving the nest and to allow easy examination of the young.

A number of different types of nest box have been the subject of experiment in recent years. There is the old type mentioned earlier in the chapter but this is not commonly used for the wire cage, although variations are. An open type box, usually measuring some 45 cm long, 30 cm wide and 15 cm high without a lid or top has some disadvantages. It is certainly cheap, but it is often overlooked that the saving of one or two young will amply repay the additional cost of a better nest box. As with other types of nest box, these can be made of various materials, including wood, plastic, hardboard and even cardboard, the latter of course being disposed of after each litter. Some are set down into the floor so that the box floor is 10 to 12 cm lower than the hutch floor, but this is only feasible with wire-mesh cages (Fig. 6.23).

A wooden, galvanised steel or plastic nest box of any configuration can be withdrawn if provision is made in the manufacture of the pen. The use of these is sometimes necessary when the rows of pens have been built too close. The withdrawal of the nest boxes certainly makes examination of the nest easier.

Probably the most satisfactory type in commercial establishments is the external

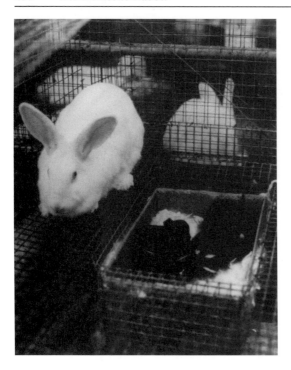

Fig. 6.23   Sunken nest box in mesh floor

metal nest box, with removable floor and hinged top. This type is attached on the outside of the hutch and the pen front wall is cut away to allow the doe entry (Figs 6.24 and 6.25).

An ideal size for such a box is 40 cm wide, 25 cm from front to back, and 25 cm high. A fairly small entrance opening from the cage, and a lid which can be fastened securely, complete the nest box. In hot weather this lid can be replaced by a mesh which must of course be well secured. Very often nest boxes are made rather too large; there is great merit in a compact nest. The side of the box facing the cage has an opening 16 or 18 cm square or round which allows the doe to enter. The lowest level of this opening should be 6 to 8 cm from the inside floor level of the nest box. When the nest box is mounted on the front of the cage it is mounted at such a height that the level of the entrance is the same as the floor of the cage. Any young inadvertently dragged from the nest into the cage can thus more easily find their way back into the nest.

The edges of the opening must be smooth or covered. A refinement is a method of closing the opening to prevent the entry of the doe, but this is not necessary. It is desirable that the base of the nest box should be removable for thorough cleaning and the floor itself can be wood which gives better insulation than steel. As to materials, galvanised sheet is preferable but plastic, or wood can be used. The nest box should be strongly made. It is desirable that some holes be punched or drilled in the base of the nest box to allow for drainage, and two or three drilled or punched at the top of the back will allow for the prevention of condensation.

Although it is not generally necessary, extra protection can be given to the nest box by packing it into a larger box with a straw lining. Alternatively, a false bottom can be installed and a low wattage bulb (15 watts) fitted beneath the false floor. These

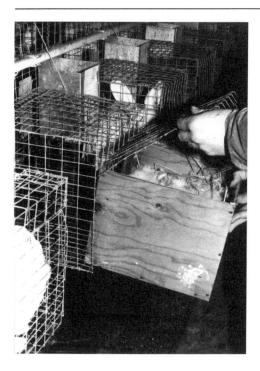

Fig. 6.24 Wooden insert which is withdrawn from the external nest cage for examination

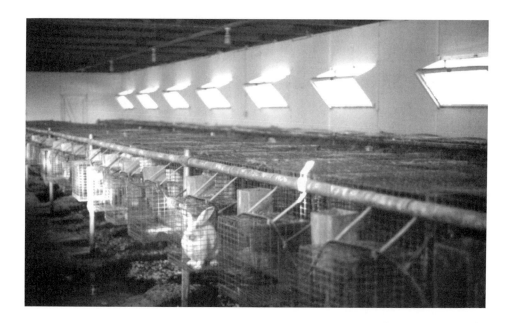

Fig. 6.25 Interior of one of the breeding sheds in Fig. 6.20. This is a flat deck system with suspended cages, external sunken nest boxes and concrete passages with chalk flooring beneath the cages for drainage. Note plenty of draught-free ventilation and the use of low energy light bulbs. (Courtesy of Tony Barber)

nest boxes can be left on the floor of the cage, or sunk into the floor. Indeed, a sunken area alone is sometimes used as a nesting site. Unless this sunken area is lined with insulating material it will be completely unsatisfactory. The advantage of the sunken area is that young will tend to fall back into the nest if they stray, or are dragged out by the doe. This sunken area – to which, of course, nesting materials are always supplied when the doe is to litter – is however, difficult to clean, and the young are difficult to examine.

Lighting

It has been known for many years that different light patterns have varying effects on the rabbit, as indeed they have on most other animals and birds. That varying the light pattern can be used to increase production has been established beyond doubt. There is some small evidence that there is an effect on growth of the young, but as the young are almost invariably in the same house as breeding does, the matter is rather academic. Until further evidence is produced there is no doubt that a 16-hour light and 8-hour dark pattern should be used. Not only should the light pattern be correct but the intensity of light should also be at a suitable level.

A minimum figure of approximately 25 lux at the level of the animals is desirable. This will allow for the losses which occur with increasing dirtiness of the lights (although when appropriate these should be cleaned). The calculations necessary to achieve any particular level of illumination are somewhat complex and necessitate an assessment of the reflective power of the building. However, a white fluorescent light will give 25 lux at 2 m below the fitting if used at the rate of 0.7 to 1 watt per m^2. Two 36 watt tubes per 10 m^2 would provide this amount of illumination satisfactorily.

Ordinary filament bulbs can be used, but the wattage per square metre has to be increased. The initial cost of fluorescent tubes is higher than that of filament bulbs, but the running costs are less.

Cleaning

The final matter to be considered is the matter of hygiene and cleaning. Constant hygiene and the routine maintenance of cages and equipment are essential in intensive rabbit farming. The ideal cleaning of equipment and cages takes place when a special area, away from stock, is set aside for this purpose. This area will contain high pressure hoses and tanks in which suitable disinfectants can be held to soak equipment. Calcium and other deposits from urine and dried-on faeces are difficult to remove unless it is thoroughly soaked first.

The usual method of removing fur by a flame, whilst satisfactory for this purpose does in no way sterilise the cage, as some people imagine. What is more it often ruins the galvanising. A more satisfactory method is to use an industrial vacuum cleaner. The animals soon become used to the noise and the results are far more satisfactory than any other method.

The procedure for sterilisation is as follows: all items are first thoroughly cleaned with hot detergent, then sterilised, then thoroughly rinsed and thoroughly dried. The drying takes longer than most people imagine. The process may sound long, but when methodically carried out is surprisingly quickly and efficiently accomplished.

Finally, it should again be stressed that whatever equipment is selected for the commercial rabbit unit, it should be of the best quality possible. Poorly designed and manufactured equipment costs a great deal more to use than does well-designed and well-made equipment.

Chapter 7

Nutrition and Feeding

The correct nutrition of the domestic rabbit is certainly one of the most important aspects of rabbit keeping. There is no rabbit so good that poor nutrition will not ruin it, nor any so bad that good feeding will not improve it. An animal which is not well fed cannot give of its best, and when it is realised that by far the greatest cost of producing rabbits lies in feed, the importance of correct feeding is very evident. The chances of a rabbit winning well at a show are always improved by it being in the best of condition as a result of good feeding.

It can be said that the range of feeds on which the rabbit will live is very wide indeed. There used to be many studs which were maintained on the waste from gardens, whilst others were maintained almost entirely on purchased feeds, and again others only on specially home-grown foods. This variety meant that the feeding programme could be adapted to the circumstances of the breeder, a fact which enabled many people to keep rabbits who would otherwise have been unable to do so.

Prior to 1950 there were very few specially compounded feeds for the rabbit, and these only manufactured for special purposes (such as laboratory investigation) or at the express wish of a particular breeder when a large batch would be required.

Today the situation is very different and many feed manufacturers compound special rabbit feeding pellets and mixtures which are supplied direct to the larger farmer or other outlet. The majority of pet shops stock many of these feeds and some even supply their own 'home-made' mixtures. Probably the majority of rabbits today are fed at least to some extent on these compounded feeds. It is therefore not strictly necessary, as it was prior to 1950, for a rabbit breeder to have a knowledge of the preparation and calculation of rations, in order that he can work out his own rations or system from the foods most easily and cheaply available. However, there are some rabbit keepers, particularly those on a large scale, who prefer to study this subject, for, without such knowledge, it is impossible to use alternative feeds – which in terms of pure cost – may be a good deal cheaper than the compounded feeds. Furthermore a knowledge of the principles of nutrition are of invaluable help to the breeder in getting the most out of his feeds and whatever is being fed there are good practices to be followed.

The first part of this chapter will then deal with the biology of nutrition, the measurement of food values and the practices of good feeding, leaving the use of alternative foods to pellet feeding and the construction of rations to the later part of the chapter.

It must always be remembered that rabbits vary a good deal, and therefore the standards of nutrition and recommendations made by manufacturers and others must be used only as a guide. The final and precise details must be based on the art of stock feeding, for the final details must be varied by the breeder depending upon any number of factors, such as weight, lactation, number in litter and so on.

THE COMPOSITION OF FEEDS

Feeds can be conveniently grouped into:

● roughages (hays and similar materials);
● succulent foodstuffs (grass, roots, and all green foods);
● concentrates (all cereals and their by-products, and animal products such as fish meal, meat meal, etc.);
● rabbit feeding pellets or compounded feeds.

All these feeds contain similar constituents in varying proportions. These constituents may be listed as:

(1) water
(2) carbohydrates
(3) proteins
(4) oils or fats
(5) minerals
(6) vitamins

Carbohydrates are composed of carbon, hydrogen, and oxygen, and include starches, sugars and celluloses. They are the main source of energy and heat in the animal body, and any surplus is stored in the body as fat.

Proteins, in addition to the carbon, hydrogen, and oxygen found in carbohydrates, contain nitrogen. Protein is the substance from which muscle, hair and all other body tissues are built and repaired. Proteins are built up from simpler substances known as amino acids, of which there are 25 known at present (of which only 11, however, are essential in the diet). Different proteins contain different amino acids in varying proportions, and thus some proteins containing important amino acids are more valuable than others, and are normally in short supply. Such protein as is not used for the building and repair of the body is broken down and used as a source of energy, but it is an unnecessarily expensive source.

Oils or fats differ from carbohydrates in that the proportion of carbon is much higher in the oils. Thus the energy value is much higher, being in fact rather more than twice that found in carbohydrates.

Minerals, of which some 14 have been shown to be essential to the healthy animal body, are necessary for the production and repair of certain tissues, particularly bones and teeth, and also as chemicals to regulate many of the normal processes of the body. The minerals necessary in the animal body (although some are required only in very small amounts indeed) are: calcium, phosphorus, potassium, chlorine, sodium, magnesium, sulphur, iron, zinc, copper, manganese, fluorine, iodine and cobalt. The first seven of these are major mineral requirements of the rabbit and the last seven are required in minute quantities only and are referred to as trace elements.

Vitamins are substances which are required in very minute quantities to maintain health. Many of these are co-factors in the chemical reactions which constitute metabolism at cellular level. Not only does a shortage of some vitamins cause abnormal disease conditions, but an excess can have the same results.

THE DIGESTIVE SYSTEM OF THE RABBIT (Fig. 7.1)

The teeth of the rabbit are very well adapted to its normal foods which consists, in the wild, of herbage, sometimes of a very woody nature. The teeth consist of two pairs of incisors (or 'cutting' teeth) on the upper jaw and one pair on the lower; three premolars and three molars (both 'grinding' teeth) on either side of the upper jaw; and two premolars and three molars on either side of the lower jaw. The incisors in the upper jaw appear from the front to be two pairs side by side, but are in fact only a single pair, with a groove down the centre of each tooth. A much smaller pair of incisors lie behind the front incisors which, together with the front incisors, form a V-shaped groove into which the chisel edge of the lower incisors normally fit. The cheek teeth, that is, the premolars and molars, are rather smaller than the incisors, but have flattened ends with prominent ridges, thus forming a most efficient grinding mechanism.

The incisor teeth (both upper and lower) of the rabbit grow continuously throughout life at a rate of up to nearly 1 cm per month. The surfaces of the teeth constantly wear down in order to maintain the correct length and the chisel edge for perfect cutting.

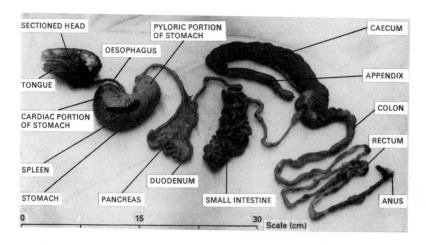

Fig. 7.1   The digestive system of the rabbit

Leading into the mouth are several ducts from the especially well-developed system of salivary glands which secrete saliva when the rabbit is eating. From the mouth, a slender tube, the oesophagus, carries food to the stomach, which is a thin-walled organ having little power of contraction. Food passes from the stomach through a muscular band of tissue known as the pylorus, which controls the entrance of the partially digested food into the small intestine. The first part of the small intestine is the duodenum, formed in a loop and within this loop lies the pancreas. The pancreas is a diffuse, irregular organ which supplies fluids containing digestive enzymes to the duodenum. Also entering into the duodenum, from the gall-bladder in the liver, is the bile duct which carries bile from the liver, where it is produced.

The small intestine continues until it enlarges into the sacculus rotundus, an enlarged sac peculiar to the rabbit. From the sacculus rotundus arises the caecum and the colon with the latter continuing to the rectum. The caecum is a very large organ with the appendix attached to the end.

DIGESTION AND THE PASSAGE OF FOOD

Digestion takes place in stages and consists of the breaking down of the complex food substances into relatively simple substances which the animal can absorb into its body. The protein of the food must be broken down into amino acids, the carbohydrates into sugars and the oils or fats into fatty acids and glycerides (although the rabbit can absorb some very small fat particles). The breakdown of food into these simpler substances is accomplished by enzymes, of which there are a number produced in various parts of the digestive system, starting with the salivary glands.

After food is cut up by the incisors of the rabbit and whilst it is being ground by the cheek teeth, the first enzymes, in the saliva, are mixed with the food. The rabbit when not unduly hungry masticates its food a good deal and therefore when the food reaches the stomach it is in a finely divided state. When a rabbit is excessively hungry it may not masticate its food sufficiently with the consequent production of digestive disturbances.

The walls of the stomach produce fluids which are of an acid nature and contain further enzymes. Digestion therefore proceeds a stage further, the food being stored in that portion of the stomach nearest the pylorus. The walls of the stomach, having little power of contraction, cannot force the food through the pylorus and this only occurs when there is additional pressure from more food (or caecotrophes, see below) coming into the stomach.

When the partially digested food is passed into the first part of the small intestine, a further series of enzymes mix with it, in addition to bile from the liver. The bile acts upon the fat of the food, which until this stage remains undigested, and breaks it up into minute droplets. This process assists other enzymes to break most of it down into fatty acids and glycerides. During the remainder of its passage through the small intestine, the food is finally digested and absorption of the food nutrients takes place. The inner surface of the small intestine is covered with minute knob-like projections called villi, which increase the surface area of the intestine very considerably. The food passes through the surface of the villi into the blood system inside them and thence throughout the bloodstream to all parts of the body for further use. The digested materials from the fat portion of the food pass through the surfaces of the villi into the lymphatic system, and by way of this into the bloodstream.

The remains of the food left after absorption, which consists both of some undigested and fibrous material, passes into the caecum, wherein bacteria attack and, to some extent, digest it. The content of the caecum is normally a thick fluid, and at certain periods contractions of the caecum force some of this material into the upper part of the colon. In this area a separation occurs between the larger fibrous material and the fluid and the smaller particles, this latter material being returned to the caecum.

The final residue of the larger particles from which much moisture has been expressed, passes through the colon and the normal faecal pellets are formed and passing through the rectum are excreted.

The simple products of digestion, having passed into the bloodstream, are transported to the various parts of the body requiring them. Any surpluses are stored in various places, as fat, for later use.

CAECOTROPHY (OR COPROPHAGY)

In 1882, a French veterinary scientist, one Charles Morot, published a detailed paper on the subject of coprophagy as it was then called and remained so for nearly 100 years. Morot showed that rabbits produced two types of faecal pellets one of which they re-ingest. It was not until 57 years later, when the work was rediscovered, that the full importance of Morot's work was revealed and the perfectly normal physiological process in the rabbit became well known.

Of the two types of pellet, one is that normally seen on the floor of the hutch, the other is never normally seen, for it is taken directly from the anus by the rabbit and swallowed whole. These pellets are known as caecotrophes.

After digestion in the small intestine, the residue of food material passes from the small intestine into the caecum where thorough mixing and fermentation occurs. Periodically, some of this caecal mixture passes into the colon which separates the fibrous indigestible material from the more finely divided digestible material mixed with fluids. This fine material is passed back into the caecum. The process is accomplished by the fibrous indigestible material being held on the walls of the colon whilst the thick fluid with the fine particles is passed back to the caecum in the centre of the colon. Once or twice a day, after the hard pellets have been evacuated, some of the caecal contents, which is now very much less fibrous, is passed into the colon where the caecotrophes are formed. These are given a coating of mucus which comes from the goblet or chalice cells in the walls of the colon. The mucus makes the caecotrophes adhere together, in small groups or bunches, which are passed to the anus from where the rabbit takes them and swallows them whole. Caecotrophes can sometimes be found in the stomach of a rabbit if the animal is examined post mortem. At least half, and probably more, of the material excreted by the rabbit is re-ingested as caecotrophes.

Several reasons for this peculiar physiological habit have been suggested. On a dry matter basis, the coprophagous pellets contain 3.5 times as much crude protein as do the normal pellets, but only a third of the fibre. In addition, the caecotrophes contain considerable amounts of B complex vitamins. There is little doubt, therefore, that part at least of the explanation of this process lies in the increased efficiency of digestion and the production of at least some of the animal's vitamin requirements. In the wild state the presence of caecotrophes keeps food in the stomach of the animal during periods when it remains in its warren. It should perhaps again be stressed that the habit is perfectly normal, and indeed can be observed occasionally during the day.

VITAMINS

As has previously been mentioned, vitamins are nutrients required in minute quantities for the maintenance of health.

Vitamin A (or substances from which the rabbit can manufacture it) is found in green foodstuffs and in fish liver oils. A deficiency may cause various nervous disorders. There is also some evidence that rabbits fed on rations which are deficient in this vitamin become more susceptible to certain diseases. The normal rations of the rabbit are, however, not deficient, and therefore trouble from a deficiency of this vitamin is unlikely.

Vitamins of the B group are also found in fresh green foods, and in oil seeds and cakes. Further, the bacterial population of the caecum manufactures these vitamins. Thus it is unlikely that any deficiency would normally occur. There have, however, been very infrequent reports of poor growth and reproductive failures due to a lack of these vitamins.

Vitamin C is found widely in green foodstuffs and, is furthermore, synthesised by the rabbit itself. No deficiency is therefore possible.

Vitamin D deficiency at one time was responsible for many cases of severe rickets and lowered growth, and in practice occasionally does so. The vitamin does not occur in any of the food normally fed to the domestic rabbit with the exception of some hays, although the amount in these foods is usually low. Normally the vitamin is produced by the animal itself, but this can only occur when the animal is subjected to sunlight. Fish liver oil is a rich source of the vitamin, and where deficiencies are likely to occur a small amount of this may be necessary. Problems have arisen with excesses of this vitamin.

Unlike the situation in some other animals, vitamin E deficiency does not affect the fertility of the rabbit. A deficiency does, however, produce muscular dystrophy. The feeding of excessive amounts of cod liver oil, by destroying the vitamin E content of the rations, may thus produce this trouble. Vitamin E itself is present in fresh green foods, in cereal grains, and particularly in the cereal germ.

Whilst it is usual to consider only deficiencies in vitamins in the feedstuff of rabbits, there have been some problems associated with excesses. These will only occur in compounded feeding stuffs and at the present time are unlikely.

THE DIGESTIBILITY OF FEEDS

Different foods, and the different constituents of foods, vary in their digestibility. Thus in order to arrive at the true value of any particular food it is necessary to know not only the chemical composition of that food, but the amount of each constituent which is digested by the animal.

Different strains, and different rabbits within a strain, vary in their powers of digestion of the same food at equivalent ages, but to a degree which is insufficient to cause significant problems with the formulation of rations. Hence, once the digestibility coefficients (that is, the percentage of the amount of food consumed which is digested) of a food are known, they can be applied to that food as a reasonable guide.

The method by which digestibility coefficients are obtained is relatively simple. Several rabbits are fed the experimental food, which is carefully analysed for the different constituents, for a period of some 10 days, after the elapse of a trial period. The faeces of the animals are similarly analysed, and the difference will be the amount of the different constituents digested.

There are a number of factors which affect the digestibility of any feeding stuff. Probably the most important is the amount of fibre it contains. As the proportion of fibre increases, so the total digestibility falls. Furthermore, as the proportion of fibre rises, the individual digestibilities of the various constituents of the food fall. The reason for this is that the fibre tends to protect the more digestible constituents from the digestive juices.

The depression of the total digestibility of a food by increasing fibre content is fairly constant. When the fibre content is about 35% of the dry matter of the food, then the total digestibility of the organic matter of the food (i.e. excluding such materials as minerals) is about 40%. This figure may rise to as much as 90% when the fibre content is eliminated (Fig. 7.2). The fineness to which foods are ground has an effect on digestibility. The finer it is ground the more digestible it appears to become. Too fine grinding, however, produces problems with digestion and disease.

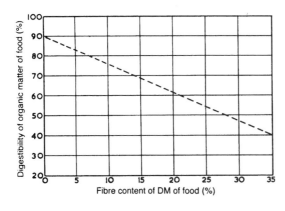

Fig. 7.2 Diagrammatic illustration of relationship between the fibre content of dry matter of food and the digestibility of the organic matter

The speed with which food passes through the digestive tract has some influence on total digestibility, as also has the amount of food fed. Thus a rabbit which is excessively hungry and in poor condition, and a rabbit which is fat and receiving an excessive amount of food, will neither digest nor utilise the food to the maximum efficiency.

The composition and values of some foods are given in Table 7.1. It must always be remembered, however, that there is sometimes considerable variation in these, depending on any number of factors and particularly the variability of the feeds themselves.

Table 7.1   Approximate composition and values of some common feeds for the rabbit

Feed	% DM	Fibre (% in food)	Fibre (% of DM)	Minerals (% in food)	Digestible crude protein (%)	Total digestible nutrients (g/kg)	Digestible energy (MJ/kg)
Mangolds	12	<1	5	0.8	<1	110	2.02
Carrots	13	1	11	0.9	1	120	2.21
Fodder beet	21	1	5	0.8	1	200	3.68
Turnips	9	<1	11	0.7	<1	80	1.47
Cooked potatoes	24	<1	4	1.0	1.4	220	4.05
Sugar beet tops	20	1.8	9	2.4	1.5	131	2.35
Clover hay	84	24	29	6.0	9	440	8.10
Meadow hay	86	26	31	6.0	6	330	6.08
Lucerne hay	89	28	32	7.5	12	440	8.10
Nettle hay	89	11	12	14	18	580	10.68
Timothy hay	89	1.8	2	6.1	2.8	318	5.86
Oat straw	86	34	39	4.9	<1	230	4.23
Young grass mixture	20	3	15	2.0	3	150	2.76
Marrow stem kale	14	2.5	18	1.8	1	100	1.84
Cabbage	14	2.5	18	1.3	<1	90	1.80
Red clover	19	6	27	1.6	2	120	2.21
Green lucerne	22	5	24	2.4	4	150	2.76
Green maize	19	6	29	1.2	1	110	2.02
Grass silage	20	7	35	1.8	3	130	2.39
Maize silage	19	5	26	1.4	2	120	2.21
Oats	87	10	12	3.1	8	680	12.52
Wheat	87	2	2	1.7	10	710	13.07
Barley	85	4	5	2.6	8	730	13.44
Maize	87	2	3	1.3	7	810	14.91
Dried grass	90	20	22	10	10	570	10.49
Dried brewer's grains	94	16	17	3.8	22	587	10.6
Bran	87	10	11	5.9	10	470	8.65
Bread – dried	95	3	2.6	7.1	15	950	17.5
Cotton cake (decorticated)	90	8	9	6.7	34	700	12.89
Ground nut cake (decorticated)	90	7	7	5.8	42	850	15.65
Linseed cake	89	9	10	5.5	26	760	13.98
Dried beet pulp	89	18	20	3.1	8	460	8.47
Soya bean meal	86	5	6	5.4	38	790	14.54

Table 7.1 *continued*

Feed	% DM	Fibre (% in food)	Fibre (% of DM)	Minerals (% in food)	Digestible crude protein (%)	Total digestible nutrients (g/kg)	Digestible energy (MJ/kg)
Fish meal	87	–	–	21	54	620	11.41
Spillers Rabbit Pellets[1]	88	14	15.9	9	13.5	–	10.5
Burgess Supa Rabbit Deluxe mix[2]	88	11	12.5	6.5	11.9	610	11.3
Burgess Supa Natural Mix[3]	88	8	9	4	10.8	730	13.6
Russell Rabbit mix[4]	88	13	14.8	8.3	16.0	–	10.25
Dengie Dried Alfalfa 6 mm pellets or Bales[5]	91	31	34	–	16.0	–	9.3

1–5: Figures supplied by manufacturers.
1, 2, 3: Designed for use with supplement such as hay.
4: Complete food.

THE MEASUREMENT OF FOOD VALUES

When this book was first written, the systems used to express the values of foods consisted of the starch equivalent system, and a system which expressed the total weight of digestible nutrients in a given weight of food. Whilst the system of *Total Digestible Nutrients* (TDN) is used in rabbit feeding in many countries, a further system to replace the old starch equivalent system has been developed. This system, the *Digestible/Metabolisable Energy* (DME) system, is now used because it has greater precision and allows the efficiencies with which the animal uses food for different purposes such as growth, lactation maintenance and the like (all of which vary), to be taken into account.

The *Gross Energy* of the food is not of course available to the animal. Some of the energy is lost in the faeces. The amount digested and absorbed is therefore the *Digestible Energy* (DE). From the food absorbed, some is lost in the urine and also, in small amounts, in gases produced. In general these losses usually amount to between 18 and 20%. The amount left in the body is the *Metabolisable Energy* (ME). For all practical purposes the DE figures are satisfactory for use.

The energy values are measured in megajoules, usually written MJ. The DE is then given as megajoules per kg of dry matter, abbreviated to MJ/kg DM, and the requirements for animals are written as MJ/day.

The DE in any food varies in itself, but it will also vary depending on its utilisation by the rabbit. The effect will also depend upon other feeds fed at the same time, particularly the amount of fibre in the diet, the temperature at which the animals are housed, the plane of nutrition at which the animals are kept, and so on. Unfortunately there have been few assessments of the requirements of DE in the rabbit, and therefore these values for different feeding stuffs have to be calculated.

The TDN of a food also varies depending on a number of factors and must therefore be used with caution. The figures in Table 7.1 do, however, give a good guide. The TDN of any food is calculated by adding together the amounts of digestible crude protein, the digestible crude fibre, the digestible crude N-free extractives (carbohydrate) and the digestible fats. It is necessary to multiply the digestible fat by a figure of 2.25 because the fat has that much more energy than the other elements. It is sufficiently accurate for general purposes to assume that 1 g of TDN will produce approximately 0.0184 MJ of DE.

It cannot be stressed too often that such figures and those of the make up of rations give a guide only, for rabbits of varying ages digest the constituents rather differently, and foods grown in different places and at different times may well vary a good deal. Furthermore the same position applies to feeding standards for different classes of rabbits, which are dealt with below.

WATER REQUIREMENTS OF THE RABBIT

Before considering the requirements for different forms of production in the rabbit the subject of water requirements must be addressed. The question as to whether domestic rabbits should be given water or not was the subject of considerable controversy amongst rabbit fanciers for many years. The reason for this was that it is possible to maintain rabbits without freely available water if sufficient green food or roots are fed, and several troubles had been wrongly attributed to the giving of water. That rabbits can be maintained on a low plane of nutrition on a green food diet which contains considerable water does not affect the fact that freely available drinking water is essential.

Rabbits can lose nearly all the fat from their bodies, and more than half the protein, and still remain alive, but a loss of one-tenth of the water of the body will result in death. Furthermore, the rabbit can live for a relatively long time without solid food, but lack of moisture very quickly produces harmful effects.

Water is essential as a constituent of all parts of the body, and without it no food could be digested. The maintenance of effective elimination of harmful products via the urine is dependent upon sufficient water, as is also the maintenance of almost all other physiological processes. A small amount of water is obtained by the animal by chemical action during the breakdown of food in its body, this being known as metabolic water, but as the total amount of this metabolic water is not great, it should be discounted.

The water requirement of rabbits is variable. It is relatively a good deal higher in the young rabbit than in the old, and thus a shortage of water in early life has a much more serious effect and even a restricted amount of water may seriously retard growth.

The water requirement also varies according to the temperature of the environment and the food being eaten. Rabbits in direct sunlight during the summer may lose nearly 30 g of water per hour, compared with an eighth of this amount when in the shade. Foods with high fibre, protein and mineral contents require more water than normal. In the case of the protein, the increased requirement is due to the necessity for adequate elimination and dilution of urea, the waste product from the utilisation of protein.

In general it is unlikely that any rabbit would ever drink excessive amounts of water, except perhaps in the case of some diseases. It occasionally happens, when animals are fed on excessive amounts of low dry matter green food or roots, that in order to assimilate sufficient dry matter, they are bound to take rather more water than might be satisfactory. This can be overcome by ensuring that excessive succulents are not fed.

The water content of different foods varies greatly, from as much as 91% in turnips (although 85 to 87% for roots is a more general figure) to as low as 10% or even less in the case of some oil seeds. Most of the concentrates and hay fed to rabbits have about 15% of moisture. The requirements by rabbits of water are of the order of three times the dry matter of the food. With some foods this will be less, with others (particularly fibrous foods) it may be more. Thus for medium-sized breeds on a maintenance ration, the requirement would be between 0.4 and 0.6 l per day. This higher amount of moisture might be given by 0.7 kg of greenstuff or roots. The requirement of young animals is much higher, being probably in the region of double that of adults. The suckling doe will require considerable amounts for the production of an adequate milk supply.

It can be seen therefore that the water requirements of the domestic rabbit are relatively high. They can sometimes be satisfied by a very high succulent ration (which is generally not desirable), but in every case a full supply of fresh drinking water is highly desirable.

FOOD REQUIREMENTS OF THE RABBIT

Whilst, over the past years, there has been considerable work done on the nutrition of the rabbit, it is only in fairly recent years that the most detailed investigation into the best feed compositions for rabbits used in intensive commercial farming has been undertaken. This work has resulted in the compilation of tables of feed compositions or analyses which meet the requirements of different classes of stock. The most satisfactory of these recommendations have been prepared by Professor F. Lebas, Director of the National Institute for Research in Agriculture (INRA) Rabbit Research Station at Toulouse (Table 7.2). It should be stressed that these re-commendations are ideal for animals of an adult weight of about 5 kg which are required to produce large numbers of young which themselves grow very rapidly. There are other circumstances which demand a modification of these feed recommendations.

Table 7.2 Nutrients required by different catagories of stock in intensive rabbit farming, recommended by INRA 1989

		Categories of stock				
Feed compositions required based on a DM of 89%	Units	Fattening or growing 4–12 weeks	Lactating does	Does in kindle	Animals on maintenace	Mixed stock
Digestible energy	MJ/kg	10.4	10.9	10.4	9.2	10.4
Fat	%	3	4	3	3	3
Crude fibre	%	14	11	14	15–16	14
Indigestible fibre	%	10	9	11	12	10
Crude protein	%	15.5	18.0	16.0	13.0	16.5
Digestible protein	%	10.9	13.4	11.0	9.2	12.0
Ratio: DP/DE		10.5	12.3	10.6	10.0	11.5

Feed compositions required based on a DM of 89%	Units	Categories of stock				
		Fattening or growing 4–12 weeks	Lactating does	Does in kindle	Animals on maintenace	Mixed stock
Amino acids						
Lysine	%	0.65	0.90	–	–	0.75
Sulphur amino acids	%	0.60	0.55	–	–	0.60
Tryptophan	%	0.13	0.15	–	–	0.15
Threonine	%	0.55	0.70	–	–	0.60
Leucine	%	1.05	1.25	–	–	1.20
Isoleucine	%	0.60	0.70	–	–	0.65
Valine	%	0.70	0.85	–	–	0.80
Histidine	%	0.35	0.43	–	–	0.40
Arginine	%	0.90	0.80	–	–	0.90
Phenylalanine + tyrosine	%	1.20	1.40	–	–	1.25
Minerals						
Calcium	%	0.80	1.20	0.80	0.40	1.20
Phosphorus	%	0.50	0.70	0.50	0.30	0.70
Sodium	%	0.30	0.30	0.30	–	0.30
Potassium	%	0.60	0.90	0.90	–	0.90
Chlorine	%	0.35	0.35	0.35	–	0.35
Magnesium	%	0.30	0.30	0.30	–	0.30
Sulphur	%	0.25	0.25	–	–	0.25
Trace elements						
Iron	ppm	50	100	50	50	100
Copper	ppm	15	15	–	–	15
Zinc	ppm	25	50	50	–	50
Manganese	ppm	8.5	2.5	2.5	2.5	8.5
Cobalt	ppm	0.1	0.1	–	–	0.1
Iodine	ppm	0.2	0.2	0.2	0.2	0.2
Fluorine	ppm	0.5	–	–	–	0.5
Vitamins						
Vitamin A	iu/kg	6 000	10 000	10 000	6 000	10 000
Vitamin D	iu/kg	1 000	1 000	1 000	1 000	1 000
Vitamin E	ppm	50	50	50	50	50
Vitamin K	ppm	0	2	2	0	2
Vitamin B_1 (thiamin)	ppm	2	–	0	0	2
Vitamin B_2 (riboflavin)	ppm	6	–	0	0	4
Pantothenic acid	ppm	20	–	0	0	20
Vitamin B_6 (pyridoxine)	ppm	2	–	0	0	2
Vitamin B_{12}	ppm	0.01	0	0	0	0.01
Niacin	ppm	50	–	–	–	50
Folic acid	ppm	5	–	0	0	5
Biotin	ppm	0.2	–	–	–	0.2

Source: F. Lebas, National Institute for Research in Agriculture, 1989.

Rabbits of different weights, ages, and conditions, i.e. resting, in kindle, suckling, etc., will obviously need different rations, both in bulk and constitution. It is customary to consider the rations of any animal in two parts. The first part is that used for maintaining the animal without loss or increase in weight, and without production of any sort. The second part of the ration is that required for growth, or production.

Requirements for maintenance

When an animal is completely at rest it still uses a certain amount of energy. This energy may be measured by suitable experimental techniques, and the amount of such energy which the animal uses is known as the *basal metabolic rate* (BMR). In the case of the domestic rabbit this basal metabolic rate has been measured on many occasions. Thus, in addition to the basal metabolic energy required, if the animal is to move about, digest its food, keep warm, etc., more energy will be required. It is common practice to double the basal metabolic rate to arrive at a figure for the amount of energy which the rabbit requires to maintain itself in good health but without increasing or decreasing in weight. The amount of maintenance energy will depend on the size or weight of the rabbit, and will decrease in proportion as the animal gets larger. Details of the theoretical amounts of energy required by various sizes of rabbits, based on double the BMR, are given in Table 7.3.

Table 7.3   Energy and protein requirements of the domestic rabbit for maintenance

Body weight		Adult BMR	Theoretical maintenance requirement	Average daily requirements		
lb	kg	MJ/day	MJ/day DE	MJ/DE/ day	Digestible crude protein (g/day)	TDN (g)
2	0.91	0.24	0.48	0.55	2.7	30
3	1.36	0.33	0.66	0.73	3.6	40
4	1.81	0.40	0.80	0.95	4.6	52
5	2.27	0.48	0.96	1.12	5.4	61
6	2.72	0.54	1.08	1.26	6.21	69
7	3.18	0.63	1.26	1.39	6.8	76
8	3.63	0.69	1.38	1.52	7.4	83
9	4.08	0.77	1.54	1.67	8.1	91
10	4.54	0.85	1.70	1.80	8.8	98
11	4.99	0.92	1.84	1.93	9.45	105

By calculating the energy values of different rations which will maintain the rabbit in equilibrium, and the various standards suggested by various research workers, a further column has been calculated, which gives the actual energy requirements. These will be seen to compare very well with the theoretical requirements.

As well as energy, the maintenance rations of the rabbit must contain a sufficiency of protein. The amounts of digestible protein for different sizes of rabbits are therefore listed in Table 7.3 as grams of digestible protein required per day. A final column of the amounts of TDN required per day is also given.

It will be noted from Table 7.3 that the protein level is of the order of 12%. It is sometimes considered that this is too high for pure maintenance but a range from 10 to 15% is quite suitable.

Requirements for growth

The growth of the rabbit is extremely rapid, and consequently its nutritive requirements are relatively high during the early period of its life. In addition to the maintenance requirement which grows with increasing weight, the amount of digestible nutrients required for any unit of growth will also increase. Thus a rabbit of a medium-size breed at weaning will require, in addition to the normal maintenance requirement for its size, just under a kilo of digestible nutrients to produce one kilo gain in liveweight. At six months of age, when it weighs nearly three times as much, it requires, in addition to its normal maintenance requirement, about two-and-a-half times as much digestible nutrient to produce one kilo of liveweight. Table 7.4 gives approximate figures for the growth of a medium-sized animal and its requirements of digestible nutrients to produce one gram liveweight gain (these of course being in addition to its maintenance requirements).

Table 7.4 Weight gain and nutrient requirements of growing rabbits of medium-sized breeds

Age (weeks)	Approx. weight (kg)	Weekly gain in weight (g)	TDN required per gram of gain in weight (g)
8	0.96	160	0.97
10	1.28	170	1.14
12	1.62	125	1.34
14	1.87	115	1.53
16	2.10	85	1.72
18	2.27	70	1.89
20	2.41	70	2.13
22	2.55	60	2.31
24	2.67	–	2.53

It must be appreciated that the requirements of digestible nutrients per unit gain in weight depend on the composition of that gain. For example, if the rabbit is laying down fat to a large degree, its requirements per unit gain will be higher than if it were not so doing, for fat, having a higher energy value, will require a correspondingly higher nutrient intake for any given weight of production.

On comparing the requirements for growth and maintenance, it will be seen that at an early age the requirements for growth are only slightly less than the maintenance requirement for an adult animal of the same weight. Thus the early nutrition will be nearly twice the maintenance requirement, but will fall considerably in relation to the maintenance requirement as the animal grows.

Although an adult animal can be maintained on a crude protein content of the rations of as low as 10%, the needs of the young growing animal are considerably higher. The initial food with which the young rabbits supplement their milk should have a crude protein content of at least 15%. In some Continental feeding standards, the recommended proportion at one time exceeded 20%, but this was both costly and found to be of no advantage.

Requirements for pregnancy

For the production of healthy, well-developed young and a satisfactory milk supply in the doe, her nutrition must be on a rising plane throughout pregnancy. The food supply should not, however, be fattening, for this will not give satisfactory results. It is particularly during the last half of pregnancy that the main requirements come. If the doe is not suckling as well as being in kindle, the most simple, and probably the most satisfactory, standard, is for a ration of 1.3 times maintenance at the start of pregnancy, rising to double maintenance at the end. The ration itself must also be modified in constituents, for a higher protein content is desirable, as also is a higher mineral content. The protein content should lie between 15.5 and 16.5% and the mineral content between 5 and 6%.

Requirements for lactation

Milk production varies greatly in different breeds and within the breed. Those breeds which have not been improved in their milking ability will yield some 30 or so g per kg bodyweight. However, improved breeds will yield between 160 and 200 g of milk per day in total in the first lactation, increasing to 180 to 240 g or even more in subsequent litters. The average energy value of rabbits' milk is of the order of 1 MJ per 100 g. The efficiency with which food energy is converted into milk varies but it is usually in the region of 75%. Thus an unimproved doe of 4.5 kg will require of the order of 1.8 MJ for her daily milk production, and the improved breeds, more. It will be seen that this is approximately double the maintenance requirement, or that level with which the doe was fed at the end of pregnancy. The total needs of the doe, allowing also a small proportion for her young when they first start eating solid food, may rise as high as three times maintenance at the end of the fourth week of suckling.

Approximately one-third of the energy value of the doe's milk is supplied by protein. Thus the first foods of the young rabbits will need to have a high protein content. Furthermore, the quality of milk protein is very good, and thus if possible some animal protein should be incorporated in the first feeds. Mineral requirements are similar to those for the pregnant doe.

Requirements of the stud buck

A stud buck, to remain vigorous and in good health, requires more than the normal maintenance ration. Approximately 10 to 15% above maintenance, both of total energy and digestible protein, is satisfactory.

Requirements for fattening

Except for intensive commercial rabbit farming, fattening rations for rabbits are difficult to establish and it is unusual for the exhibitor to require fattening rations for his stock. Furthermore, the normal practice of 'storing' animals and then fattening, as occurs in other animal husbandry, is never used, except to a modified extent when prime pelts are being produced and the animals kept on a fairly low plane of nutrition throughout their lives. Even in these cases they are rarely specially fattened before pelting. Thus the standards for growth, which will provide a suitably fattened carcase, are satisfactory, although the proportion of protein in the ration may be slightly reduced.

Requirements of bulk

Apart from supplying sufficient energy, protein and minerals, a ration must supply sufficient bulk to satisfy appetite, but not more than the animal can comfortably consume. A ration containing the different requirements but in a bulk of dry matter which the animal could not consume, could easily be devised. On such a ration correctly balanced except for bulk, the rabbit would starve.

Appetite varies greatly and thus it is difficult to lay down standards for bulk of dry matter, but a generalised statement is given in Fig. 7.3, where approximate maximum and minimum amounts of dry matter to be fed per day are given for different liveweights. In general the higher amounts are usually given to developing and pregnant stock, whilst the lower limits are suitable for maintenance. Heavily lactating does will often exceed these figures by nearly twice.

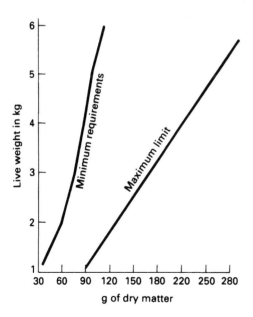

Fig. 7.3   Minimum requirements and maximum limits of dry matter in rations per day

Requirements of minerals

Although minerals are required in much smaller quantities than other food nutrients, they are no less important. They are particularly important for the high producing does and growing young, for without an adequate supply of minerals serious troubles can arise, and production will certainly be lowered. Although a number of different minerals are required by the rabbit, those most likely to be deficient are calcium, phosphorus, sodium and chlorine, the last two being found together as salt. The maintenance requirements will be met if the ration contains some 4% of appropriate minerals, but a higher level of 5% or so is quite satisfactory for pregnant and suckling does and growing young. The requirements of different minerals vary a good deal and it is therefore necessary that the total mineral content of the feed should contain all the minerals required. In addition, the balance between different minerals is important. Each mineral, in its correct proportion is required. The need for supplements is eliminated when high quality pelleted feeds are used.

Requirement of fibre

The importance of fibre in the rations has always been recognised and when rations were composed largely of roughages, considerable quantities of fibre were incorporated. In fact, in some cases the amount of fibre was so large that the animals were very poorly nourished or even starved. It is now clearly recognised that some fibre is easily digested, whilst other fibre elements are not. A lack of indigestible fibre causes digestive disturbances, in many cases leading to mortality. Too great a preponderance of digestible fibre (fibre from root crops is highly digestible) also causes digestive disturbances, although a gradual introduction (as in all foods) tends to lessen this. When the fibre is fed in pelleted form the coarseness of the grinding of the fibre has an important influence on the rabbit. Excessively fine grinding causes digestive disturbances.

When the ration is high in fibre, rabbits tend to increase their consumption of the food and thus, to an extent, compensate. However, if a high level of energy is required then the animals may not be able to eat enough to satisfy the requirements for their best production, whether it be growth or lactation, and consequently this will suffer.

The problem, then, is that it is necessary to incorporate in the ration enough indigestible fibre to ensure that the digestive tract of the rabbit has sufficient, but to ensure that the total energy content and protein content of the ration will also be sufficient for the rabbit's needs when it consumes as much as it is able. The current food compounders producing rabbit feed pellets in general do this.

PELLETED FEEDS

Originally pelleted feeds were used only in laboratories but during the last 40 years their value in producing consistent and sound feeding and in reducing the labour of feeding became recognised. Today all commercial rabbit farmers and probably the majority of non-commercial rabbit keepers use only pelleted feeds. Sometimes indeed the very large user in the commercial field can obtain such feeds compounded to his own formulae. Apart from consistency and ease of feeding, pelleted foods allow the easy introduction of supplements of vitamins, minerals, medicinal additives and the like.

The pelleted feeds tend to be very consistent in their composition and (certainly if produced by good feed companies) are usually based on the latest findings of research into rabbit nutrition. Provided that the pellets are well made and do not disintegrate, there is little waste and usually they are palatable to rabbits, which do not like finely ground meals which tend to cause irritation. The ideal size of feed pellets is 4 mm in diameter by 6 or 7 mm in length, although larger, and smaller pellets and cubes are sometimes used.

There are two schools of thought on the use of such rations. The first suggests that different types should be used for different types of stock, e.g. pregnant does, weaners, stud bucks and so on, whilst the second school of thought considers that a standard ration may be used and variations produced by restricting the amounts fed to different types of stock or by supplementing the pellets with other balancing feeds. Which of these two systems is used must of necessity depend upon the pellets available and also whether the rabbit keeper has the time to selectively modify the rations with supplementary feeding.

Quality in pellets is difficult to assess, except in the case of the physical characteristics, the most important of which is the hardness and the withstanding of crushing and abrasion. In modern commercial conditions it is often necessary to use bulk delivery systems to reduce costs, in which case pellets are blown into silos. Dusting indicates a lack of quality.

There are two apparent disadvantages to pellets. The first is that they tend to be expensive, but when their cost is balanced against the ease of feeding and the saving in labour, in addition to the fact that feeding is consistent and production is therefore usually increased, this disadvantage is seen to be more apparent than real. The second disadvantage is that non-commercial stock often tend to get too fat unless the feed pellets are restricted and supplements fed. Particularly in the case of a single feed pellet available in the rabbitry of an exhibition breeder, the answer is to feed supplementary roughages.

There are, apart from pellets, feed mixes made up for the home user. Sometimes these contain some pellets and sometimes not, but they all have in common the use of feeds, usually whole, of which rabbits are fond. There is little doubt that their composition and nutrient analysis varies more greatly than do pellet batches, but in the circumstances in which they are fed, this is of little importance.

Some compounders manufacture a single type of pellet, whilst others have two or more formulations. Where supplements are fed or where there are less than 100 or so breeding does in a commercial establishment, it is doubtful whether two different formulations are necessary, particularly if rapid remating systems are used.

There are two general methods of feeding in the farming of rabbits, ad lib feeding in which hoppers are filled with pellets which last several days, and the system of feeding a standard weight per day for each class of stock. This second system is sometimes criticised with the argument that it requires more labour than the ad lib feeding system. This argument overlooks the fact that the hand-feeding system does ensure that the stockperson checks his or her stock daily and that a very good indication that all is not well is that the animals are not eating.

The ad lib feeding also has a slight benefit in the nature of the feeding of the rabbit. The rabbit naturally has a large number of small meals throughout the day. The wild rabbit may have small meals up to 70 or 80 times throughout the 24 hours. The domestic rabbit, however, has fewer, probably only half as many, although younger rabbits eat more frequently and over slightly longer periods. If food is before it at all times it can comfortably practice this habit. If, however, it consumes the last of the hand-fed food relatively soon after it has been hand fed, then obviously it cannot.

A general rule for daily allowances for the typical commercial meat producing breeds (with an adult weight of some 4 to 5 kg) are:

- adults on a maintenance ration: 115 to 130 g;
- stud bucks: 130 to 140 g;
- growing young (5 weeks onwards): average 100 to 130 g but usually ad lib feeding;
- lactating does: 340 to 400 g.

With exhibition animals, which of course have very variable weights, these general allowances would not be correct. Certainly the smaller breeds would be overfed.

ADDITIVES

One of the benefits of pelleted feeding stuffs is that additives of various sorts can be simply and accurately included. In any other form of feeding, the incorporation of medicines, for example, is difficult. The animal may receive the correct dose, but this is unlikely. With pelleted feeds the dose per pellet is reasonably accurate.

There can be many additives to rations, such as growth promoters and coccidiostats (that is, chemicals used to keep down the level of coccidia), and even antibiotics. The question of coccidiostats is dealt with in Chapter 12. One important point should however be stressed. At the present time, most pelleted feeding stuffs with an additive (e.g. a coccidiostat) are so formulated that the amount of coccidiostat is incorporated at the correct dosage level only if the pellets are fed at the correct level. If, therefore, in such a case only half the level of the ration is supplied by the pellets, then the animal does receives only one half its correct dose. In such cases, not only does this mean that the disease is not being kept under control, but it means that with the under-dosing, the coccidia are being accustomed to the drug and a resistance to its correct use in the future is being built up.

Antibiotics are the products of certain micro-organisms, and their use has been widely developed in animal feeding. The first antibiotic was penicillin, and this was followed by aureomycin, terramycin and many others. Although the addition of a certain amount of some antibiotics to the foodstuffs of some animals has resulted in increased growth rate and improved conversion ability, experimental work with the rabbit has not shown these results, except in a few cases.

In recent years, particularly in America, investigations into the use of yeasts and acid-producing bacteria incorporated into the feed have shown considerable improvements in the reduction of mortality from enteritis complexes and also improvements in growth rates. These are not as yet incorporated into feeds in the UK, but advances in this technology are continuing.

In all cases of medicinal additives, there are certain legal restrictions when the additive is being used for meat animals and whatever the formulation, feeding stuffs with additives (apart, of course, from those solely used in the feed or for its manufacture) must be discontinued for the withdrawal period given for the feed and an additive-free pellet used for the last appropriate number of days before slaughter.

FEEDING PRACTICES

No matter what feed is fed, be it pelleted or home-grown roughages and cereals, there are certain practices which should be followed.

Changing rations should be carried out slowly and gradually. Very often a rapid change of foods will lead to digestive disturbances. It is important that the appetites of stock should not be affected, and sudden changes, particularly to unpalatable foods, will easily do this. For example, some stock refuse to eat a new type of pellet until this is slowly mixed in increasing quantities with the old. If a change has, however, to be made rapidly, then the amounts of the new ration fed should be slightly reduced for a week or so.

Force feeding by starving the animals in order to make them eat an unpalatable food is a very unsatisfactory procedure. On occasions molasses and other very palatable feeds are used to encourage stock to eat food they do not like.

Regularity of feeding, as with other aspects of management, is very important, unless the rabbit is being fed ad lib. A hungry rabbit will not utilise its food to the best advantage, and will use up considerable energy in its restlessness whilst waiting for its food.

Individuality in their feeding habits occurs amongst domestic rabbits. Although some consideration may be given to these individual characteristics, the rabbit feeder should take care to ensure that his stock do not become subject to 'fads'. Apart from encouraging an animal with lost appetite with an appetizing morsel, the feeder should adjust the amounts of food only. When an animal goes off its food then the amounts should be reduced until it regains its full appetite.

Cleaning: Pelleted feeds are never required to be cleaned, but the subject of dusting should be mentioned. Some pellets, that are not as well manufactured as others, do suffer from excess dust, which is not only expensive to the breeder but also is disagreeable to the stock. If pellets are excessively dusty they should be sieved before feeding.

The use of alternative feeds and the construction of rations

Statements have been made on the various requirements of different classes of stock for different purposes. It should again be stressed that these statements and the analysis of feeding stuffs given can only be taken as a guide. It should also be stressed that the various requirements given are only applicable when the rations are correctly balanced for all constituents and bulk of dry matter.

A mineral supplement made of equal parts of salt, feeding bone flour and finely ground chalk is quite suitable, although if a small amount of fish-meal is fed in the ration such a supplement is hardly necessary. There are also a number of proprietary brands of mineral mixtures. It should perhaps be added that an excess of minerals is likely to cause as much trouble as a deficiency. Mineral supplements may be added to grain which has been slightly dampened immediately prior to feeding, or incorporated in a wet or dry mash.

QUALITY IN FEED

It is important that the rations for rabbits should be of good quality, as well as providing the necessary nutritional requirements. Foods vary a great deal in this respect, especially the proteins. Freshness is always important for if food is not fresh it is likely to be unpalatable and also to cause digestive upsets.

Proteins are composed of various amino acids, some of which are essential to the animal, whilst others are not. Protein from different sources will not be equally valuable to the animal. In general the proteins from vegetable matter are of poorer quality than are the proteins from animal feeding stuffs such as fish-meal, meat and bone-meal, milk, etc. Thus, to overcome the difficulty of inferior quality in proteins, as far as possible a variety of them should be incorporated in the rations, in particular some of the animal proteins.

Obviously food which is dusty or dirty will be inferior to the same food when it is clean. The appearance of different foods will often give a fairly reliable guide to its quality. For example, a thin oat is of less value than a plump oat. Hay which is of poor colour and feel is not satisfactory. It has previously been said that digestibility is correlated closely with the percentage of fibre in the food. Thus as foods increase in the percentage of fibre, they become of lower value. All plants as they grow increase in fibre, and consequently the older the growth the lower the quality of feeds made from them. This is particularly so in the case of hay and dried grass. Hay made from grass which has flowered will prove of much lower value than hay made from grass before it flowers.

Palatability of foods also varies and is not much guidance as to the value of the food itself. In some cases rabbits will not find a food palatable at first, and indeed it may take some weeks before they will eat it readily. Nevertheless unpalatable foods should not be given over long periods unless stock begin to like it, for it will lead to lowered production. Some breeders endeavour to increase the palatability of food by sprinkling it with such things as molasses or by mixing the unpalatable food with palatable. This method is excellent provided the foods themselves are satisfactory. It should always be remembered that a mixture of foods is usually more palatable than single foods. Thus it is not really satisfactory to feed wheat by itself, but a mixture of oats and wheat is quite suitable.

There are some foods which are definitely harmful to domestic rabbits. Under commercial conditions it is not likely that these will be used, but the fancier who may be feeding a proportion of home-collected foods may encounter them. In many cases plants which are poisonous when fed fresh, lose their harmfulness when dried. Buttercups, for example, are perfectly harmless in hay but are deleterious when fresh. Contrary to general belief, rabbits will not reject poisonous plants themselves. Amongst the more harmful wild plants are such species as nightshade, bryony, nearly all plants from bulbs (daffodils, bluebells, etc.), buttercups, celandines, figworts, foxgloves, fool's parsley, hellebore, hemlock, poppies, ragwort and spurges.

Some of the cultivated plants are also harmful, although many others are very useful foods. The harmful ones include antirrhinums, dahlia, nearly all plants from bulbs, lobelia, garden lupin, most evergreen trees (except conifers), ivy berries, laburnum, privet and yew. Potato leaves and tomato haulm are also harmful.

At one time the gathering of wild plants, grass, dandelions, plantains and many others was quite normal. Today, however, with the widespread use of insecticides and weed-killers and the presence of potentially lethal contaminants, many rabbit breeders no longer collect such foods. If they do they must also ensure that the food collected is not contaminated by wild rabbits, dogs or sheep. There are occasionally cases of poisoning resulting from the use of cereals which have been dressed with mercurial dressings, and foods contaminated with fertilisers and sprays are also harmful. Contrary to popular belief, rhubarb leaves, poisonous for many other animals, are a perfectly safe and indeed a useful food for domestic rabbits.

Young clovers and lucerne when fed in excessive quantities will often give rise to bloat.

Because the rabbit has a fairly high tolerance of poisons, the inclusion of small quantities of harmful foods, although they should be eliminated if possible, should not cause undue worry. Provided a variety of foods is available to the animal, little harm should come to it.

Different foods may produce different effects in the carcase. For example, rabbits fed on rations containing strong smelling plants like wild onion have a tainted flesh when killed. In the same way, high levels of fish-meal may produce the same effect. Some feeding stuffs such as maize, when fed in excess, produce a soft fat, but most other cereals produce a hard fat. The quality of the fat in the carcase will also depend upon the materials in the food from which it is built up. Fat built up from fatty foods tends to be less satisfactory than fat built up from carbohydrate foods.

PURCHASING FEEDS

The cost of producing domestic rabbits lies very largely in the cost of food. Thus it is important to feed cheaply. This should not be taken as a recommendation for foods which cost least, for often this type of 'cheap' food is very expensive in terms of results. Feeding stuffs should be compared on the basis of their content of TDN and digestible crude protein, or on the basis of DE in MJ. For foods with similar protein contents, the cheapest food will be the one which supplies one unit of TDN or DE at the cheapest cost. If the cost per ton is divided by the TDN or DE, then the cost of one unit of TDN, or DE, is obtained. Protein is always more expensive than other digestible nutrients, and therefore the cost of one unit of protein should also be determined. In addition, other characteristics should be considered. Compounded foods should have some allowance made for the cost or the value of this compounding. Similarly, antibiotic-supplemented foods should be credited with the value of this. Some foods are to be preferred because they are more palatable or give a better carcase. Thus if one unit of maize costs the same as one unit of oats, the oats would be selected, for they have a slight advantage apart from simple nutrient value.

FEEDING SYSTEMS

There are several different types of feeding systems employed by rabbit breeders. Undoubtedly the most common, after pelleted feeding, is that in which a wide variety of green food (and/or roots) is fed, with hay and usually a small concentrate feed. Hay is often left before the stock at all times, and this method has much to commend it. Usually the rabbits are fed twice per day, and young rabbits which are to be grown rapidly may be fed three times per day. The rabbit, being a more-or-less continuous feeder, can, however, be fed only once each day. In its natural state the rabbit feeds over an extended period and may take as many as 70 or 80 small meals during a 24-hour period.

For the production of the highest quality pelts, the rabbits must usually be kept for a minimum of about seven months. Thus they can be maintained on a low level of nutrition in order to economise cost. The system used generally in this case is to feed greenstuff, roots and hay, thus eliminating all or nearly all concentrate feeding. On the other hand, for young meat production, where the cost of liveweight, and hence carcase weight, rises steeply in terms of feeds, the fastest growth possible is desirable, which means concentrate feeding.

FEEDING PRACTICES WITH ALTERNATIVE FEEDS

Variety in feeding is most important except of course where a complete compounded pellet is fed, which supplies all the nutritional requirements of the rabbit. The major advantage of feeding a variety of foods is that any deficiencies in one will usually be compensated by the constituents of another. Furthermore, a variety of foods is usually more palatable than any single food making up the mixture. This does not apply to pelleted feeding.

Regularity: Again as with pelleted feeds, regularity of feeding is important.

Preparation of food is not often necessary, except for wet mashes, and for ensuring cleanliness. Wet mashes, which during the 1939–45 war were made largely from kitchen scraps, potatoes, etc., dried off with bran, have the disadvantage that they deteriorate rather rapidly and are now very rarely used. Some foods, such as sugar beet pulp, should be soaked before feeding, and other foods, particularly of a dry, fine nature such as dry mashes, may be improved by damping. This should, however, only be done immediately before feeding. Peas and beans are sometimes soaked before feeding.

Meals: Finely ground meals are disliked by rabbits and are of less benefit when coarser material is used.

Cleaning of food is sometimes necessary. Roots are best scrubbed, and although greens can be washed by dipping in a water tank, the most satisfactory way of washing them is under a running tap. It is rarely necessary to chop or pulp feeds as is sometimes done for other animals. It is, however, sometimes necessary to split the stems of kales and cabbages in order to allow the stock to eat the soft cores. Furthermore, it may be necessary to cut up the larger leaves of kales and cabbages, if they are being fed in a rack, in order that the rabbits can pull them through the wires of the rack.

Changing feeds: As with pelleted feeding, gradual changes in food should be made.

Mixing of concentrated foods after grinding must be very thorough if the ration is to prove satisfactory, for unless the mixing is thorough, the resulting mix will not be uniform and some rabbits will have too much of one constituent and a deficiency of another. The most satisfactory way of mixing mineral supplements is to mix them with a small amount of meal and then mix this with the main bulk.

NOTES ON COMMON FEEDS

Below are given brief notes on different foods which are commonly used for rabbit feeding. It is unfortunate that the majority of rabbit breeders do not normally investigate the many foods which are at their disposal at probably cheaper cost than many that they use. The cost of rabbit production can be materially lowered by the judicious selection of foods.

Cereals

The commonly used cereals are oats, barley, maize, and wheat, in that order. Oats have been one of the most popular foods for domestic rabbits, and produce an excellent hard condition. Good oats should be plump, and should feel solid when a handful is squeezed. Whole oats are to be preferred to crushed oats, particularly for adult stock. Rabbits tend to pick out the kernel and leave the husk when oats are crushed, though this may not be considered undesirable in young stock growing fast. Oats should be crushed only just sufficiently to split the skin.

The other three cereals are all useful but are usually fed in mixtures rather than alone. In the past some publicity has been given to the use of sprouted or germinated cereals as a food. The cereals are allowed to grow sprouts up to about 20 or 25 cm; there is a slight loss of nutrients when cereals are so sprouted, and no advantages have been found. Wheat has a tendency to be 'pasty', and thus is only fed in mixtures. Maize, containing the highest amount of nutrient of any of the cereals, is a safe and excellent food for all classes of rabbits.

Beans and peas

Beans and peas have a high protein content, the protein also being one of the more valuable vegetable proteins. Old beans are preferred for feeding, as new beans, when ground, are very liable to heat and to become very unpalatable and even dangerous for feeding. When the old season's beans are ground and used fresh, however, they are a safe and excellent food.

Bran

Bran was the only foodstuff of all rationed materials to be allowed the rabbit breeder during the 1939–45 war rationing. Bran is only suitable for drying off wet mashes, and, because it enjoys a reputation for stimulating milk production and is also laxative in nature, is usually more expensive than its mere feeding values merit.

Concentrates of animal origin

Feeding stuffs of animal origin, such as meat and bone-meal, blood meal, fish-meal, dried milk, whale meal, etc., are all high protein concentrates, the protein being the most valuable of all forms of this nutrient. Fish-meal is the most commonly used and has the advantage of supplying minerals as well as protein, having some 21% mineral content. It is necessary to use the best quality of fish-meal, i.e. white fish-meal, for other types have excessive oil. Fish-meal is usually limited to at most 10% of the rations, owing to the high amounts of protein available and also to cost. As with all feeding stuffs, but particularly with meals of animal or fish origin, freshness and freedom from rancidity or 'off-smell' is absolutely essential.

Meat meals are very variable in composition, but generally contain in the region of 40% of a very high quality protein. They are useful as protein additions to the rations, but a meat meal with a low oil content should be selected. Meat and bone-meal differs from meat meal in that it contains a much higher proportion of minerals. Blood meals are similar but have a higher proportion of protein (usually about 65%) and very low minerals. Dried skimmed or separated milk and occasionally dried whole milk is used in some rations. Both have excellent protein contents, but the oil content of dried whole milk is rather high (usually about 26%).

All the concentrates of animal origin, then, are of high protein value. They are invariably used by mixing in mashes, either wet or dry, or incorporated in compounded pellets.

Grass

Grass, both fresh and dried, is an important food for the domestic rabbit, although it varies very considerably. During the spring the grass grows rapidly, and at this period the plant is leafy and is rich in protein and low in fibre content. During summer when the plant flowers, there is a great increase in fibre and a reduction in protein and other digestible nutrients. The grass improves slightly in autumn, and then tails off again during winter. Thus young, quickly growing grass is an excellent food for all classes of stock, although older grass is not so valuable, and rank old growth is not at all satisfactory. These variations are important, for young rabbits may easily starve if fed on old growth.

Hay, dried grass, and grass silage are all of value when made at the correct age, but these feeding stuffs must be made from grass which is itself valuable, that is, before it flowers in the case of hay, and at an earlier age in the case of the other two. Generally speaking, the grass fed to rabbits consists of a mixture of grass and other plants, and this is often of advantage.

Dried grass is a particularly valuable food and can be made even by the rabbit breeder on the smallest scale. Lawn cuttings, if allowed to dry without heating, can be stored for winter use, and give rather better results than most hays. It is essential to stress that only young grass should be used for drying; that of one month's vigorous growth is ideal, but older growth than this produces poorer results.

Green foods and roots

There is an infinite variety of green foods which are useful for feeding purposes, and many breeders on a small scale rely for the bulk of their food supply on wild plants. On a larger scale some breeders will grow green food crops, of which cabbage, chicory, kale, red clover, lucerne, maize, oats and tare mixtures, and sainfoin, are probably the most satisfactory.

There are a number of crops for human consumption which supply consider-able amounts of food for rabbits. For example, mishappen or damaged roots, carrot tops, waste cabbage leaves, and rhubarb leaves (contrary to popular belief) are all valuable.

Roots take the place of greenstuffs during the winter months. Most of the roots fed to rabbits (which include carrot, sugar beet, fodder beet, mangold, swede, kohlrabi, and turnip) have a low dry matter content. Fodder beet and sugar beet, however, have a much higher content, and weight for weight are nearly twice as nutritious as other roots.

It is most important that, when roots are first introduced, they should be fed in limited quantities. If given in too great a quantity they will almost certainly scour the rabbits. Potatoes should be considered separately from the other roots, for they have a very high dry matter content compared with the others. Potatoes are normally fed cooked and incorporated with other ingredients to form a mash. They are an excellent fattening food.

Hays

Hay of all types is a roughage, and different types, and indeed the same type, are very variable in composition. A good quality hay is an excellent food for rabbits, and most breeders are agreed that it should be fed when available. Many breeders also make a practice of leaving hay before the stock at all times. All types of hay should be leafy, for it is the leaf that is the most nutritious part. Clover hay is probably that most preferred by the majority of rabbit breeders, and good results are usually obtained with it. Nevertheless, nettle hay, made by drying the common stinging-nettle (rabbits will not touch the fresh plant), is the best of all hays, if made with relatively young nettles, and produces excellent condition and growth. Having a very high protein content, this type of hay is extremely useful for young stock. Good quality hay will have a good 'nose', that is to say, it does not smell musty or unpleasant. It should be of good colour, and should above all be made from young material, thus having a good proportion of leaf to stem.

Oil cakes and meals

Oil cakes and meals are never fed by themselves, except in the case of a linseed mash, which is now not often fed. Depending on the method used to extract the oil from the original seeds, the various cakes may have an oil content of from under 2% to over 8%. When the oil is extracted by means of a solvent, the oil content is reduced to 1 or 2%; with the expeller type of extraction, the oil content is usually 3%; and with the crushing type of extraction, the oil content may be 8% or more. The method of extraction must be stated on samples. The higher oil contents are not entirely desirable. Some of the oil cakes have had a proportion of the fibre removed from them, when they are known as decorticated cakes. The undecorticated cakes contain a high proportion of fibre and are not desirable.

Linseed cake is extremely popular. It is slightly laxative, and gives an excellent bloom to the animal. Usually, however, the price is rather higher than is merited by its nutritive value. The linseed mash so much liked in pre-war days for toning up stock is prepared by boiling linseed vigorously for 15 minutes (to destroy an enzyme which produces prussic acid), and then allowing it to stew for some time. The linseed should be stirred during boiling to prevent it from sticking to the pan.

Groundnut cake, when decorticated, is a valuable and palatable food. It is usually much cheaper than linseed cake.

Soya bean cake and meal are extremely rich in protein and are very palatable. They are one of the most popular protein supplements used in rabbit feeding. They can be used safely in moderation to balance the rations, but added calcium is necessary.

Most of the oil cakes and meals are employed in the manufacture of pelleted foods by compounders. It is usually difficult for the average rabbit breeder to compound his own foods in this way, but often cubes of oil meals may be used to supplement grain rations, to give the concentrate part of the ration.

There is a very wide variety of different foods available for the rabbit breeder, and details of books in which he or she can find further particulars are given in the bibliography. A knowledge of different foods will enable the breeder to purchase to advantage, and thus to reduce his costs considerably.

Chapter 8

Reproduction and Breeding

THE REPRODUCTIVE SYSTEMS

The functions of the male reproductive system are to secrete, store, and then transport into the female system the sperm or male cells. The sperm are very minute tadpole-like organisms, with a head which contains half the inheritance of the future animal, a short body, and a relatively long thin tail. With rapid movements of the tail the sperm can move about freely in the fluids which are ejaculated with them at each mating.

The sperm are produced in coiled tubes which make up each of the two testicles. These are carried in the scrotal sac or purse, which is attached to the abdominal wall. The testicles in the rabbit may be withdrawn on occasions into the abdomen, when the animal will become sterile, due to the increased temperature of the testicles. In the wild rabbit the testicles descend into the scrotum before the breeding season, but are withdrawn at the end.

The sperm are passed, at mating, through a tube in the penis. The penis consists of muscular tissue and is protected by the sheath or prepuce. Included in the male reproductive system are a number of glands which produce fluids to carry the sperm when ejaculated.

The function of the female reproductive system is to produce eggs, and to carry the developing embryos until birth. The system consists of the ovaries, two small organs lying within the abdominal cavity which produce the eggs (ova), and the womb, which is concerned with the carrying of the embryos. The womb consists of two uteri (singular, uterus), each having a muscular band of tissue (a cervix) at the mouth. Two Fallopian tubes which have wide funnel mouths lead off from the other end of the uteri. The funnel-shaped mouths embrace the ovaries and receive the ova when they are shed. The uteri lead into the vagina, which opens into the vulva.

Ova are almost continuously being produced in the ovaries. When a doe is stimulated, usually by the actions of a male, then she will ovulate. That is to say, eggs are shed from the ovaries, and pass into the Fallopian tubes. Here, if the mating is successful, they will be met by the sperm, and on the union of a sperm and an egg, a zygote will be formed. This will later become the embryo.

The ovaries produce hormones which control a number of functions. There are of course a number of other glands in the body which produce hormones, and one of these, the pituitary gland, is responsible for the hormone which causes the egg to be shed. This gland is stimulated by excitement caused in the doe by the behaviour of the buck, and one hour after mating has occurred, i.e. the pituitary gland being stimulated, some hormone is released. This hormone causes the shedding of the eggs about ten hours after mating.

Within the cavities left by the shed ova, yellow tissue is formed. Each small mass of tissue is known as a corpus luteum, and one of its functions is to maintain the rest of the female reproductive system in a suitable state for pregnancy.

PREGNANCY

Pregnancy starts when an egg is united with a sperm. The fertilised egg starts to divide into new cells, at the same time passing down the Fallopian tube. After about four days the dividing egg which becomes the embryo reaches the uterus where it remains until birth. During these four days, and immediately afterwards, the uterus is preparing to receive the embryos. By the eighth day the outside cells of the embryo attack the walls of the uterus, and the uterine wall produces new cells. Thus the placenta is formed, part from the embryo, part from the uterus. Through the placenta oxygen and nutriment pass from the blood of the mother to the blood of the embryo, although the blood of both never mix.

Until about the middle of pregnancy, that is, about the 15th day, there is relatively little increase in the size of the doe's organs or the embryos. During the last half of pregnancy, however, the increase is very great, and the future of the litter, and certainly the milk supply of the doe, are greatly influenced by the doe's feeding during this period.

Pregnancy in the rabbit usually lasts some 31 days. There are many factors which may influence its duration; for example, the time of year, the size of the doe, and the size of the litter, all have an effect. Rabbits born on any day between the 28th day and the 34th day after mating usually survive. These extremes are, however, rare.

Usually a few days before the young are born, the doe will make a nest from her bedding. She will line this with fur plucked from her breast and belly, and there is some evidence that the time and the amount of nest building are influenced by inherited characteristics. It is, therefore, important to note the maternal characteristics of does and take these into account, with all other factors, in selecting future breeding stock. There is a tendency for the quality of nest building to improve from the first to the fourth or fifth nest, and this factor also should be taken into account when assessing the general level of nest building.

LACTATION

It is often said, with some truth, that the quality of rabbits is made in the nest. The first three weeks of the rabbit's life, when it should feed on milk from the doe only, are very important, and will affect its future growth, development and ability to thrive. The mammary glands which manufacture the milk start their development, for lactation, early in pregnancy. This development is relatively slow until about the last week of pregnancy when they develop rapidly, and milk may be produced by about the 29th day.

The growth and development of the mammary glands are much affected by the improvement in the physical condition of the doe throughout pregnancy. A doe which is in high condition at the start of pregnancy, and remains in that condition throughout the period, will not have such well-developed mammary glands as one which improves throughout the period. It is this improvement which is important. It must also be noted that there is an increased tendency to foetal atrophy or resorption in over-fat, or in poorly nourished, does.

During the lactation period, which usually lasts, at the most, about seven weeks (although the young may occasionally suckle after this period), the milk yield of a doe varies. It not only varies to some extent from day to day, but the average amount given varies. The milk yield varies also between does. Some does of the same size and breed, under the same conditions will give appreciably more than others. Part of the milk yield variation is due to inherited factors, the milk yield characteristic being of medium heritability.

The peak yield is reached at about three weeks and it remains at this highest level for a very short period before it begins to decline. The rate of decline is dependent on several factors. These include the level of nutrition of the doe, including the amount of water she is able to drink, the size of the litter she has been suckling, the age and number of litters the doe has previously had, whether she is pregnant and when she became pregnant.

The amount of food she is given and the level of the water intake are obvious factors, for they form a limiting factor to milk yield, particularly the water intake. The size of the litter has an important influence, for the larger the litter the larger the total milk yield is, although each youngster does not usually receive as much milk as would be the case had the litter size been smaller. The first lactation or two of the doe is lower than her average, and after a variable number of litters her average milk yield also declines. Whether the doe is pregnant or not has an important influence on the final level of milk yield, but more importantly on length of the lactation period.

It is unusual for an exhibition breeder to remate a doe whilst she is suckling young. This is, however, the reverse of what occurs in the intensive farming of rabbits, where the does are remated at any time from immediately post-partum (i.e. the day or the next day on which she kindles) to 21 or even 28 days after kindling. In the old type of rabbit farming, when does were rarely mated before the litter was weaned the doe was never lactating and pregnant. Indeed there was usually a rest period between the end of lactation and mating. In the case of the exhibition breeder there is usually such a rest period. To sum up these different states – in the most intensive forms of rabbit farming, the doe is pregnant and lactating for at least three-quarters of the time; in the case of the old type of farming, she was pregnant for slightly less than half of the time; and in the case of the exhibition breeder she may be pregnant for one-third of the time, but usually less.

If the doe is mated immediately post-partum, then the milk yield will commence to decline, at the latest, by the end of the third week, but usually earlier, and cease by about the end of the 26th day. In the case of the doe who is mated after two weeks post-partum, the decline will be slower and will cease at about the end of the sixth week. In the case of the doe who has had an interval of rest between late weaning and remating, the lactation period will continue to the seventh week, or even a few days longer.

Suckling by the young rabbits keeps the mammary glands in active operation, and therefore if they reduce their suckling, or if their number is reduced, the milk production will be lessened. The doe usually only suckles her young once a day, and then only for the very short period of three or four minutes. It is sometimes suggested that a system whereby the doe is prevented access to her nest except for a short early morning period might have benefits. There is, however, little point in such a system, for if the youngsters are properly fed by the doe they do not leave the nest and the doe does not enter it.

The milk of rabbits is the richest of all domestic animals. It contains from 13 to 15% of protein, 10 to 12% of fat, 2% of sugar, and 2 to 3% of minerals. The gross energy is about 8 to 12 MJ per kg, and this compares with about 2.8 to 4.2 MJ per kg for cow's milk and 6 to 9 MJ per kg for milk from the bitch. The very high value of rabbit's milk explains the rapid early growth of the animal, but it means also that the doe will require a good deal of food for the manufacture of the milk.

The amount of milk produced each day by the doe varies from as little as 40 g or even less per day, to over five times this figure or even more in the larger breeds. The richness and the volume of milk produced, coupled with the fact that, if she is pregnant the doe also requires nutrients for the developing embryos, means that her level of nutrition must be excellent. It is not surprising also that it is usual in cases of high producing does, that they are almost invariably called upon to supplement the feed which they get with the reserves in their bodies.

The yield of milk from the doe and the length of the lactation period is influenced by several factors, including inheritance. For this reason it is important that the yield of milk should be considered when selecting animals for future breeding. Unfortunately there is no simple direct method of measuring this yield, although a fairly reliable indirect method is the measurement of the weight of the litter at three weeks. There is also the fact that if the doe is not giving sufficient milk the young rabbits leave the nest early in search of other food. The reason why the total weight of the litter is a fairly reliable index is that the major limiting factor in growth is the supply of milk. There is, however, an important point which must be taken into consideration when this index is being used. The same doe will yield different amounts of milk with different sized litters, for although the amount of milk will increase with increasing size of litters, the amount of increase will not be in direct proportion. Further, the age of the doe will have some effect. The milk yield with the first litter of a doe will almost invariably be lighter than that with an equivalent litter which is her second or third, and an old doe will yield progressively less milk.

Prior to the introduction of high-level nutritional regimes (with the use of pelleted feeding stuffs) it was rare for a domestic rabbit to become pregnant whilst suckling, a condition opposite to that which occurs in the wild rabbit when feeding conditions are good. Under a low nutritional diet, although does might be mated and become pregnant up to about 10 days after kindling and again after the 30th day, between these dates she would rarely mate. Post-partum mating, i.e. mating within a few days of kindling, when the does are on a low plane of nutrition, are still almost invariably successful in that the does became pregnant, but they rarely carry the youngsters to full term, the litter being reabsorbed by the doe.

On a high plane of nutrition, this situation is changed. In order to obtain very high levels of meat production, that is to say, 50 or more youngsters per year reared to meat weight, or say a minimum of 80 kg of liveweight gain per doe per year, early re-mating and early weaning is used. Re-mating within 10 days of kindling with weaning at 24 to 28 days may be employed as one system. Alternatively re-mating at 21 to 28 days and weaning shortly thereafter can be used.

Some commercial farms insist that post-partum mating, that is, immediately after the doe litters, is necessary. These early re-mating systems are used only in commercial husbandry to produce large liveweight annual production. They undoubtedly shorten the productive life of the doe and necessitate very high feeding levels, as well as increasing the percentage of early mortality.

SEXUAL MATURITY AND PUBERTY

Puberty is reached when the rabbit is capable of producing viable ova or sperm, although rabbits may attempt to mate as much as two months before this stage of development. Puberty occurs a month or two or even more before the rabbit attains full sexual maturity, that is, the age when it attains full reproductive powers. As an example, a doe of a small breed might stand to the buck as early as three months, but be incapable of producing a litter until four months. She might then reach her full maturity at about six months. A larger-breed buck might reach puberty at 3.5 months or so but will not normally become fully sexually mature until about seven months of age. Age is not, however, the best criterion of sexual maturity, or of puberty. It is better to use weight as the most reliable measure. This naturally varies greatly from breed to breed, and indeed between strains of the same breed.

Different breeds and strains will reach puberty and sexual maturity at different times. The most important factors influencing these times are breed size and nutrition. The larger the breed the later, in general, it reaches puberty. As a rough general rule, puberty might be said to be reached when the animal is between 75 and 80% of its full normal adult weight. On this basic pattern, determined by weight, is imposed a good deal of variation due to the nutrition of the animal. The well-fed animal will develop much more quickly than the poorly fed specimen of the same breed. Maturity in body growth is closely related to maturity in sexual development, and therefore general development is a much better guide to the correct time for first mating than is any other.

BIRTH WEIGHT AND SEX RATIO

The birth weights of rabbits are rather variable, but it is in the interests of the rabbit breeder to strive towards as high birth weights as possible. The reason for this is that there is a considerable relationship between high birth weight and subsequent growth, development and ability to thrive.

There are a number of factors which affect birth weight. Of these, that having the greatest influence is the size of the mother. A doe weighing, say, 1.36 kg will on average have young weighing about 28 g, whilst a doe weighing, say, 5.44 kg may have young weighing as much as two-and-a-half times this weight.

The number in the litter also affects the weight of individuals. Young from a small litter may weigh twice as much as those from a large litter, other things being equal. Does fed well produce larger offspring than does fed badly. In the same way as milk yield is increased by an improving condition, so are the birth weights of the young. It might be stressed again that it is the improving condition in the doe which is important, not a high condition throughout pregnancy.

The length of time for which the young are carried, and the age of the mother, have some slight influence. The shorter the gestation period, and the younger the doe, the lighter will be the individual weights of young produced. It is sometimes said that males are heavier than females at birth. This is not so, and all evidence tends to prove that there is no difference in birth weight related to sex.

The secondary sex ratio (that is, the number of males per 100 females at birth) may vary, but it is almost certainly influenced by inherited tendencies. Figures for very large calculations of the secondary sex ratio have in two cases given results of 95 males per 100 females and 105 males per 100 females. Generally speaking, however, it is often found that slightly more males than females are produced. There is evidence that rather more males are produced at conception than females, for it is known that the pre-birth death rate is usually slightly higher for males than females.

There appear to be many factors which influence this sex ratio. In one experiment, numerous repeated matings at the same time by the same buck showed a great decrease in the number of males produced in the litters from these matings. In the first matings the ratio was 129 males per 100 females, but this dropped to 28 males per 100 females in litters resulting from the 20th mating on the same day, by the same buck. When two pure breeds are mated together, the number of males may be high, as also it will be during the early part of the spring and summer. The proportion of males may also increase as the doe produces further litters.

FERTILITY AND STERILITY

The ability of animals to produce living young is obviously of the greatest importance. Although rabbits are often the subject of jokes about great fertility, the rabbit breeder may sometimes be faced with difficulties in getting his stock to produce regularly. On occasions permanent sterility, from one of a number of causes, may occur, but this is generally not of such importance to the rabbit breeder, for the animal may be eliminated without serious loss. Even more occasionally a strain may become infertile, when of course there is little which can be done except to introduce new blood, or recommence with another strain. It is generally temporary sterility with which the breeder must contend.

Fertility and good bodily condition are closely related. One of the first bodily functions to suffer from poor management and, in particular, poor feeding, is the reproductive system. Excessive fatness and very poor condition both lead to sterility, but it must be remembered when the reasons for sterility are being sought, that sterility itself will often lead to excessive fatness.

Apart from nutrition, probably the most important factor (excluding disease) is under- or over-use. In the buck, periods of rest may result in a temporary sterility which, however, usually ceases after the first services. Long rests, or more frequently very much delayed first litters in does, may result in difficulty in getting the does pregnant. It often occurs that a doe being shown for a year or possibly two is then unsuccessfully mated. The reason is that the ovaries do not function normally and the solution in both cases is to ensure that the animals are bred at the proper times.

A doe will be extremely fertile immediately after kindling. Conception rate therefore tends to be much higher with immediate post-partum mating than at any other time. She will be of above average fertility immediately following the termination of pseudo-pregnancy, and she will conceive more easily immediately after weaning. A difficult doe should therefore be bred at one of these times.

As to the causes of other types of sterility, there are abnormalities of the reproductive system, but these are rare. Inbreeding may cause one of two types of sterility. In one type sterility is permanent, and the majority of the animals produced are completely infertile. In the other type, some early breeding is possible, but then a permanent sterility occurs. An inbreeding degeneracy to sterility should therefore be closely watched.

A buck whose testicles have failed to descend into the scrotal sacs is known as a cryptorchid or rig, and is invariably sterile. In some cases only one testicle descends and then the animal, a half rig, may or may not be sterile, although usually he is capable of producing sperm. Temporary sterility may be produced in bucks by high temperature. In Britain temperatures are rarely high enough for this to occur (except in houses with poor ventilation in hot weather), but it is a fairly common cause of temporary sterility in other countries with a hot climate.

There are infrequent cases of sterility between two particular animals. That is, a doe may never hold to a particular buck, but is fertile to other bucks. The buck itself is fertile to other does. A rare type of sterility in which the embryos do not survive until birth is inherited. There is some evidence that sterility in a strain may be associated with some forms of vices such as cannibalism or desertion of young, and also that good maternal characteristics usually go together. Good mothers are, generally speaking, highly fertile. It is probable that hormone treatment may result in the clearing up of some cases of sterility, but generally speaking this approach to the problem would be expensive, and the better way to tackle the matter is to breed for good fertility in the same way as for other desirable characteristics.

Apart from the question of permanent or temporary sterility, there is the problem of infertile matings. In some studs, where the standard of management is high, the number of matings per 100 litters may be as low as 110, whilst in some studs the average may be about 300. On average throughout the year probably half the matings, or rather less, are infertile, in the average stud. In commercial farming, where the does are mated post-partum or at weaning, at latest, conception rates are higher, usually averaging over 75%.

Infertile matings are a great inconvenience to the rabbit breeder, no matter what his or her ultimate aim. In the case of the commercial breeder there is loss due to decreased output with the same overheads. For the fancier there may be a missed chance of exhibiting at a particular show. For the laboratory there may be some disarrangement of experimental work.

The highest percentage of fertile matings occurs during the early summer. This is probably the result of improved nutrition, which gives an indication of the methods of maintaining good fertility, and also the light patterns under which the animals are kept. Good feeding, good management, and regular use are the most important.

PSEUDO-PREGNANCY

It will be remembered that the small yellow bodies or corpora lutea left in the cavities of the ovary after the eggs are shed produce certain hormones which maintain the rest of the reproductive system in the right condition for pregnancy. Now, if a doe is mated, and the mating is not fertile, then the eggs will have been shed and the corpora lutea formed. The hormones released by the corpora lutea will stimulate the remainder of the reproductive system and the doe will behave as though pregnant, although she is not.

This condition is known as pseudo-pregnancy. The mammary glands are stimulated to activity, the uterus increases in size, and so on. During proper pregnancy the corpora lutea, after the 16th day of pregnancy, are themselves maintained by other hormones from the placenta. If there are no placentas, as occurs in pseudo-pregnancy, then the corpora lutea of pseudo-pregnancy degenerate, the doe acts as though she were about to give birth to young, i.e. she makes a nest, and the mammary glands may even secrete some milk.

Pseudo-pregnancy continues for 16 to 18 days, and after this period the doe is highly fertile, and opportunity should be taken to mate her. It is only when the doe ovulates, but the eggs are not fertilised, that pseudo-pregnancy occurs, thus not every infertile mating results in this condition. Nevertheless in some studs the percentage of matings which result in pseudo-pregnancy is high, and as many as one-third may produce this result.

The nest building at the end of pseudo-pregnancy may be very slight, but any such signs as early as the 16th or 17th day after mating (or indeed sometimes quite a few days earlier) may be taken as a fairly reliable sign that the doe has been pseudo-pregnant.

The stimulation which causes the doe to shed eggs and thus produce this condition is usually the behaviour of a buck. It may also be produced, however, when one doe 'jumps' another, and for this reason does should not be run together if it is intended that they should be mated within three weeks.

Some cases of pseudo-pregnancy might be prevented by double matings, i.e. a second mating within at most five hours after the first. A mating later than this will have no effect. When the services of a buck are freely available, that is, when spare bucks are in use, then a second mating could be given and can be done to very good effect almost immediately after the first.

LITTER SIZE

No matter for what purpose rabbits are kept, the size of litters is a matter of some concern. In the commercial field the largest litters consistent with good growth are obviously desirable. Whilst fertility is a measure of the ability to produce viable young, fecundity is a measure of the number of young produced. Litter size is controlled by two different sets of factors. The first set are those of an inherited nature. The second include those of environment. Obviously the environmental factors will influence the doe only, but the inherited characters will affect both the buck and the doe.

Litter size is affected at ovulation, at fertilisation, and during pregnancy. At ovulation a certain number of eggs are shed. Some of these may not be fertilised, and some of the fertilised eggs may die during pregnancy. The potential fecundity of the doe is therefore the maximum number of eggs shed at ovulation, whilst the actual fecundity is the number of young born in each litter.

There are two basic hereditary influences. In general, the larger the breed, the higher the number of young produced in each litter. But at the same time, in strains of the same size, some hereditary factors occur for high or low fecundity. In the rabbitry where management and breed are the same for all animals, and large litter size is desired, preference should be given when selecting breeding stock to animals which have a high average litter size.

This applies to the bucks as well as the does, for inheritance of fecundity (which has a heritability lying between 0.2 and 0.3) can be transmitted through the male line as well as through the doe. Inheritance of fecundity is not controlled in a simple way by one or two genes. Thus the inheritance of this characteristic blends over a wide range.

Occasionally, when extra-large animals are desired, the breeder may unconsciously select breeding stock for smaller and smaller litter size. This is because he or she will often select for future breeding on the basis of size alone, and most frequently the size of young in small litters is greater than that of those in large litters.

Apart from inherited characteristics, nutrition, age of doe, number of previous litters, and disease all have an effect on the final litter size. Of these factors nutrition is the most important. A rising condition will produce the largest litter, and poor nutrition, over fatness, a falling condition and so on will lead to small litters. Litters born during the spring and summer are often larger than those born at other times of the year. But this is probably correlated with the better feeding condition then, for when nutrition is standardised throughout the year these variations tend to be reduced.

There is almost invariably an increase in litter size between the first and second litters, but thereafter, depending on the strain, variation occurs. In some strains the litter size continues to increase for some litters, in others it remains more or less stationary, in others it decreases. In some strains an increase may be noted up to an age of some three years, but eventually litter size decreases. It is rather the number of the litter than the age of the doe. Thus it might be truer to say that litter size increases for the first few litters and usually, but not invariably, decreases with increasing number of litters.

During the course of pregnancy, embryos may die for several reasons. Poor nutrition will cause the death and reabsorption of the litter. Apart from this, there are one or two diseases which cause death, but the most important factor is an inherited one which causes foetal atrophy. This factor is recessive, and when present in a homozygous state in the doe (for the character occurs in the doe and not in the embryos) the majority of embryos die. Following the death of the embryo it is either resorbed or aborted, depending mainly on the stage of pregnancy. In the early stages the embryos are reabsorbed whilst later on they are aborted.

Fertility (the ability to produce living young) and fecundity (a measure of the number of young produced) are closely connected. Strains showing high fertility are usually also highly fecund. But this general rule does not of course apply to the relationship between weight of adult and litter size, for in this relationship the small breeds (early maturing sexually) have smaller litters than do large breeds (late maturing sexually).

BREEDING PRACTICES

There are many lessons in correct breeding procedure to be learnt from a study of reproduction in domestic rabbits. Good breeding practice must be based on a knowledge of reproduction. One of the most important, as has been so often stressed before, is that concerned with the proper nutrition of the doe to produce the desired result.

The selection of animals for breeding, ignoring their inherited characteristics for the moment, depends on health, condition and age. No matter how good an animal may be because of its ability to transmit a good inheritance to its progeny, unless it has good health, and is in the right condition, it is not suitable for breeding. A sick doe cannot possibly be a good mother, and will almost certainly infect all her offspring if the sickness is due to a contagious condition.

Condition suitable for breeding is rather more difficult to define. The doe should not be fat, but should be well fleshed, and most important, she should be improving in condition. There is no doubt that over-fatness in does causes the death of many more embryos than is the case with does in good but lean condition.

AGE AT WHICH TO BREED

The correct age for first breeding is important. It is often wise to breed slightly before the age of sexual maturity, and in this the breeder should be guided by the bodily development of the animal rather than by a question of months. Too early an age is not desirable, but neither should an animal be left too long, except for some special reason such as showing, before it is mated.

Does will continue to breed in some cases for a number of years, but in general a three-year-old doe will often be discarded unless she is above average quality. In commercial rabbit farming, does on average are probably discarded after little more than a year's production.

In the case of the smaller breeds, for the exhibition breeder, four months at the earliest, and usually five or six months, is the age at which breeding should start. For the largest breeds, it is not usual to commence before six or seven months. In commercial farming, much earlier ages are the rule.

NUMBER OF LITTERS

The number of litters which a doe should be allowed to have during the year is often the subject of argument. In general the fancier will usually breed the doe twice and occasionally a third time. The aim of the commercial breeder should be to take anything between six and eight or even more litters a year from each doe. There is little harm likely to result from frequent breeding. Indeed, the reverse is true: if feeding and management are satisfactory, then frequent breeding is desirable.

A method sometimes adopted to obtain as many offspring as possible from a particular pair of animals is the repeated mating of the doe and the fostering of the young on to foster does. In this way as many as 11 litters can be taken in the year, the doe being remated immediately after kindling. Contrary to general belief, such a system imposes less strain on the doe than does intermittent pregnancies and suckling.

A similar system is sometimes used to increase average litter size and fertility. In some of the smaller breeds, the Netherland Dwarf in particular, difficulty may be experienced with breeding. Thus several does are mated at the same time, and average litters of five or six fostered on to some does, whilst the others are rebred. This assists in getting fertile matings, and also assists in keeping youngsters small, a desirable characteristic in these breeds.

MATING

The doe should never be mated in her own hutch, for this may lead to her resenting the intrusion of the buck and consequent fighting. She should always be placed in the buck's hutch, or in a special service hutch. It is of advantage to allow a buck at least his first services in his usual surroundings. Some bucks may refuse or be slow to serve in strange conditions.

The doe should not usually be left with the buck for any considerable period, and the mating, which should normally be accomplished in a very short time, should be observed. If no mating takes place within a few minutes then the doe should be removed and retried later, or immediately tried with another buck. By placing his hand in front of the doe, a breeder may sometimes make her stand to the buck instead of running from him.

As soon as the mating is completed, the buck falls backwards or, in the case of a less vigorous buck, scrambles from the doe. The falling of the buck is due to his becoming unbalanced. Often, when mating is accomplished, a scream will be heard. This is usually uttered by the buck, although it may occasionally be made by the doe. It is the result of some pain but is perfectly normal.

A method of assisted matings has been developed for use with reluctant does, and also in cases of shy bucks. The doe is grasped by the loose skin on the shoulders whilst with the other hand the hindquarters are slightly raised, the vulva being pressed backwards and upwards with the finger and thumb. The doe thus adopts the normal mating posture and is available for the buck. This system does not, in most cases materially affect the number of infertile matings, but is of assistance in procuring more matings than would otherwise be the case. In well managed commercial farms it is, however, rarely used.

The stud buck is a most important animal in a rabbitry, and should be used carefully. There is little doubt that young bucks are easily spoilt by over-use, but on the other hand it is equally true that fully mature bucks are not often given sufficient work. The first few services of a young buck should be well spaced; that is, one or at most two a week. When the buck is fully mature, and well managed and fed, he can accomplish six matings a week with ease. It has previously been mentioned that the first services of a buck which has been rested for a long period may be infertile, and in these cases a double mating should always be made.

Some authorities advocate regular double matings. This method is to mate a doe and then an hour or two later to mate her to a second buck. The system has usually little to recommend it, for a vigorous buck should accomplish all that is desired, and when two bucks are used the parentage is not known – a serious disadvantage for future selection. Double matings are, however, much favoured by some commercial breeders who believe that their percentage of infertile matings are reduced and their average litter size increased.

A buck should not be put to service immediately after feeding, for mating at such times imposes an unnecessary strain upon him. Similarly, it is better to space matings on the same day as much as possible. It must always be remembered that a stud buck used reasonably frequently is being worked hard, and should be well fed and looked after.

It is frequently said that the quality of the young is affected by the age of the buck. There is no truth whatsoever in this statement. Many breeders will discard a buck solely on the grounds of age. Such a practice should be strongly condemned. The older a buck gets, provided he still remains capable of service, the more valuable he may become, for the breeder will have a greater knowledge of his capabilities as a stock-getter. This argument also reinforces the desirability of the reasonably early use of a buck. The more young a buck begets, the more able is a breeder to assess his qualities, for the value of a stud buck lies entirely in his ability to transmit good characteristics to his progeny.

FOSTERING YOUNG

Fostering is the art of transferring offspring from one doe to another. There are advantages in using this art, but in some cases there may also be disadvantages. One disadvantage is that unless the newborn animals are well marked their true identity may be completely lost unless whole litters are transferred and the young of the foster doe destroyed. Secondly, the true value of the mother cannot be assessed unless she is left with a full-sized litter. Fostering enables a breeder to obtain young from a doe with particular characteristics, but very often her qualities as a milk producer and rearer of young are ignored. In general this is not very satisfactory.

On the other hand fostering does enable a breeder to produce a large number of young from a particular mating, and it also enables litter size to be averaged out, thus getting the best results. Sometimes when it is only desired to rear a particular type of animal, as for example reasonably well-marked patterned animals, fostering is of value. All the does are mated, the desired youngsters selected from all those produced and fostered on to one or two does, the remaining does being again mated. This same procedure may be adopted when animals of a particular sex are required, for example for laboratory use. When a doe dies, or produces her first litter, fostering may be of use. If, however, she dies from disease the young should not be fostered. Thus the decision to foster must depend upon the particular requirement of the individual breeder, and provided the objections are considered and overcome then fostering can be extremely useful.

Young rabbits up to the age of three weeks may be fostered, although at this late age it will not always be successful. When it is proposed to reduce a litter it is best to reduce it only after a few days. This is because suckling stimulates milk secretion, and consequently, by fostering only after a few days, the maximum activity of the mammary glands will have been achieved. As far as possible, however, fostering should be carried out within at most ten days of birth. Litters as much apart as three, or even more, days can be successfully amalgamated, although usually it is preferable that the litters should be as close in age as possible. When differently aged litters are being amalgamated it is of advantage to foster the younger animals and not the older.

Fostering is accomplished by transferring the young into the nest of the foster doe. It is advisable to remove the doe for a short period and then give her some tit-bit when she is returned to her hutch. Care should also be taken to observe that she takes to the youngsters and does not attack them. When a doe is being used as a foster for the first time, or her maternal characteristics are uncertain, it may be desirable to refuse her access to her nest for an hour or two, a practice which is perfectly satisfactory. Indeed in some cases does are barred from their nests for a number of hours at a time during the day.

DETERMINING WHETHER A DOE IS IN KINDLE

It is desirable for the breeder to be able to tell as soon as possible after a mating whether the mating has been successful. If the doe is not in kindle she can be remated, or a watch kept for signs of her being pseudo-pregnant. If the doe proves to be in kindle then she can be managed and fed accordingly.

The most reliable method, and that giving the earliest confirmation of pregnancy, is palpation of the abdomen. The method consists of feeling the abdomen to decide whether developing embryos are present in the uterus. The tips of the fingers should gently press the abdomen just in front of the pelvis, when, if the doe is pregnant, the embryos can be felt. These are about the size of marbles (between the 12th and 14th day), but care should be taken to make sure that the faecal pellets are not mistaken for the embryos. If a pregnant doe of about 12 days duration is sacrificed and opened, then the relative position and size of the organs can be determined easily. It is important when palpating the abdomen that the doe should be relaxed, for tightened abdominal muscles make the task more difficult. Does cannot be palpated easily before about the 12th day of pregnancy.

A method, which, although widely considered of value, is not at all reliable, is that of test mating. The doe is returned to the buck some days after mating and it is assumed that if she accepts the buck then she was not pregnant, whereas if she refuses the buck it is assumed that she was. A pregnant doe will often accept the buck during pregnancy, and a doe not in kindle may sometimes refuse him.

The third method which may be employed on about the 24th day of pregnancy is quite reliable and consists in noting the increase in thickness of the mammary glands. The mammary glands start to increase in thickness about the middle of pregnancy, and by the 24th day are sufficiently different from mammary glands in non-pregnant does to be easily distinguished. It is of advantage to feel the thickness of the glands in a known non-pregnant doe at the same time as testing the supposed pregnant doe, until the breeder becomes experienced.

ARTIFICIAL INSEMINATION

The domestic rabbit has been widely used to develop artificial insemination (AI) techniques and thus the correct techniques are well known and available, although they require experience and skill.

AI has been used in some cases on very large farms and may have advantages for the specialist breeder. There are a number of advantages in special circumstances. These include:

- one buck can be used to service considerably more does than is possible with normal matings;
- possible disease transmission is eliminated, provided the strictest hygiene precautions are taken;
- large batches of does can be mated at the same time, thus allowing much easier management in the commercial field, with larger batches of uniform animals being available;
- animals which are very different in size can be easily mated;
- there is no need to make certain that all does to be mated are in the right condition, for an injection of a chemical to induce ovulation is given;
- in with sufficient numbers there is a saving in the time required for the mating operation.

For the small breeder, however, it is doubtful whether it has advantages.

Briefly, the technique involves the collection of sperm from the buck in an artificial vagina, consisting of a glass tube about 30 mm in diameter into which is fitted a rubber sleeve. This sleeve terminates in a small tube. Warm water is introduced into the large tube and thus warms the rubber sleeve. The artificial vagina is held between the legs of the doe or in an artificial muff, and the buck induced to serve into it. The semen is collected in the small tube and is examined micro-scopically to check that it is a good sample, that is that the proportion of good and active spermatozoa is high and that the concentration of spermatozoa is good. The semen is then diluted up to about 15 times its original volume with a suitable solution and then kept under carefully controlled temperature conditions. Each good diluted sample can be used to inseminate five or six does.

Before insemination the doe must be made to ovulate, that is to shed eggs which must be fertilised. In the earliest AI procedures this was sometimes done by mating with a buck which had been made sterile by surgical operation. Now, however, the doe is ovulated by injection of an appropriate synthetic hormone. The semen is then introduced into the vagina with the aid of a glass syringe or pipette.

Conception rates obtained by AI differ little from those obtained by normal mating. When well performed, both conception rates are about the same.

Chapter 9

Genetics and Improvement

The development of each of the physical characteristics of the rabbit is controlled by one or more units of its heredity. That these characteristics may be altered in life, even to a fair degree, by the environment in which the rabbit lives, does not affect this basic law.

Some of the major controlling 'units' or genes, as they are termed, have been identified, as well as the mechanism by which the characteristics produced are inherited. There are, in addition, many others which have not been identified, and many more which produce too small an effect by themselves for their identification to be possible. Nevertheless, when a breeder is selecting stock for a particular character or characters, a knowledge of how these are inherited will make the work easier and more interesting, and may in many ways save the breeder time.

THE MECHANISM OF INHERITANCE

The entire inheritance which a rabbit receives from its dam and sire is contained in the egg from the doe and a single sperm from the buck which unites with this egg. Both the sperm and the egg contain a minute body known as the nucleus, and these nuclei each contain 22 sausage-like bodies known as chromosomes. All cells of the body contain 22 pairs of chromosomes, but each egg and each sperm contain only one of each pair, that is, 22 single chromosomes. Thus when the sperm and the egg unite, forming the new body, the 22 single chromosomes from one join with the 22 chromosomes from the other, once again forming the 22 pairs in the new individual.

On each chromosome are located a very large number of even smaller bodies, the genes. Normally the same genes are present at the same point on the same chromosome. This point is the locus of the gene. As the chromosomes are in pairs, one gene on one of the chromosomes will become the pair to the gene on the other chromosome.

Each gene pair which has been identified is usually labelled with a letter, and the capital is used to denote the dominant gene, whilst the recessive gene is labelled with the smaller letter. Originally each pair of genes was identical, but in many cases they have changed (that is, mutated) and when this occurs, and the mutated gene produces a change in a characteristic of the rabbit, the 'changed' type of rabbit is spoken of as a mutation, or a mutant. The mutant gene, of course, is still a pair with the original gene, and the animal produced may or may not show the mutant characteristic, depending on whether the mutated gene is dominant or recessive to the original gene. An example will make this clear.

The original Agouti rabbit contained a gene *A* which produced the distinctive Agouti pattern. This gene mutated at one time to a gene which produces a self pattern. Thus if a germ cell containing the original gene *A* unites with a germ cell containing the mutant gene *a*, the resulting rabbit will contain in its body-cells the gene pair *Aa*. As gene *A* is dominant to gene *a* (see below), the rabbit will look like an Agouti but will carry the gene for self pattern.

This *Aa* rabbit will produce germ cells containing either gene *A* or gene *a*. The doe will produce eggs which may be *A* or *a* and the buck will produce sperm which are either *A* or *a*. If rabbits of this genetical constitution are mated together there will be four possibilities:

- the *A* gene in the egg may combine with the *A* gene in the sperm giving a pure Agouti *AA*;
- the *A* gene in the egg may combine with the *a* gene in the sperm giving an Agouti-looking rabbit which carries the gene for self colour *Aa*;
- the *a* gene in the egg may unite with the *A* sperm giving an impure Agouti *Aa*;
- the *a* gene in the egg may combine with the *a* gene in the sperm giving an animal which is self coloured, being of the constitution *aa*.

This can be shown diagrammatically by using a system of squares or checkerboard (Table 9.1).

Table 9.1 Segregation of genes *Aa* + *Aa*

		The sperm from the buck must contain	
		either large *A* gene	or little *a* gene
The egg from the doe must contain	either large *A* gene	New individual *AA*–pure Agouti	New individual *Aa*–impure Agouti
	or little *a* gene	New individual *Aa*–impure Agouti	New individual *aa*–pure self

When a rabbit is pure for a particular gene pair, that is, when each of the genes of a pair is the same, the rabbit is known as a homozygote, and it is homozygous for that gene. When a rabbit is impure for a gene pair, that is, it contains different genes in the gene pair, it is known as a heterozygote and it is heterozygous for that gene. The physical appearance of any rabbit is called its phenotype, and its genetic constitution is known as its genotype. The *AA* rabbit and the *Aa* rabbit are both phenotypically Agoutis, but the *Aa* rabbit has the genotype *Aa*.

In the above example homozygous rabbits *AA* if mated together will always breed true for Agouti colour, and homozygous *aa* rabbits will always breed true for the self colour, but the heterozygote *Aa* will not. If bred together the *Aa* rabbits will produce pure Agoutis, impure (heterozygous) Agoutis, and selfs, in the proportion of 1:2:1. The proportions of the phenotypes of the animals will be 3 Agoutis to 1 self.

If the heterozygote *Aa* is mated to the homozygote *aa*, then the proportions of the progeny will be different again. Half of the animals will be heterozygous Agoutis, and the other half homozygous selfs. This can again be shown on a checkerboard (Table 9.2).

Table 9.2   Segregation of genes *Aa* + *aa*

		Germ cells from *Aa* parent must contain	
		either large *A*	or little *a*
Germ cells from aa parent must contain	little a	New individual *Aa*– heterozygote Agouti	New individual *aa*– homozygote self

It will be noted that the homozygote *AA* and the heterozygote *Aa* will both be Agoutis. This is because a single gene *A* will produce the Agouti pattern, irrespective of whether the other gene of the pair is *A* or *a*. The *A* gene is said to be dominant, as it dominates the expression of the character, whilst the *a* gene is said to be recessive for if it is combined with a dominant gene in a pair, the character it normally produces is suppressed. Thus it will be seen that an animal homozygous for a pair of recessive genes will always breed true for the character produced by those genes.

To summarise, each individual contains very many paired sets of genes, having received one gene of each pair from each of its parents. In turn the individual passes on to its progeny only one or other of the genes of each pair, which combines with the other gene of the pair from the other parent. In this way a number of different combinations of genes is possible in each generation. The separating of the gene pairs and their recombination in each new generation is known as segregation.

In some cases the mutation from the original gene mutates again. This has occurred in the Agouti gene *A*. In addition to the mutant form *a*, there is another mutant form *a^t*, which produces a tan pattern. These different genes are also called alleles. In the Agouti allelic series there are therefore three genes. It is important to remember, however, that in any series of genes, only two can be carried by any animal. A rabbit in the above example can be either: *Aa*; *AA*; *Aa^t*; *a^t a^t*; *a^t a*; or *aa*.

In the case of genes which show complete dominance, there is no difference in the appearance of the homozygote or the heterozygote carrying the dominant genes. Not all mutated gene pairs, however, have one gene which dominates the other. In some cases the heterozygote has a completely different appearance from either of the homozygotes. This is well illustrated in the case of the inheritance of the English pattern.

The English pattern is controlled by a gene *En* which is not completely dominant to the recessive form *en*. The homozygote *enen* is a self-coloured rabbit with no spots. The homozygote *EnEn* is a very lightly spotted English, known in the exhibition world as a 'Charlie'. The familiar exhibition English is the heterozygous form *Enen*. If exhibition type English are mated together, only 50% exhibition type are produced, together with 25% Charlies, and 25% self coloured. If Charlies are mated with selfs, then 100% English type are produced; if Charlies are mated to Charlies, only Charlies are produced; and selfs mated together will give selfs only. This is shown diagrammatically in Table 9.3.

Table 9.3   Segregation of the English pattern genes

Crossing English with English — English genes

English genes	En	en
En	EnEn Charlie	Enen English
en	EnEn English	enen self

Crossing Charlie with self — Charlie genes

self genes	En	En
en	Enen English	Enen English
en	Enen English	Enen English

Crossing Charlie with Charlie — Charlie genes

Charlie genes	En	En
En	EnEn Charlie	EnEn Charlie
En	EnEn Charlie	EnEn Charlie

Crossing English with Charlie — English genes

Charlie genes	En	en
En	EnEn Charlie	Enen English
En	EnEn Charlie	Enen English

Crossing self with self — self genes

self genes	en	en
en	enen self	enen self
en	enen self	enen self

Crossing English with self — English genes

self genes	En	en
en	Enen English	enen self
en	Enen English	enen self

SEX CHROMOSOMES

One pair of the 22 pairs of chromosomes carry genes which are responsible for determining sex. In the male, this pair of chromosomes is not identical, as it is in the female. One of the male sex chromosomes is known as the Y chromosome, and the other as the X chromosome, these two forming the pair. In the female, both sex chromosomes are identical, both being X. Thus the male will give germ cells which carry either the Y chromosome or the X chromosome, whilst the female will give eggs which all carry the X chromosome. Thus when a sperm containing a Y chromosome unites with an egg containing an X chromosome, the resulting individual will be a male XY, whilst when a sperm containing an X chromosome unites with an egg, which must contain an X chromosome, a female XX is produced. In some animals certain genes which lie on the sex chromosomes have been identified, and the characters which they produce are therefore linked with sex. That is, the genes on the male chromosome (the Y chromosome) will always produce the characters in the male, and vice versa. As yet no sex-linked characters have been recorded in the rabbit.

EPISTASIS

Epistasis occurs when there is one gene on a chromosome which prevents another gene on the same chromosome from having its full effect. For example, an Albino rabbit has gene *c* which prevents its true colour from being developed. Thus an Albino is a coloured animal which shows no colour because of an epistatic gene.

LINKAGE

Each chromosome contains many thousands of genes, and it follows therefore, that genes lying on the same chromosome would apparently always remain together. When two genes lie on the same chromosome they are said to be linked, and they do in fact remain linked to a much greater degree than genes lying on different chromosomes. They do not, however, invariably remain so linked.

The reason for this is that during the process when the sex cells are being formed, the chromosomes of each pair join together. Segments of each chromosome in the pair may be exchanged, and thus genes previously lying on one chromosome may, after this process, lie on its pair. This crossing-over of chromosome pairs does interfere with the normal segregation ratios. Thus the gene producing yellow fat is linked to the gene producing albinism, and therefore these two characters are more often associated together than they would be if they were carried on separate chromosomes. Obviously the more closely together on the chromosome that the two genes lie, the more unlikely are they to be exchanged,

In the rabbit some 10 linkage groups have been identified, together with over 100 gene variations, although many of these are of little concern to the rabbit breeder. Before discussing those of interest to the rabbit breeder, some reference should be made to modifying genes.

POLYGENIC INHERITANCE AND MODIFIERS

If a Lop-eared rabbit with an ear length of some 30 cm is crossed with a rabbit having a short ear, the first generation will have ear lengths approximately between the two. If the animals of this first generation (known as the F1 generation) are mated together, the second generation animals (known as the F2 generation) will have ears varying in length from that of the short-eared parent to that of the Lop. This is due to the fact that ear length is controlled by a number of minor genes or modifiers. Such a type of inheritance is known as a blending or polygenic inheritance.

In the same way, although a number of different rabbits may be blue, the actual shade of blue may vary considerably. The inheritance of the blue colour is basically controlled by one gene, but many modifying genes act upon the colour to produce the particular shade. This to some extent explains why a skilled breeder is able to select his stock to produce a particular result. The breeder is (albeit unconsciously in many cases) selecting for stock which carry the modifying genes which he or she desires in the progeny. Again, the original wild grey Agouti colour of the Belgian Hare has been greatly modified to the rich chestnut colour of the present day by the accumulation of modifiers in the genotype of the breed.

It can be seen that if the effect produced by a single gene is too small to identify, then it is probably produced by a modifying gene, but when a number of modifiers act together, the result may be appreciable. These modifiers may be linked to the major gene, the result of which they modify, although it is believed that in general they are more often transmitted independently of the major gene.

Probably the majority of what might be termed the utilitarian characteristics of the rabbit, that is, reproductive capacity, growth rate, milk yield, carcase conformation, food conversion ability, coat density and so on, are controlled by modifying genes. The inheritance of these characteristics is therefore termed polygenic, that is, controlled by a number of genes.

It is necessary to appreciate the very important role played by modifying genes. The art of all breeding consists in increasing the number of desirable genes, modifiers or otherwise, in future generations of animals. As the domestic rabbit gains in economic importance, so it becomes more desirable to improve its efficiency and its products. Only by a thorough grasp of the basic essentials will the breeder be able to do this in a satisfactory fashion.

HETEROSIS OR HYBRID VIGOUR

A phenomenon, known as heterosis occurs when two lines of relatively different genetic purity are crossed. That is to say, the cross produces animals which are significantly better than either of the two parent lines. In general, the greater the genetic difference between the two lines, the greater the effect of heterosis. This is of course the basis on which pure lines are sold to rabbit breeders, the animals being used as the breeding stock. The progeny or F1 generation are only of use for utilitarian purposes and not for the selection of future breeding stock.

The measurement of heterosis is by the difference in the particular characteristics being considered (e.g. litter size, weight at weaning, etc.) of the average of the two parent lines against the value for the F1 generation. The magnitude of heterosis may sometimes be as high as some 20% for some characteristics. Heterosis, however, is of use only in the matter of the production of 'utility' products of the rabbit.

Very similar to heterosis, is the nicking of some breeds or individual pairs. Nicking means that particular crosses, whether it be of breeds or individual pairs produce a result which is much better than is usually produced by either breed, or either parent, with other breeds, or other individuals. It might be regarded as selective heterosis, but its use to rabbit breeders of particular breeds, can be substantial.

COAT COLOUR AND TYPE

Table 9.4 gives details of all the genes affecting coat colour and type which have so far been identified. There are a number of other mutations which are of less interest to the practical rabbit breeder. These control such things as the inheritance of blood groups, changes in body structure, various abnormalities and so on. From Table 9.4, particulars of the genes which any breed must contain, i.e. its genotype or genetical constitution, can be determined.

Table 9.4 Identified genes for colour and coat. The table gives details, with gene symbols, of those genes which have so far been established and which are of use to the rabbit breeder. In all at the present time, some 100 different gene pairs or allelic groups have been identified. Because in many parts of Europe, German gene symbols are used, these are added in a second column. It is to be greatly regretted that there is no single international set of symbols

Series	Gene symbol		Gives rise to
	English	German	
Agouti	A	G	Agouti pattern
	a^1	g^o	Tan pattern
	a	g	Self colour
Black pigmentation	B	C	Black colour, found in normal Agouti; when combined with a^t gives black tan; when combined with a gives self-coloured black
	b	c	Brown (chocolate) colour; when combined with A gives brown Agouti; when combined with a^t gives chocolate tan; when combined with a gives self brown
Dilution	D	D	Dense colour
	d	d	Dilute colour; when combined with B gives blue colour; when combined with b gives lilac colour
Colour	C	A	Full colour
	C^{chd}	a^d	Dark chinchillation, i.e. elimination of yellow from Agouti pattern; blue eyes; produces normal chinchilla
	C^{chm}	a^{chi}	Medium chinchillation; not normally seen
	C^{chl}	a^m	Light chinchillation; brown eyes, as found in sables
	C^h	a^n	Himalayan character; an albino with colour developed at the extremities
	c	a	Albinism; prevention of development of all colour
Extension of black	E^D	B^{ee}	Dominant black, increases development of black in Agouti pattern, preventing nearly all ticking; and dark colour to belly; not completely dominant to E, thus $E^D E^D$ produces darker animals than $E^D E$, which produces steel
	E^s	B^e	Steel grey
	E	B	Normal extension of black as found in Agouti
	e^i	b^i	Harlequin pattern
	e	b	Exclusion of black which in Agouti animals thus produces yellow animals with white bellies; when combined with homozygote BB produces tortoiseshells
Vienna white	V	X	Normal colour; the heterozygote is a coloured rabbit with white nose or feet as v is incompletely recessive
	v	x	Blue-eyed white
Wide band	W	$Y^1 Y^2 Y^3$	Normal Agouti band of yellow
	w	$y1\ y^2\ y^3$	Yellow band in Agouti pattern increased producing an Agouti more yellow than usual

Table 9.4 continued

Series	Gene symbol		Gives rise to
	English	German	
English spotting	*En*	*K*	English spotting; *En* is incompletely dominant to *en*; heterozygote *Enen* gives exhibition type English; homozygote *enen* selfs, and homozygote *EnEn* lightly spotted animals
	en	*k*	No spotting, i.e. self colour
Dutch pattern	*DU*	$S_1 S_2 S_3$	No markings
	*du*w	$s_1 s_2 s_3$	Dutch markings; incompletely recessive; the inheritance of the pattern is not entirely understood but certainly several major genes and a number of modifying genes are involved
	*du*d		
Silvering	*Si*	$P^1 P^2 P^3$	Non silvered ⎫ Inheritance of silvering not completely
	*s*i	$p^1 p^2 p^3$	Silvered ⎭ understood; certainly polygenic
Rex coat	R_1	Rex	*R* is the normal coat and r_1 is the Rex coat; r_2 is the German (short hair) Rex coat and r_3 is the Normandy; the three pairs of genes producing the three Rex coats (which are not distinguishable in appearance) are quite distinct; r_1 and r_2 are borne on the same chromosome, but r_3 is on another; to produce the Rex coat the animals must be homozygous for any recessive pair; the Rexes found in this country are r_1
	r_1	rex	
	R_2	Dek	
	r_2	dek	
	R_3	Nok	
	r_3	nok	
Angora coat	*L*	*V*	Normal coat
	l	*v*	Angora coat or long hair
Satin coat	*Sa*	*Sa*	Normal coat
	sa	*sa*	Satin coat
Waved coat	*WA*		Normal coat
	wa		Waved coat; only produced in very fine coated Rex; with modifiers the homozygote is the Astrex

A knowledge of the genetical constitution of the rabbit, and the mechanism of the inheritance of the characters produced, will enable the breeder to combine in one strain of rabbits particular characteristics which he or she desires, with the least waste of time and material. The breeder can select the colour from one variety, the coat type from another, and even the coat length from another.

THE OBJECTS OF IMPROVEMENT

When the first simple laws of genetics became widely known amongst rabbit breeders, it was thought that a knowledge of them would solve the breeders every problem. This was not of course the case, and it is necessary to consider the art of improvement as a whole.

Improvement entails the selection of suitable animals in order that in the future generation genes for desirable characteristics will be encouraged, or brought together, and genes for undesirable characteristics will be eliminated. The average quality of the stock will then progress towards the ideal.

The ends to which breeders strive vary widely. On the one hand a breeder may wish to produce, at no matter what expense, several animals which conform closely to an artificial standard of excellence. On the other hand, the aim may be the improvement of the average animal in the 'utilitarian characteristics', such as increased litter size, better milking qualities, better pelts, better food conversion or quicker growth.

The ideal animal will not be the same for all breeders. One may wish to keep the stock under a particular environment, another may wish to produce high quality pelts, another flesh at the cheapest cost. No two aims can be identical, and no single method can achieve them. The breeder must understand the general principles and adapt them to his or her own circumstances. The selection of two animals for mating to give a desired result is still an art, based though it be, or should be, in most cases on the measurement (generally by eye) of the desired characters, or a knowledge of the constitution of the parents.

Generally speaking, breeders cannot select for one character alone. They must base their selections on a number of points. The breeders will bring together in their studs the qualities which exist in different animals in the breed. The concentration of good points and the elimination of bad ones is the essence of livestock improvement. But improvement must be balanced. To aim for the concentration of good points whilst forgetting the elimination of bad ones may destroy the work of years. A difficulty arises in that the larger the number of characteristics the breeder wishes to select for, in general the slower the improvement will be.

As will be seen below, characteristics in an animal are the result of its inheritance and its environment. The improvement in the genetical quality of stock can only be made if the environment allows the full expression of the genetical characters. Thus there are two aspects to the improvement of stock – the improvement of the inherited characteristics of the animal and the improvement of the environment.

ENVIRONMENT AND INHERITANCE

The environment of an animal consists of all those factors which influence it in any way but which are not inherited. The major group of environmental factors include diet, housing, management, and contact with disease, but there are many others. All factors that cause stress in any way are part of the environment of the animal as also are such things as the size of the litter into which the animal was born and so on. The importance of these environmental factors are very little appreciated although they have a profound effect on the animal.

Some characteristics of the rabbit are more affected by inheritance than by environment, and others more by environment than inheritance. For example, the coat colour of a rabbit is determined by its inheritance. Certainly it may be slightly changed by some external influences (sunlight may fade it) but the colour and the pattern are fixed by the animal's genetical constitution. On the other hand, such a character as milk yield in does, although again influenced to some extent by inheritance, is affected by environment, especially diet, by the suckling of young and the parity of the litter.

The environment of animals may limit the expression of some inherited characteristics. For example, if the rabbit has a genetic constitution for large size, that size cannot be fully attained unless the environment (particularly diet, housing, and management) is sufficiently good. Nowhere is this relationship between environment and inheritance more clearly seen than in the reproduction of rabbits. The broad pattern of fecundity, for example, is determined by inherited factors, but superimposed on this pattern are a number of limitations and modifications due to environment.

The age of sexual maturity is a matter of both inheritance and environment. Generally speaking, the larger the breed, the later it becomes sexually mature. But young born in the spring of the year have an older age of sexual maturity than do those of the same strain born in the late summer and autumn.

It may be that sometimes a breeder will not wish to improve the environment under which the stock are kept. He or she may, for example, wish to rear young meat rabbits on a roughage-only diet. The ideal animal which the breeder will select will not be the same as that selected by a breeder who wishes to rear meat animals very intensively, with the fastest growth rate.

In the first case, the breeder will select stock which thrive best on the roughage diet. For the second, he or she will select animals which have the quickest growth rate on concentrate feeding. The animals having the best growth rate under good conditions may not have any ability to grow well under poor conditions. In their case, growth rate will be masked or hidden by the poor diet. It is likely to be impossible to select the animals with the best growth rate when a poor diet is fed.

The rabbit breeder is fortunate amongst livestock breeders because he or she can control the environment to an extent. One breeder may wish to breed the best possible stock under a certain rather poor environment. Another may wish to breed the best stock under the best environment he or she can establish. The two aims are quite different. In the first case, the breeder will simply select the animals which fare best under the poor environment. In the second case the breeder must continually seek to improve the environment. The breeder may achieve the maximum possible genetic improvement under the environment, and then only when he or she improves the environment will further improvement, genetically, be possible.

Although improved environment can achieve a good deal of short-term improvement, long-term benefits can only be achieved by genetic improvement. The changes made in an animal during its life, which are due entirely to environment, affect only that one individual animal. The improvement is not passed on to the progeny. But good conditions will allow the breeder to see the good qualities of the stock. It is necessary to improve both inheritance and environment to allow the full expression of the genotype.

One word of caution should be added. Apparent improvement, say in growth rate, may not be real when economic considerations are taken into account. For example, the ability of a strain to grow fast might be greatly improved, but the needs of the 'improved' stock in the way of concentrated rations might be more costly kilogram for kilogram of flesh produced, than the needs of the 'unimproved' stock.

It can be seen, then, that the breeder is faced with two problems. The first is to supply the animals with an environment which will allow them to develop to the full the inherited characters which the breeder wishes to select. The second is to distinguish between the effects of the inheritance of the animal and the effects of its environment.

HERITABILITY

In those cases most familiar to rabbit breeders, the inherited characteristic in the young is the same as in the parent. That is the characteristic is controlled by a single gene. For example, the basic colour of the young is the same as the parents. But there are other characteristics of the rabbit which are inherited to different degrees. For example, such things as litter size and wool yield in Angoras are to some extent inherited, but the degree is sometimes difficult to establish.

The amount by which any characteristic is inherited is called the degree of heritability. The degree of heritability is calculated by measuring the resemblance for the characteristic (or phenotype) which occurs in the general population on the one hand and the doe/young group on the other. The scale on which this is calculated runs from 0 to 1. Some characteristics, for example coat colour, have a degree of 1, that is to say, that characteristic is totally inherited. Other characteristics are not inherited at all and therefore have a degree of 0. A low degree of heritability runs from 0.01 to 0.10. A high degree of heritability runs from 0.40 upwards.

The higher the degree of heritability of the characteristics for which selection is made, the faster will be the rate of improvement. It is therefore desirable in a commercial unit to select those characteristics which have a higher degree of heritability, and of course only those characteristics which have an economic value.

Possible selection criteria for commercial meat rabbits, with their degree of heritability, are given in Table 9.5.

Table 9.5 Possible criteria for selection of commercial meat stock (degree of heritability in brackets)

- Number of teats on doe (Low)
- Temperament of doe (Med.)
- Life performance of doe, i.e.
  - number of litters (Low)
  - number of young in total (Low)
  - total weight of all young at 21 days (Med.)
- Pregnancy rate (i.e. % pregnancies resulting from all matings or AI (Med.))
- Young:
  - number born alive/dead (Med.)
  - number surviving to 7 days (Low)
  - number alive at 21 days (Low)
  - number alive at slaughter (Low)
  - weight at 21 days (Med.)
  - weight at slaughter (High)
  - total feed consumption to weaning (Med.)
  - total feed consumption to slaughter (Med.)
  - carcase conformation and quality (High)
  - carcase fat-distribution and colour (High)
  - carcase dressing-out % (High)

SYSTEMS OF BREEDING

There is a variety of different breeding systems adopted by rabbit breeders. The commonest is 'like to like' matings. No system is ideal for all purposes, and the particular system the breeder adopts will depend upon his or her requirements.

Inbreeding

Inbreeding is a mating system in which animals more closely related than the average are mated. Usually the term is reserved for close inbreeding, that is to say, brother to sister, or parent to offspring. Inbreeding leads to a greater degree of genetical purity in the line in which it is carried out, and the animals of that line or family will tend to become more uniform in genetical constitution. If (as is almost certain) undesirable genes were present in the stock when inbreeding was commenced, then the characters produced by these genes will quickly appear. There is therefore a tendency for inbred stock to degenerate initially. This degeneracy may be overcome after a few generations, when a strain genetically pure for certain characters would have been established. Some inbred lines, however, die out and because inbreeding leads quickly to the appearance of undesirable characters in the stock, culling must be severe.

   Close, consistent inbreeding may be a valuable breeding system in the hands of the experienced and relatively large-scale breeder, but in general its disadvantages to the average breeder outweigh its advantages. True close inbreeding is a system rarely found in rabbit keeping, although many breeders practising other breeding systems believe that they are using it.

Line breeding

The majority of breeders who claim to inbreed are probably line breeding in some form or another, and this system is often the most satisfactory. Line breeding itself is a form of inbreeding, but is less intense. The object of all line breeding is to keep the strain related to particular animals, or their direct descendants. Usually the animals to which stock are line bred are bucks, but may just as easily be does. In line breeding, animals are mated together which are both descended from the particular animal, but otherwise are as distantly related as possible.

   The pedigrees below show two forms of line breeding. A is mated to B to produce C, which is mated to A to produce D, which is mated to A to produce E. This is the closest possible form of line breeding. In the second pedigree F is mated to G to produce H, and F is mated to I to produce J. H and J are mated together to produce K which, having F as both its grandsires, is nearly as closely related to F as to its parents (Table 9.6). Line breeding will therefore increase the purity of the stock in relation to the qualities of a particular animal and its descendants. Selection of the right animals, with good culling, is of course of great importance.

Table 9.6   Two forms of line breeding

A × B   F × G   F × I
   C × A   H × J
      D × A   K
         E

Like-to-like breeding

Like-to-like or assortive mating means the mating of animals which are similar in appearance, but not necessarily (or even usually) similar in genetic constitution. It is therefore unlike inbreeding. Assortive mating does not 'fix' characteristics in a stud as does any form of inbreeding. On the contrary, it tends to keep the stud genetically variable.

The similarity of the progeny to their parents is increased and with good culling the uniformity in appearance of the animals in a stud can be increased. But this uniformity can only be maintained by severe selection and can only be 'fixed' by some form of inbreeding.

Corrective mating

Corrective mating, that is, the mating of unlike to unlike animals, is also much used by the rabbit breeder. It is a system in which animals with certain excellent characteristics and certain weaknesses are mated to animals with the reverse characteristics. Thus the failings of the one are compensated by the good points of the other. Any particular type can be held uniform by this system, but again that type cannot be 'fixed' unless some form of inbreeding or line breeding is resorted to.

Both assortive and corrective systems keep the stock genetically variable, and therefore tend to produce one or two excellent animals. These, however, do not necessarily breed true. For the production of one or two 'flyers' from a stud in which the average quality, apart from the occasional really good ones, is not of great importance, the system works satisfactorily.

Cross-breeding

Cross-breeding implies the mating together of animals from two distinct and pure, or relatively pure, breeds. It sometimes happens that the first generation progeny of these matings may be excellent, in fact the average quality is usually better than the parents. This is due to the fact that generally, good dominant genes from one breed, acting together with good dominant genes from the other, suppress the effects of undesirable recessive genes which might have been homozygous in one or other of the parents. It may also be due to the combination of the good characteristics of both parents.

The disadvantage of the system, however, is that if the cross-bred animals from the first generation are mated together, a very variable, and often very unsatisfactory, second generation is produced. The undesirable recessives segregate out after being temporarily covered up in the first generation.

For any satisfactory system of cross-breeding, therefore, two distinct lines or breeds must be maintained, and only animals from these lines used for breeding, with all the cross-bred stock being utilised for other purposes or, particularly if different breeds are being used, 'back crossed' to a sire of the first breed. This system is adopted with success in some cases, but it is doubtful whether such a system would greatly commend itself to rabbit breeders, except those producing large numbers of animals for meat.

It should perhaps be added that the majority of the present breeds of domestic rabbits have been produced by cross-breeding in some form or another, but after the initial type of animal has been produced, it is usually many years before the new breed is improved to a reasonable standard.

SELECTION AND CULLING

The severity of culling, that is, the elimination of unwanted animals from the breeding stud, does, to a certain extent, influence the rate of improvement. The more drastic the culling, the sooner undesirable animals and genes are eliminated. There is, however, a limiting factor to the number of animals that can be culled, and that is the need to maintain the breeding stock at the appropriate level required.

Obviously culling can be more severe in the case of bucks than in the case of does. In a large stud, where the number of animals remains more or less constant, the proportion of does which must be kept as replacements will vary depending a good deal on the number of young per doe produced in the year and the purpose for which the establishment is maintained. In a rabbit fancier's stud, possibly 8% of the bucks might be retained until mature, and possibly 15% of the does. Further culling would take place later. In a commercial establishment the figures would be slightly less, for whilst the does, certainly, are replaced more quickly than in the fancier's establishment, there are more young to choose from.

There are several difficulties in the process of selection with which the breeder must contend. One of these is that the breeder has to attempt to distinguish those animals which are most suited for the production of future generations, from those which are not so suited. It is not the animals that the breeder has before him or her which are of such importance, it is their progeny.

Then the breeder has to distinguish between the animal which appears suitable because of its genetical constitution, and the animal which appears suitable because of a different environment. The final difficulty is the selection for several characters at a time. No animal should be selected for one character alone; it must be chosen on the basis of all its characteristics which tend to make it a good animal for breeding.

When a stud is being improved for several characteristics (as is almost invariably the case) the breeder has three methods of selection open to him or her:

● selecting animals which attain more than a certain level in each character;
● selecting for one character at a time; or
● selecting animals on their total merit, or total score as the method is known.

An example will make these three systems clear.

Assuming the main characteristics on which the breeder bases his or her selection are:

Good litter size	(L)
Early maturity	(M)
Good food conversion	(FC)
Good meat quality	(MQ)

If the breeder classifies each character into ten grades, recording each animal from the group being considered for selection into one of the grades for each character, the maximum possible score for any character being ten, then of six animals so recorded, the scores might be as in Table 9.7.

Table 9.7 Total score assessment. Scores given to six animals on four different characteristics

Animal	L	M	FC	MQ	Total
A	9	9	10	8	36
B	5	10	10	9	34
C	10	5	7	10	32
D	6	10	7	7	30
E	7	7	7	7	28
F	5	3	8	9	25

If the breeder wanted to keep three animals, he or she would select A, B and C, i.e. those with the highest score, if using the total score method. If, the breeder however, was using the system of rejecting those with less than, say, six marks for any particular characteristic, he or she would select A, D, E, and if selected on the basis of the best animals in any one characteristic, he or she would select those as follows:

Litter size	A, C, E
Early maturity	A, B, D
Food conversion	A, B, F
Meat quality	B, C, F

If the results of this example of the three systems are amalgamated, it will be found that the breeder would select:

A	five times
B	four times
C	three times
D	twice
E	twice
F	twice

That is to say, by combining the various systems we find that the three best animals on average are A, B and C. These are given only by the method of the total score.

The great advantage of this system is that it does balance one characteristic against another, and selects out the best rabbit on average. The system can of course be modified by allotting more marks to one particularly important characteristic, which would thus give more emphasis to this characteristic in the selection.

It will be appreciated that if the breeder is endeavouring to improve several characteristics at the same time (and there is no doubt that improvement should be balanced) then the improvement in each characteristic in each generation will not be as great as if the breeder were selecting for one characteristic only.

Although the preponderance of selection at the present time is based on the appearance of the animals, the most reliable guide is given by their performance, i.e. the production of good stock. Before considering this point, however, it is as well to consider the question of selection by pedigree.

PEDIGREES

A certain amount of confusion exists as to exactly what a pedigree is, and the importance to be attached to it. A pedigree, to be of any value, must contain details of all the ancestors. Incomplete pedigrees giving details of certain individuals only (always the best!) are biased and often quite misleading. Unless a pedigree contains more than a simple list of names it has little value. To the names should be attached details of their particular characteristics and performance.

The use of pedigrees will, however, emphasise the need to think more in terms of families or strains than in terms of individuals when selection is being practised. That breeding stock should be selected from families which give consistently good results rather than from families which may produce one or two spectacular specimens, is obvious. But it must always be remembered that the nearer relatives of an animal are more reliable guides to its value than the more distant ones. The performance of a litter from an animal will give more valuable information on which to base selection than will the performance of the animal's parent, and so on. An average animal from a really good strain may, and very often does, produce much better breeding results than a good specimen from a poor strain.

The use of pedigrees, when they are accurately compiled, quite unbiased, and when they give sufficient detail, is an additional aid to selection, although culling of undesirable stock cannot be based upon them alone.

PERFORMANCE AND PROGENY TESTING

It is obvious that the only sound and reliable test of the breeding worth of an animal is the quality of its offspring. No matter how good a show specimen a rabbit may be, or how nearly perfect a coat it has, unless it can reproduce these characteristics in its progeny, it is of little value as a breeding animal. Performance testing implies the measurement of the efficiency with which a rabbit, or a group of rabbits, produce meat, pelts, young stock, etc. Progeny testing implies the estimation of the breeding value of an animal by the performance of its progeny.

In the breeding of rabbits solely for exhibition purposes, the criterion of the breeding value of a rabbit differs from the criterion to be used in the economic production of, say, meat rabbits. In the latter case a breeder will want to produce a uniform set of good quality meat rabbits, whilst the exhibitor will want to produce several outstanding animals. It does not really matter to the exhibition breeder whether the stock produced are variable, so long as one or two really good animals are produced. As the breeding of show specimens can never be an exact science, but rather more of an art, performance and progeny testing cannot be used to such advantage as they can in the production of 'utility' rabbits.

Economic production of rabbits for meat depends on large litter size, good and cheap growth, and freedom from excessive mortality. Certain does will be found to have a larger than average litter size, and to feed their young so well that their growth rate is high. Clearly progeny from such does will be selected for future breeding stock.

If the records of the progeny of a group of does, mated to different bucks, are examined, it will be found that the average of the different groups sired by the different bucks will vary. One buck may consistently produce progeny which have perhaps a better carcase and a better growth rate. Clearly again, the progeny of this buck should be selected for future breeding rather than the offspring of another buck, the average quality of whose youngsters was not so good.

The most important factor to be recognised in any progeny test is that the progeny should be unselected for the characteristics considered. That is to say, it is of little value to pick out, say, the six best animals sired by one buck for comparison with the six best sired by another. Ideally, all the young sired by all the bucks should be compared, but when this is not possible, the animals to be compared should be picked quite at random.

Since, also, the qualities of an animal are made up from both its genetic constitution and the effects of its environment, comparisons should be made of the progeny of different bucks reared under exactly the same conditions.

With progeny testing it is essential that the qualities or characteristics which are measured and compared should be due to heredity to as great an extent as possible. To record that the progeny of a buck have inferior growth rates due to their inheritance, when in fact the cause is faulty feeding or disease, immediately makes the test useless.

There are unfortunately some difficulties in the way of complete progeny testing. To begin with, accurate recording is absolutely essential, and although it is of great advantage to all breeders to keep full sets of records, few do so. Secondly, the number of progeny which must be kept and recorded until the test is concluded is usually rather larger than is maintained in the average stud or herd. As culling cannot be practised until the test is complete, there is also a certain amount of expense.

Nevertheless, by the recognition of the fact that the breeding value of an animal lies in the quality of its progeny, the breeder will be encouraged to select his breeding stock on a more rational basis than simply by its external appearance.

TEST-MATING

The purpose of test-mating is to endeavour to eliminate, as efficiently as possible, a particular characteristic (or more than one) which occurs in homozygous recessive animals. When the characteristic which is to be eliminated is produced in this way then the number of heterozygote animals, i.e. those not showing the condition but carrying it, is of course much higher than the number of animals showing the condition. If it is possible to detect those animals which have the recessive gene in their make up and prevent their use in breeding, no animals with the recessive gene will remain in the breeding programme.

The importance of the detection of heterozygosity is that the elimination of recessive genes simply by not using animals which are homozygous for the recessive, i.e. those animals which show the characteristic which it is hoped to eliminate, is very slow and takes a number of generations if it is to be eliminated. Indeed it is unlikely that it would ever be eliminated by this method.

A good example of such a condition in the rabbit is malocclusion, in which the lower teeth do not meet correctly with the upper and hence continue to grow. The incidence of this condition has increased a good deal in some breeds in recent years and whole strains have been discarded because of it, although its elimination by test-mating is possible and relatively quick.

Test-mating is a system employed to determine whether an animal carries one or more particular and undesirable characteristics; that is to say, whether the animal is heterozygous for certain undesirable recessive genes.

There are two methods of test-mating. In the first method the animal to be tested is mated to another which is homozygous for the character. For example, a breeder may wish to test whether a buck carries the factor for long hair. The breeder will thus mate the buck to an Angora doe. If the buck is heterozygous for woolly, then approximately half of the progeny will be woolly, but if the buck does not carry the gene for long hair, as short hair is dominant to long hair, all the progeny will be short-haired. In the same way, to test whether an Havana carries the dilution factor, the rabbit would be mated to a Lilac, which is of course the homozygous dilute brown. If no Lilacs are produced, then the Havana does not carry the dilution factor.

Certain undesirable recessives are lethal or semi-lethal when present in the homozygous form. In this case the rabbit must be tested with a known heterozygote for the factor, when approximately one-quarter of the progeny will be homozygous for the recessive character if the buck carries it.

The second method of test-mating is by breeding back to his daughters the buck in question. If the buck is heterozygous for any gene, obviously approximately one-half of his daughters will be homozygous or heterozygous for that character, depending on the constitution of their dam. Therefore a mating between the buck and his daughters will always yield approximately one-quarter of the progeny as recessive homozygote in approximately half of the litters. If, then, a buck is mated with, say, 6 or 7 of his daughters, and in all the litters, say 40 young, none is homozygous for the undesirable character, then the buck can safely be considered to be free from that recessive gene.

This second method of test-mating is more laborious than the first, but it has the advantage that not only does it test the buck for one particular gene, but it tests for many others at the same time. Any undesirable recessive genes in the buck's constitution are likely to be shown up. This method, however, reduces the available breeding life of the buck after testing, for some months are wasted waiting for the daughters to reach breeding age.

In both systems, enough young must be produced before the test can be considered reliable. In the first method two litters (say 12 young) from does showing the recessive character to be tested would be sufficient. In the second system at least 6 daughters, and preferably more, should be mated back to the buck.

Test-mating a stud buck will prevent the phenotypic appearance of any unwanted recessive characters, even though the does are not tested, for the buck will only pass on dominant genes which will prevent the appearance of the characteristic. It will also reduce the proportion of heterozygotes in a stud by 50% in each generation, but will not eliminate the recessive gene from the stock.

Test-mating should not be confused with progeny testing, which is of course the estimation of the breeding worth of a buck (or doe) on the basis of the value of his (or her) progeny.

NATIONAL IMPROVEMENT SCHEMES

From time to time the domestic rabbit has been the subject of improvement schemes on a national basis. In such schemes breeders either keep certain specified records which are submitted to, and analysed by, a central body, or send a selection of animals to a recording station which records each animal's actual performance. In either case the sponsoring body has the duty of accumulating valuable information on rabbits as a whole, and of advising the individual breeder on which animals are the most suitable for future breeding stock.

Angora testing in Germany

Performance tests were first instituted in Germany in 1933, when two centres were set up, one at the University of Halle and the other at the Poultry Experiment Station of Kiel-Steenbek. Later, other centres were established. Breeders sent their Angoras to these centres for an 8-month, or 12-month test (although later it was established that a 4-month test would probably yield as satisfactory results). Various characteristics such as total wool yield, quality, market value, food consumption, and so on were recorded. Individual breeders were advised on the most suitable animals for further use and excellent results were obtained. Quite apart from the improvement in individual strains, however, the accumulation of accurate production figures, and the setting up of standards of production, greatly assisted all breeders in the country.

The CIS

During the 1930s a Rabbit Breeding Research Institute was established in Moscow to assist the development of the domestic rabbit industry. After very extensive surveys, the Institute issued a number of recommendations for increasing production, together with standards of efficiency produced as a result of testing various stocks. It was particularly stressed that accurate recording should be established on the farms, and this was in fact carried out with a good deal of success. The facts that the recording was practised on most farms (and still is) and was carried out by the stock people tend to show that it has a very real value and is not such a difficult task as is often thought.

The Danish rabbit recording station at Favrholm

The General Rabbit Production Board and the State Livestock Production Board collaborated to establish, in 1943, a 'Control Station' for domestic rabbits at Favrholm under the general management of the Danish National Institute of Animal Sciences. Progeny testing continued to be done at Favrholm until 1961 when the work was transferred to Nordrup. Until 1963 breeders forwarded young stock (four per litter) and these were reared to slaughter weight. In 1963 the system changed from performance testing to progeny testing proper, in which bucks were sent to the station and mated to the station's does, in order that their breeding potential could be evaluated. The bucks were of course returned to the breeders after the initial matings. The young were weighed every two weeks and calculations of each buck's fertility, mortality of the young during growth to slaughter, growth ability of the young, food conversion, and carcase evaluations were all carried out.

To give some idea of the value of such a programme it should be said that something like 2000 animals per five-year period between 1944 and 1979 were tested. During that period the following results were obtained (Table 9.8).

These remarkable results show the very great value that can be obtained by such programmes.

Table 9.8   Improvements achieved at Favrholm between 1944 and 1979

Parameter	Average for period	
	1944–60	1976–79
Average days to slaughter weight	167.0	83.0
Daily gain in weight (g)	18.0	37.0
Feed units per kg weight gain	5.7	2.6

In 1974 the station started breeding experiments on its own stock with particular emphasis on growth rates and liveability of young. A rule was developed under which only bucks whose offspring had a greater liveability than the average for the whole station could be used for future stock. This has produced excellent results. It might also be added that in more recent years the station has done a good deal of research on the nutrition of the rabbit.

The American record of performance

The American Rabbit Breeders' Association set up, in 1946, a Committee to organise a programme which 'represents a serious attempt to increase the efficiency at which the rabbit (collectively) reproduces itself and produces the highest quality of the products for which it is valued – namely, 'meat, wool, fur and laboratory stock', to quote Dr P. B. Sawin, one of the originators of the scheme. In this scheme, individual breeders instead of sending their stock to a central station, maintained an accurate recording system, sending their records periodically to a central body for collation and analysis. The rations for participating stock were the subject of recommendations to ensure that all animals were fed the same. The analysis of some of the earlier records proved most interesting.

The American Rabbit of Tomorrow Contest

Although this scheme was not, in the sense in which it is used above, a recording or testing scheme, it was a method of accumulating information relating to production, and also assisting in the way of publicity. Breeders sent does in kindle to a central unit where the does were maintained until the young were slaughtered for meat. Their food consumption was accurately recorded, and eventually each doe was allotted marks in proportion to her performance, the weight and quality of her progeny, etc. The owners of winning does were rewarded by cash prizes, and there was a fair amount of publicity for all concerned and for the domestic rabbit. The scheme also focused the attention of all breeders on the necessity for accurate recording and the selection of future breeding stock on the basis of their performance.

Great Britain

At the end of the 1920s an attempt was made in Great Britain to start an Angora Wool Test. Meetings were held, but no tests were ever started. It was not until 1960 that a test was begun by the Commercial Rabbit Association, but this was a test of carcase production.

In 1962, however, British Oil & Cake Mills, at that time the leading rabbit food manufacturers, at their station in Selby started the first Rabbit Litter Test, into which some 41 does were entered, although only 20 litters were reared to 56 days. The second test produced an entry of 33 does but the results were greatly improved, due probably to weather conditions. This second test was the last in the first series, but others followed.

PERFORMANCE RECORDING – THE PRESENT DAY

In 1994 the performance recording of breeders' stock on a multiple breeder basis was mostly in abeyance. There are, however, particularly in France, stations which do considerable work with large batches of families in improving the genetic constitution of the animals.

There are also some large breeding firms, who have established specialised relatively genetically pure lines, which are purchased for production of meat by rabbit farmers. These farms have usually invested large sums of money to establish these lines, usually carefully controlled by geneticists.

It is difficult to say which type of schemes are the best to produce the most desirable results, but that they are important is beyond doubt. They have the result not only of demonstrating impartially how various strains perform but also the great benefit of confirming to breeders the idea that stock improvement by scientific methods is both desirable and possible.

MYTHS AND LEGENDS

In animal breeding there have always been false beliefs held so strongly, that they become widely regarded as fact. These myths, in many cases, become so widely entrenched that they are adopted as true by the most unlikely people to be so taken in. For example, there is the false belief that if a doe is remated at 10 days, she will accept the buck if she is not in kindle, but not if she is pregnant. Another is that one mating with one buck will affect the doe when she is mated for another litter to another buck. Then there is the idea, often accepted, that what happens to an individual animal during its life can affect what it passes on to its progeny. Not one of these myths are true. The greatest of all myths, however, concerned the crossing of true rabbits with true hares. The history of the leporid or Hare Rabbit cross lasted many years and both sides had dedicated adherents. This matter was, however, further confused because the name leporid so closely resembles the family name to which the rabbit and the hare belong – *Leporidae*.

For nearly 150 years it was believed by many, and sometimes with the strongest passions, that the rabbit and the hare when mated produced young of a type slightly different from both parents. It was believed that the Belgian Hare (undeniably a rabbit) was indeed derived from such a cross. Even in the days when it became known that the chromosome number of the rabbit was 44 and that of the hare 48 it was said, even by geneticists, that the interspecies cross had been seen or produced by them. The evidence it was said was absolutely certain.

The existence of the leporid, and the name, was first announced by one Paul Broca in 1858, who stated that he had examined a number of animals produced by a cross between hare and rabbit by A. Roux, President of the Agricultural Society of Angouleme in France. These crossbreds had been produced since 1847 up to the fourth generation. Crosses back to the original species were also obtained and in 1858 alone Roux sold 'about one thousand' on the local markets.

No matter that the differences between hare and rabbit were numerous, size, gestation period, fecundity, state at birth – eye open and furred in the hare as against the reverse in the rabbit – and many more, these were ignored. A number of very detailed studies of the bones of both species provided much 'evidence' for and against the mythical hybrid.

Darwin considered that the cross was 'possible, though not probable', but Haeckel, in 1874, being certain, took the opportunity to name the 'new species' *Lepus darwinii*.

Any number of papers were presented to learned societies, for or against the existence of leporids for some 40 years. But, although the debate tended to die out after the turn of the century there were still people who were convinced that the cross could be made. Hagedoorn, an internationally known animal breeding scientist very interested in rabbits, maintained until his death in 1953 that he had produced leporids. He described them in detail but admitted that he could not account 'for the failure of his colleagues to produce leporids'. E. C. Richardson, a leading rabbit geneticist and a past President of the BRC, until the late 1940s firmly believed in the existence of leporids, but finally agreed that they were impossible. The debate was eventually terminated by numerous attempts to breed the two species by artificial insemination. All attempts failed.

In addition to the sincerely held but mistaken beliefs in the leporid there were other people who used the belief for fraudulent purposes. Some very high prices were paid for such supposed animals. To an extent also it formed part of the basis for the American Belgian Hare craze.

Whilst this particular myth was so widely spread and held there are numbers of others which often militate against good selection and breeding practice. The more the breeder learns to eliminate them from his thinking, the greater will be his success.

Chapter 10

Uses of the Rabbit to Man

The variety of uses to which the rabbit is put by man has been touched upon in the first chapter. Here these points are further developed. In summary one may say that the rabbit is used by man to:

- supply food;
- supply a very high grade wool;
- supply furs;
- supply miscellaneous products;
- assist in laboratory and experimental work;
- be used in educational work of varied sorts;
- keep as exhibition, pet or companion animals.

The most extensive of these is in the supply of food.

THE RABBIT AS A SUPPLIER OF MEAT

There are less than 20 countries in the world in which the domestic rabbit is not kept, the majority of which lie in the Middle East. In some countries domestic rabbits form almost a staple meat supply for a large proportion of the population, whilst in others they form a not inconsiderable trade. In some countries the majority of domestic rabbits are kept in small family units or holdings, but in others the tendency is towards larger intensive farms.

World production has been estimated by Lebas and Colin (1992) to be of the order of 1 200 000 tonnes per annum. Those countries producing 5000 or more tonnes annually are listed in Table 10.1.

SUBSISTENCE RABBIT PRODUCTION

The domestic rabbit has truly been called the poor man's pig, and, that it is, probably accounts for the extremely wide recognition of its value. The fact that a few domestic rabbits can be kept for an infinitesimal cost, but yet produce a fair quantity of highly

Table 10.1   Major rabbit meat producing countries. The figures below, taken from Lebas and Colin, Proceedings of the 5th WRSA Congress, 1992, include only those countries which produce 5000 or more tonnes of rabbit meat per year. Column 3 gives the % of rabbit meat produced by rabbit farmers, the balance being produced by non-commercial farmers and column 4 gives the percentage for each country of the total world production (1 200 000 tonnes)

Country	Annual production (t)	% produced by rabbit farmers	% of total world production
Italy	300 000	83	25.00
CIS (ex-USSR)	150 000	33	12.50
France	150 000	67	12.50
China	120 000	58	10.00
Spain	120 000	67	10.00
Czechoslovakia	30 000	10	2.50
Poland	25 000	20	2.08
Portugal	20 000	20	1.67
Germany	20 000	50	1.67
Belgium	20 000	75	1.67
Hungary	19 000	26	1.58
Rumania	18 000	44	1.50
Philippines	18 000	5	1.50
USA	17 000	59	1.42
Egypt	15 000	13	1.25
Brazil	12 000	83	1.00
Morocco	12 000	8	1.00
Netherlands	12 000	83	1.00
Yugoslavia	10 000	30	0.83
Mexico	10 000	10	0.83
Indonesia	9 000	5	0.75
United Kingdom	7 000	57	0.58
Algeria	7 000	7	0.58
Columbia	6 000	17	0.50
Venezuela	6 000	17	0.50
Greece	5 000	40	0.42
Ghana	5 000	20	0.42
Total	1 143 000		95.25

nutritious and palatable meat, is widely recognised. But in recent years the situation throughout the world has been changing, in some cases dramatically. During the past 50 years there have been both increased production of the meat rabbit and a vastly increased awareness of its potential as a meat animal.

In the case of the developed countries, particularly those in Europe, the Food and Agriculture Organisation (FAO) suggests that in the 15 years to 1980 rabbit meat production increased by nearly double in those countries for which it had information. It is interesting that it was in 1980 that the FAO first recognised the real potential of the rabbit as a meat animal and it held its first Rural, Poultry and Rabbit Production Consultation in Rome in 1981.

The reasons for the usefulness of the rabbit are not far to seek. The human world population is calculated to increase from 4415 million in 1980 to 6199 million in the year 2000, with by far the largest proportion of increase taking place in the developing countries, where in general the food supply is currently the worst and the standard of living the lowest. An increase in the standard of living almost inevitably calls for an increase in the proportion of animal protein in the diet.

There are of course two possibilities in the matter of consumption. Crops can be grown and eaten directly by people, where consumption is direct, or the crops can be fed to animals which then provide food for people. This latter, indirect feeding of people is inefficient, and the rabbit, being able to utilise food that cannot be used by humans, can therefore help greatly to reduce the enormous shortages that are likely to occur in the future, particularly of animal protein.

Pigs and poultry, which are comparable in some ways to the rabbit, cannot to any great extent utilise foods which man cannot use and it is to pigs, poultry and rabbits that the greatest increase in meat production must come. The reason for this, basically, is that the productive cycle of larger animals is too slow to have a great deal of effect. Indeed, the FAO studies indicate that almost one-third of the total meat production in the year 2000 must come from poultry, pigs and rabbit. Because, as noted above, the rabbit is so able to utilise, to better effect than pigs or poultry, foods which man himself cannot use, the importance of the rabbit is likely to be great.

It is generally considered that an average daily food requirement per head of population is just under 2500 calories, with some 90 g of protein, of which roughly a quarter ought to be of animal origin. There are not many developing countries in which even half the required supply of animal protein is available. The reason for the growing interest in the use of the rabbit in developing countries is not hard to seek. The answer lies in the use of the rabbit to produce meat. An examination of the reasons may be of interest.

It is now realised by very many people and organisations that the rabbit has a number of features which make it peculiarly useful in contributing animal protein. The reasons are:

● The rabbit can produce meat from crops which cannot be utilised by people.
● The rabbit can use green crops and other vegetation more efficiently than most animals.
● Food conversion rate of crops to meat is high.
● Both energy and protein requirements in food per unit liveweight gain are lower than for most other animals.
● Some vegetation is eaten by rabbits which is unpalatable to all other livestock, and which they will not eat.
● There is a considerable degree of diversity in the gene pool of rabbits, which means that selection for required characteristics can be simply carried out to allow for good and speedy adaptation to different environments.
● Because of its fast reproduction rate and quick growth, a doe will produce more meat per unit liveweight than any other animal, except poultry. This means that when foods are scarce a small number of animals can be kept, to take the greatest advantage at a later stage when the supply improves.
● Rabbits reach their breeding age in a very short period, hence the cost of food to first breeding is low.
● Rabbits can be kept in some areas in undeveloped countries where other forms of livestock cannot, for reasons of disease, e.g. tsetse fly areas.

- Rabbits are of such a size that no storage difficulties arise on slaughter.
- Growth rate is fast and meat is therefore produced very quickly.
- Rabbit meat is highly nutritious and of excellent quality.
- There are usually none of the religious problems which occur with other forms of livestock.

Apart from the above, other important considerations are that the rabbits can be maintained by a family group which could not keep other livestock, the food for the rabbits can be collected by all the members of the family and surplus rabbits can contribute to the family income.

There is no doubt that varied and numerous problems will arise in the development of, at first, rabbit keeping on a family scale and then commercial rabbit farming in developing countries. These can only be solved by the widespread distribution of information, firstly between scientific workers in the field and then to the rabbit keepers themselves. Part of this was started by a Workshop on Rabbit Husbandry in Africa, which was held in Tanzania in 1978, and was organised by the International Foundation for Science, the University at Dar-es-Salaam and the Tanzanian National Scientific Research Council. More is being done by the government-sponsored establishments in different countries.

Finally, the World Rabbit Science Association, which was formed in 1976 as an international body for the exchange of scientific information, has held a number of discussions in collaboration with the FAO, in an attempt to further the use of the rabbit in developing countries, and has widely spread its ideas.

COMMERCIAL RABBIT FARMING

It is only in fairly recent years that large-scale commercial rabbit enterprises have begun. The largest of these are probably in Eastern Europe where farms of up to 10 or 12 000 breeding does have been established. In this country, some farms run purely for meat production have reached 1000 or more breeding does, but this is the exception. Throughout the whole of Europe, the small farmer has often kept rabbits to sell meat as part and parcel of his general farming activities, and lastly there is the small family farming unit where quite often a good deal of the produce is kept for home consumption, although in total, because there are enormous numbers of these family units, the actual production of rabbit meat is very large. The proportion of meat production in the three groups varies greatly from country to country.

Table 10.1 indicates the percentage of meat produced in different countries by the rabbit farmer. In some cases (Italy, the largest producing country in the world, Belgium, Brazil and the Netherlands), over 75% of all meat produced comes from the commercial farmer, whilst in some countries less than 10% comes from the farmer and the rest comes from the very small farmer or the family producer for home consumption.

The composition of the meat will, of course, depend upon the age of slaughter, the method of feeding, etc., but nevertheless, domestic rabbit meat of all ages is of high value for human consumption. It has in general a rather higher percentage of protein than any other meat and it is considered to be highly digestible, and for that reason is very often recommended for sick people.

The production of Angora wool

One of the oldest known breeds of rabbit is the Angora and for hundreds of years its wool has been plucked or sheared and then spun and woven or knitted. The French Angora, where the Angora industry was developed, is usually plucked, whilst other varieties (German and English) are usually sheared. The world production in recent years has exceeded 7000 tonnes annually and again in recent years the price has been very volatile. In 1971, the price per kg for first grade French wool averaged about £4.80 per kg. In 1978 it reached an average of £25 per kg. It peaked in December 1984 at £95 per kg, but then dropped to £35 a kg, owing to very large exports from China, where an industry had been slowly growing (Table 10.2).

Table 10.2 Approximate annual production of Angora wool in countries producing over an estimated 100 tonnes

Country	Amount (t)	% of total world production
China	6000	78
Chile	500	6.5
Argentina	400	5.2
France	200	2.6
Hungary	180	2.3
India	150	1.9
Total	7430	96.5
Estimated total world production	7700	

Production in Great Britain was fairly small and the best grades fetched only about £5.50 per kg in the 1950s, rising to some £22.20 per kg in the late 1970s. However, there are now no true commercial buyers in this country and all the production is used for small-scale hand spinning of wool for knitting garments.

Angora wool is usually spun pure but sometimes it is mixed with fine sheep wools. It may be plucked to obtain a super grade but more commonly it is sheared or clipped every three months or so. The yield of wool is not affected by the method of removing it. A skilled operator will be able to shear one Angora in 10 to 20 minutes, but for plucking it is almost invariably necessary to pluck the animal over several days.

There is no animal fibre which has the same lightness, softness and purity of fleece as Angora. The tex number indicates the weight of 1000 m of any spun material. With good grade Angora wool it is possible to spin 1000 m with 7 g of wool, i.e. a tex number of 7, although a tex number of 10 is more usual. The tex number for a fine grade sheep's wool would be of the order of 20.

These qualities mean that the wool has been in great demand in the fashion industry, being catered for by manufacturing facilities largely in Italy, France and Japan. The wool produces garments which are extremely warm and comfortable, and in recent years there has been the development of what might be termed therapeutic garments and aids. These are manufactured as a help for arthritic conditions and the like. The reasons that Angora wool should act in this way appears to be due partly to its heat retaining properties, partly to its ability to let the skin 'breathe' very easily and partly due to its peculiar electrical properties. Whatever the reasons, sufferers using these garments, gloves and sleeves mostly, testify to their great benefit. They are now manufactured in a number of countries.

The production of furs

Rabbit furs for clothing purposes have been used for many hundreds of years. In the earliest days these were from rabbits kept in warrens. But for the last few hundred years they have been those of hutched rabbits. France was the earliest and principal country for the production of high quality furs and the Argente Champagne the principal breed.

Under the stimulus of a new fur industry which started in this country in the very early 1920s, new fur breeds of rabbits were developed. These added impetus to this very promising industry, which grew throughout the decade, albeit on a fairly small scale. The industry concentrated on the production of high grade, mature moult-free skins, which could be manufactured into various garments. The rabbits usually had to be kept for at least six months before the pelt became a first grade fur. It was thought that the rabbit could compete easily with other fur animals kept in captivity, and for a time (and still to a small extent) this was so. The industry was however killed off in the depression of the early 1930s coupled with the imports of enormous quantities of competing furs from Russia. Apart from this period, furs were always a by-product of meat production and pelts from young meat animals are of a poor grade. Although there is no longer a fur industry in this country, several countries still produce rabbit furs and continue research into the production of the mature high grade pelt.

Furs may be grouped into three categories – Rex furs, Normal furs and Satin furs. The Rex furs are undoubtedly those which fetch the best prices for furrier work, and they are much liked by the fur trade. The Rex furs, together with the Satin furs (of which very few are now used due to the rarity of the breed), are normally used in their natural state. The Normal furs on the other hand are often sheared or pulled (i.e. guard hairs removed) and dyed.

The prices to be obtained for different rabbit furs depend upon the breed, the quality (i.e. density, length, etc.), the care with which it has been selected (in order that it is prime with no moult), and the care with which it has been taken and handled.

Miscellaneous products

Rabbit hair

Poor quality rabbit skins which are not suitable for fur work are used for the production of rabbit hair. The hair of the rabbit is used for making high grade felt, although a small proportion of hair is also used for spinning with sheep wool. Felt from rabbit hair was particularly used in the manufacture of hats. In fact all bowler hats were made of this material. The wild rabbit skin was preferred by the hatting fur manufacturers, but vast numbers of domestic skins are also used, particularly following the great reduction in the numbers of wild rabbit from the main producing areas.

Skins for felt production are almost invariably cased skins, and the manufacture of the felt is briefly as follows. The cased skin is split open and the guard hairs (which are of no value for felt making) removed by machines which pull them from the skin. The pelts without the guard hairs are then carrotted. Carrotting consists of treating the fur with chemicals to assist felting, and to produce added strength in the final felt. After carrotting, the fur is cut from the skin by revolving knives which in effect cut off the skin in thin strips. The resulting fur is blended and cleaned. The fur is then built up, layer by layer, and pressed against heated rollers by vibrating rollers. Under this mechanical vibration, pressure, and moist heat, the felt is formed.

The quality of the felt depends on a number of factors, but the most desirable skins are those which are very dense (and thus yield a good weight of fur) and in which the fur fibre has good strength and a small cross-section. White fur is preferred (although it does not make such good felt) because it can be dyed to pastel shades. It is extremely doubtful whether domestic rabbits would ever be bred for the use of their skins in the manufacture of felt, but as a by-product of meat production, the sale of skins for fur felt manufacture adds a useful additional income.

Rabbit skin glue
The skins from which hair has been removed are utilised to produce a special glue which is used for a variety of purposes. As yet it has not been found possible to produce a synthetic glue which replaces to the fullest extent rabbit skin glue.

Rabbit novelties
Everyone will have heard of the lucky rabbit's foot and in many countries consid-erable numbers of preserved feet are sold. Also in many countries tanned ears are used as novelties and for tags on such things as key rings. One unusual item is the requirement of rabbit tails by plant breeders. Apparently the rabbit tail is ideal as an artificial pollinator.

Organs for research
Many otherwise waste parts of the rabbit, including blood and a number of organs are required for experimental work and these are produced by some processors as a specialist service to laboratories.

THE RABBIT AS A LABORATORY ANIMAL

Medical, biological and some agricultural research has necessitated the use of experimental animals. Attempts are of course made to reduce this number and to find alternatives to the use of laboratory animals. But some are quite essential. The licensing of the use of laboratory animals, by the Home Office, is extremely stringent and the greatest emphasis is placed on the welfare of experimental animals. Their care, treatment and procedures have to be of the very highest quality. For the past few years the number of rabbits used in the UK for research of various types approaches 100 000 per year.

The domestic rabbit has been found to be most useful in many fields, for it has qualities that make it particularly valuable. It has the right range of sizes, it is easy and not expensive to maintain, it is placid by nature and easy to handle. In many ways its physiology and reaction to disease is similar to man, it is easily obtained or bred within the laboratory facilities and its life span is suitable for most procedures. For example, much of the early work on animal genetics was conducted on the rabbit, as also was work on artificial insemination and reproductive studies. As the rabbit ovulates some 10 hours after mating, the time of ovulation can be determined exactly, which is impossible with most other types of animal.

In the field of human medicine the rabbit has been of value for a wide range of studies. Rabbits have been used as models for research in a wide variety of bacterial and viral diseases of man in ways which are impossible to change to non-animal procedures. In the field of atherosclerosis (thickening of the arteries) research, the rabbit has always been widely used as the animal of choice. The bold eye of the rabbit means that it is one of the best animals to use for a whole range of research into problems related to eyes. It is now sometimes used as a pilot test animal prior to the use of more expensive larger animals. It is also used for the actual production of some medical products. There are many other spheres in which it is ideal.

The use of the rabbit as a test animal for the safety of medicinal products is well known and whilst attempts are constantly being made to find non-animal alternatives, until such time as they are, regrettably animals must be used.

A survey made some years ago indicated that about one-third of the animals used in laboratories are bred by those laboratories, whilst the remainder are purchased through suppliers. After the demise of the Laboratory Animal Centre, a quasi-government body, in order to ensure the highest quality of care and welfare of animals bred for medical research, the Laboratory Animal Breeders Association of Great Britain was formed. Members work to a strict code of practice for the production of laboratory animals and their welfare is thus guaranteed.

THE RABBIT – ITS USE IN EDUCATION

In the school

The rabbit has a great deal to offer schools. At one time many schools went even to the extent of having small rabbit clubs, the members of which maintained rabbits for the benefit of teaching in the school and as a hobby or interest to many of the pupils. At that time the teaching of rural studies was held to be of particular value in school work. It allowed the teaching of all nature subjects and the relations between plants and animals together with practical work which developed a responsible attitude towards all animal life and a respect for the necessity of its welfare. The combined care of the rabbits taught a sense of shared responsibility and teamwork. The emphasis on some of this work has diminished, but much of it remains.

Including animals in a lesson increases children's interest and curiosity which is so necessary to successful teaching. When animals are used to illustrate points in the lesson, those lessons are very well remembered. There are few animals so appealing to children as the rabbit and its size and temperament make it an excellent example. For probably the majority of children, school will be the only place where it is possible for them to get 'hands on' experience of animal life (Fig. 10.1).

Whilst there is at present less emphasis in the use of rabbits in schools at all junior and secondary levels, the present day curriculum for the General Certificate of Secondary Education in Rural Science does include a section on rabbits with a wide coverage of the subject.

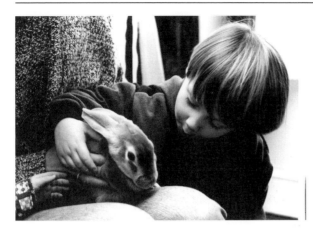

Fig. 10.1 This Essex playgroup has its own Orange Rex 'house rabbit' named Mary who is a firm favourite with all the children

In further education

Some years ago, when what might be termed the orthodox teaching of biology and zoology at schools was more in vogue than it appears to be today, the rabbit was of great use. Some of the classic anatomical and physiological texts, such as Bensley, Borradaile, Craigie, and Whitehouse and Grove, required the use of rabbits in the biology laboratory and numbers were so used. At the present time individual dissection, for example, by pre-A-level students, is unusual, and if any is to be done, then single demonstrative dissection by the teacher is carried out. The use of the rabbit for such studies occurs in more advanced education, from A-level to Medical School.

In other places

Rabbits are a popular addition to many zoos, nature parks and the like. In some cases an added attraction is an area with suitable rabbits which the children can handle. Whilst some of these establishments present a satisfactory show, there are others which could reap much benefit by obtaining advice from such organisations as the British Rabbit Council.

AN EXHIBITION, PET OR COMPANION ANIMAL

This use of the rabbit in this aspect is the subject of much that has hitherto been written in this book. As an exhibition animal there is little more to say than the rabbit gives enormous pleasure and interest to some thousands of specialist breeders.

Under the right parental guidance the pet rabbit can give a great deal of practical instruction in many fields. The rabbit, being dependent upon its owner, needs constant and regular attention. In this way the child learns lessons in reliability and regularity. The biology of life is illustrated in all its facets. The Victorians, to whom character was all important, realised this and it was largely for this reason that the increase in pet keeping was so greatly developed.

There are many well-documented cases of the rabbit being used, as it were, as a therapeutic companion. In some hospitals, for example, a well-trained house rabbit is of great value in the children's ward. One recently ended its sixth year of such work.

Chapter 11

The Commercial Rabbit Industry at Home and Abroad

HISTORY OF THE RABBIT INDUSTRY AT HOME

There has, from the early part of the 1800s, and even earlier, been some sort of commercial rabbit industry in this country. In those very early days it consisted in most cases of semi-tame animals kept in warrens, but there also existed a number of hutch-bred animals. When the rural population started to drift to the towns, they kept rabbits for their own use, but sold some for extra income.

In some cases by the mid 1800s there were one or two quite surprisingly large farms producing rabbits from hutches for the London markets, but these generally failed to continue for very many years. From that period until the early 1920s there were sporadic attempts to establish rabbit farming as a viable industry, but these met with little success.

Following the 1914–18 war and indeed just prior to that time, a number of fur breeds of rabbits, such as the Beveren, Havana, Chinchilla and Argente, were imported or became popular and vigorous attempts were made to found a rabbit industry. The 1920s were a period of considerable growth and it looked as though a strong and viable industry was to be established, although on a smaller scale, the Angora was also starting to be farmed in numbers. A Fur Board was formed as a co-operative exercise, which to an extent controlled the sale of furs for its members, and prices became such that very satisfactory profits were to be made. It was successful for a number of years, but eventually ceased when the fur industry fell on hard times. During the early 1930s depression enormous numbers of skins of various sorts were imported into the UK at ridiculously low prices and the fur trade collapsed. Some stalwarts continued, and with the aid of the sales of breeding stock at prices a good deal higher than the carcase and the pelt would command, a living was made. This, then, was the state of affairs until the outbreak of war in 1939.

Shortages of meat during the war greatly encouraged the keeping of rabbits on a wide but small scale. As has always occurred in all countries at war, the Government stimulated and encouraged rabbit keeping. The numbers produced for food in this country were vast, although it might be added that, large as it was, the number produced was dwarfed by the production in Germany during the same period.

The stimulus given by the war encouraged people to attempt rabbit farming afterwards. But these attempts were only successful when the enterprise was a part of a smallholding, and the breeder developed his own local market, usually processing the animals himself and selling the carcases to local outlets, thus cutting out the middleman and making a fair return.

This was the situation until the mid 1950s. Myxomatosis, having eliminated many millions of wild rabbits, had tended to establish a market for both domestic rabbit meat and cheap grade skins for hatting fur to replace the wild rabbit products. By the late 1950s a small number of commercially minded farmers looked at rabbit farming, and some reasonably large farms of some hundred of does each were established. Supported by one or two of the larger feed companies, and with the encouragement of one or two of the larger chain stores (who considered a quality meat, with perhaps some novelty about it, would be a useful addition to their sales), a definite approach was made to a commercial rabbit industry.

Whereas the old fur and meat farming system required mature animals, on average probably six-months-old, which therefore had to be fed on bulk feeding stuffs which were cheap, the new approach was quite different. It was based on several principles:

- The meat had to be of the highest quality and was therefore to be young, between 8 and 10 weeks of age. This young age was also necessary as after this age the cost in feed for each kg produced increased.
- To produce a high revenue per breeding doe, and to get young to the required weight in such a short period, compounded feeds had to be used.
- Because labour was expensive, systems having the lowest possible labour content had to be devised, which necessitated in most cases single-tier wire cages, which it was also considered would reduce disease.
- As the meat was to be regarded as a quality product, the highest possible standards of modern packing were to be used.
- A combined team of farmers, processors, feeding stuffs manufacturers and retailers (or wholesalers) had to work together.

THE COMMERCIAL RABBIT ASSOCIATION

These principles met with almost universal agreement and it was, therefore, in 1960 that the Commercial Rabbit Association (CRA) was founded. It was the earnest hope of all the founders that an integrated industry could be established using the central association as a link between all parties.

The objects of the CRA were (and, indeed, still are):

- to represent the interest of members to the government and its agencies;
- to promote, develop and generally assist in the conduct of the commercial rabbit industry;
- to draw up and operate an accredited breeders scheme and any other scheme for the improvement of stock;
- to encourage research relating to the rabbit and rabbit industry, and to collate and disseminate technical information;
- to promote and encourage the setting up and maintenance of marketing facilities

for the products of the rabbit industry, including meat, fur and ancillary products;
● to do all such other things as are incidental, conducive or ancillary to the attainment of the above objects.

The CRA has had a chequered career, although a great deal of excellent work has been done. At the start of the new organisation, producer groups were encouraged. These groups allowed the smaller farmer to combine his animals for slaughter with the consignments of other members. The processors were then able to collect worthwhile numbers of animals for slaughter at an economic rate. These producer groups were affiliated to the CRA.

In 1980 a number of the larger rabbit farmers in the CRA became dissatisfied with the activities of the Association, which they considered was dominated by small producers. They therefore formed another Association, the British Rabbit Federation, or BRF.

Unfortunately, neither organisation was able to establish a strong, viable industry. In 1988, both organisations realising that two organisations for an industry that would barely support one, was an absurd situation, amalgamated, with the same objects as the CRA above, and was named the British Commercial Rabbit Association.

PROBLEMS OF THE COMMERCIAL RABBIT INDUSTRY

The basic problems of the rabbit industry are the cost of capital for the housing and equipment in relation to the total output of meat rabbits; the relatively low production per doe; mortality of young rabbits; the short production life of the does; and the prices for meat rabbits obtained by the producer in relation to the price of feed.

It is unusual for special housing to be built for a controlled environment unit as the cost of this is usually prohibitive. The cost of adapting buildings is a good deal lower, although the result is not entirely satisfactory and the cost is still rather high. This has led some producers to use non-controlled environment housing, with a plastic-type cover. Whether this system will be widely adopted it is still too early to say.

Production per doe is very variable, with the best producers averaging less than 50 or so young per year. The average in the country is a great deal less than this. It would be fair to say that a production figure for all does of less than 45 young per year is, with the present costs of feed and the prices obtained, likely to mean that very little, if any, profit is made. It is fortunate that with the crossing of pure lines, the reduction in mortality, etc., and the genetic improvement which is constantly being made, such figures are likely to be achieved by the competent stockperson.

Mortality is in some cases a continual bugbear, with mortality figures of young rising to 20 and even 25% in some units. Mortality, being influenced by environment, feeds, stockmanship and so on, must be kept under constant review and steps taken to reduce it at all times. The mortality, or rather the replacement level of breeding stock, also has an important influence on profitability.

The prices received from processors in this country are a good deal less, in relation to the cost of feed, than those received by other European producers. As the cost of feed is on average over 75% of the total costs, it can be seen that the relationship of feed costs and selling prices is very important. There is a strict correlation between the cost of feed and the price obtained for the meat rabbits. If the feed cost per kg is less than 8 times the price per kg of liveweight sold, then, with reasonable management, satisfactory profits can be made. If the ratio is less than 1 to 6, it is extremely difficult to make a profit.

Unfortunately, the number of processors in the country has shown a steady decline and the attention of many producers, particularly the smaller ones, is being drawn to local markets. There is therefore likely to be a growth in home processing, except for those producers who are lucky enough to have units close to active processors.

The situation at the present time, then, is that a number of producers are attempting to make a viable industry out of rabbits. It is certain that the commercial side of rabbit keeping is no easier than any other form of livestock production, although it has the advantage that when carried on as a sideline to other agricultural or horticultural endeavours, a great deal of waste material can be converted into saleable products. It can also, of course, be a part-time activity with little land being required.

An instinct or understanding for livestock keeping, together with knowledge and experience, are essentials for success. Knowledge can be gained by education, but there are only a few courses, of short duration, held each year. There have in the past been a few schemes whereby pupils would be taken on established rabbit farms for training, but these arrangements are very limited and thus the main training ground for rabbit breeders is the hard school of practice. A certain amount can be learnt from education and books, but the final polish and experience can only be obtained by actual work. It is for this reason that the soundest advice possible is that beginners should start in a relatively small way and expand as and when they gain their quite invaluable experience. Their early errors are then less costly, and they are building on a firm foundation.

It is difficult to estimate the number of rabbit farms (in the true sense) in the UK, but it is unlikely to exceed 1000 to 1500.

The regulations relating to the commercial slaughter of meat are very rigorous, although not applying to the very small producer. For this reason the farmer almost invariably sells live direct to a processor, although better returns are made from limited farm gate sales.

THE RABBIT INDUSTRY ABROAD

The picture of the rabbit industry in many countries abroad differs considerably from that in the UK. Table 10.1 gives estimates of the production of rabbit meat in those countries producing more than 5000 tonnes annually. The total estimated world tonnage is 1.2 million. These countries therefore produce 95.25% of all domestic rabbit meat world wide. The five largest producers, Italy, the CIS, France, China and Spain, produce between them 70.0% of the total world production. Whilst the CIS has intensive farms producing only one-third of their production, the remainder have farms which produce at least 58%. Italy, indeed, the world's largest producer with 300 000 tonnes produces most of it (83%) in modern intensive farms, leaving only some 50 000 tonnes being produced by very small producers, much of which is for home consumption.

Traditionally the Latin countries, Italy, France, Spain, Belgium and Portugal have always had the highest consumption of rabbit meat per head of population, being

5.3 kg per head in Italy, Spain with 3 kg, France with 2.9 kg, Belgium with 2.6 kg, and Portugal with 2 kg. The only other country which exceeds most of these is Malta which has a per capita consumption of 4.3 kg per head, but being only small has a production of about 1500 tonnes annually. The intensive production in those countries with a well developed industry have highly professional farms, with a high standard of management and excellent qualities of pelleted feeds.

France

France was traditionally the chief producer of domestic rabbits in the world, but she has now lost this rating to Italy. In France prior to 1939, the production varied between 80 and 100 million carcases for sale per year, that is to say, up to probably 150 000 tons. During the 1939–45 war the numbers increased considerably, but mostly in small units to something just under 300 000 tons per year, but by 1980 the total tonnage was reduced to 180 000, this being produced by some 4.5 million breeding does. This total herd in France was therefore reduced by some 35%, and the distribution had also changed. Whereas at one time the production came from a very large number of small units, in 1980 the unit size was increasing. For example, there were some 440 000 units having less than 10 does, but producing 35% of the total tonnage; 35 000 units with between 10 and 20 does, producing 25%; 10 000 units with between 20 and 100 does, producing 20%; and the better farms of over 100 does, which numbered 5000 and produced 20% of the total production. Since that time the total production has decreased to 150 000 tonnes and the truly commercial farms are slowly increasing in size and numbers, with the total of commercial farms now producing two-thirds of the production. The traditional picture of the very small unit consuming a good deal of their own produce and selling the rest to meet much of the cost, is changing. There is also some revival in the Angora wool trade, which suffered a good deal of depression. The French consumption of rabbit meat is just less than 4 kg per head per year.

The technical improvements in France have been surprisingly good during the 30 years from 1950 to 1980. According to M. Lebas, Director of the French Rabbit Production Research Station, the improvements for the best farms can be summarised in Table 11.1.

Table 11.1 Improvements in best technological results in France in good farms between 1950 and 1980

Parameter	Average for year	
	1950	1980
No. of young per doe per year	20–25	60.0
Interval between litters (days)	95	42.0
Food conversion rate (1960 as concentrates not usual in 1950)	6	3.6
Hours of work per doe per year	16	7.5
Minutes to produce 1 kg carcase	27	6.2
Breeding does in larger farms	80–100	350–1000

The farms producing these results were always in closely controlled environ-mental conditions with either flat deck or triple- and even quadruple-tiered wire cages, with 15 to 16 hours of lighting per day, year-round production, with weaners often in collective cages of 5 to 10 young, and automatic watering and feeding of complete pelleted rations.

In more recent times there has been a good deal of interest in 'Open Air' systems, that is in tunnel houses (Chapter 6) with some excellent results, but the great majority of farms have standard housing. The French rabbit industry is well supplied with technological and economic information, with regular surveys giving useful information. The collection of this information is facilitated by the fact that the French industry is, to a large extent, organised in producer groups with a central body. Details of one such analysis is given in Table 11.2.

Table 11.2 Specimen average technological/economic results for the years 1991–93 (group basis)

Parameter	1991	1992	1993
No. of farms in survey	922	1101	1108
No. of breeder cages	170	180	186
% replacement of does	135	131	122
% conception rate	71.5	73.3	75.5
No. litters per doe per year	7.28	7.16	7.14
No. born per litter	9.97	9.08	9.33
% mortality – birth to weaning	19.4	19.1	18.9
% mortality – weaning to slaughter	12.7	12.9	12.5
No. young per doe per year	45.5	46.0	47.1
No. young in life of each doe	33.7	35.1	38.6
Average liveweight of young (kg)	2.34	2.36	2.38
Feed conversion index (rate)	3.97	3.95	3.92
Cost of feed (francs/kg)	1.52	1.53	1.47
Selling price (francs/kg)	12.84	11.99	10.69
Margin of cost of feed/sales per breeding cage/year (francs)	1029	918	813
Margin cost of feed/sales per kg liveweight (francs)	6.61	5.94	4.93

France is fortunate in its institutions which concern themselves with rabbits. Research Institutes include three research stations which are part of the National Agriculture Research Institute (INRA), the three being at Toulouse, Tours and Magneraud; an Institute for Aviculture (ITAVI); the Experimental Station for Aviculture (SEA, CNEVA) at Ploufragan; and the National Syndicate for Angora Quality (SNAQ) at Angers. As for Associations, there are four national organisations dealing with specialist fields. For the education of rabbit breeders to all levels there are 18 institutes/colleges.

Since 1970, producer groups have been expanding. The largest have over 200 members, but many have less than 50. There are about 100 of the producer groups which are brought together in regional groups, with a single central body, FENELAP, which looks after the interests of all and acts as a central co-ordinator with a number of specialist services. Most of the production from the intensive farms go through processors, of which there are about 900, although there are only 30 major processors with a throughput of more than 5000 rabbits per week.

There are over 400 manufacturers of feeds, but many of these are relatively small. The total production of special rabbit feeds is somewhat greater than 700 000 tonnes per year. There are numerous equipment manufacturers, and there are a number of services which supply analyses of data from the industry, and computerisation and computer programs are freely available. A number of public and private veterinary investigation laboratories exist of veterinary services.

As for the market, modern distribution takes 39% of the output with supermarkets taking 19% and hypermarkets taking 17%. Traditional markets take a total of 61% of the output, with farm sales accounting for 22%, butchers 11% and markets (of which there are many in France) 10%. The presentation of the meat is taken seriously and many attractive packs made up, from whole carcases to special cuts. A further development is the sale of pre-cooked rabbit dishes to many classic recipes.

One specialist field which does not exist in the UK is producers of special hybrid lines of various sorts. There are 14 major hybrid line producers, with their associated multipliers.

The CIS

The other intensive rabbit farming countries follow the same pattern and in some respects Italy can be said to be even more advanced. The CIS is an interesting example of the considerable development which is possible. In the late 1920s there were reported to be less than half a million domestic rabbits in the CIS. At that time the government planned to greatly increase domestic rabbit production. The success of the scheme is shown by the fact that by the early 1930s meat production was probably of the order of 75 000 tons. A Rabbit Breeding Research Institute was established in Moscow at this time and a report from this Institute in 1946 stated that although commercial rabbit breeding had become very widespread, its efficiency was not high, and research was being undertaken to improve it. An interesting report shows that in 1951 in the Molotov Province, some 88% of the collective farms bred rabbits, and this accounted for some 15% of the total monetary profit of those farms. At the present time the CIS is amongst the world leaders in the production of rabbit meat, with a production of some 150 000 tons per year.

Germany

Whilst Germany has the largest rabbit fancy in the world, with some 170 000 members of its central breeders organisation, it is not a major rabbit meat producer. Nor is it one of the major Angora wool producers although a particular variety of Angora has been produced there which has spread to many parts of the world, China in particular. The German Angora produces heavy yields of wool which has a lesser tendency to matt than does either of the other two and it can be sheared successfully. The German Angora is probably the basis of the bulk Angora wool production. Germany was also the first country to establish central stations for testing Angoras.

Denmark

Denmark has a well-established rabbit fancy and farming interests, similar to that in this country. One of the most interesting features, however, was the establishment in 1943 of the Government Rabbit Testing Station at Favrholm (details of which are given in Chapter 9). This continues to the present time and indicates the value placed on the industry by the government.

The USA

The essential basis of the modern intensive system of commercial rabbit farming with wire cages, the use of complete pelleted feeding stuffs, intensive breeding and the sale of young meat animals began in America. Certainly part of the reason for this was the foundation of the Rabbit Experiment Station at Fontana in California in 1928, with a nutritional scientist and animal husbandry professor as its director. Unfortunately it was closed down in 1960. The only work of a similar nature is now carried on by a Centre for Rabbit Research established at the Oregon State University.

Whilst the rabbit fancy in America is well developed and the central organisation, the American Rabbit Breeders Association, has something over 30 000 members, the early promise shown by the young industry did not materialise, and for the size of the country the rabbit industry remains very small, with an annual production of approximately 17 000 tons. The larger feed compounders in the US also helped in the early establishment of the industry. At one time, they were selling approximately 125 000 tons of feed per annum, and one or two established their own rabbit research centres, but this tonnage is now less.

The US Department of Agriculture was the first government to issue inspection regulations for meat processing in domestic rabbit meat plants. These regulations laid down standards of hygiene, etc., and arranged an inspection system of all rabbits slaughtered at each regulated plant. This function is now well developed in the EU.

China

China has always had a fairly large domestic rabbit population. Exports of rabbit meat from China exceed 50 000 tons per annum and there is little doubt that the internal consumption is large. In the rural type of production, typically the animals are kept in tiered hutches, usually of primitive design, and in some cases in pits. The feeding is also completely different on such farms in that the majority of the food is green forage or hay. The age at which the animals are slaughtered is usually a good deal older than in other countries. The carcases themselves have usually very little fat. The production of Angora wool is a very large industry, for it generates some three-quarters of the entire world supply, although the quality is not usually high. This production of Angora wool is also closely associated with the meat production, as numbers of young Angoras are slaughtered when their wool is sufficiently abundant.

Chapter 12

Welfare and the Maintenance of Good Health

Since the first edition of this book in 1957 there has been – and rightly so – an increasing emphasis on the welfare of livestock. During the past ten years this emphasis has increased and the domestic rabbit has received its fair share of attention. Whilst there have always been, and in the future will unfortunately always be, a very small proportion of rabbit breeders who do not give the rabbit the attention and care that it deserves, the great majority of rabbit breeders devote much of their time to ensuring that their stock is kept in comfort and health.

It is, therefore, unfortunate that in some cases people who are not keepers of rabbits and whose knowledge and understanding of the animal leaves a good deal to be desired, attempt, sometimes successfully, to impose restrictions on rabbit keeping which are certainly not in the best interests of the rabbit. An example of this has been the introduction of several rather absurd legal requirements for rabbit breeders. Amongst others was a regulation relating to hutch sizes, which gives a minimum floor space requirement being currently approximately four times as great as that laid down by the UK Ministry of Agriculture.

Those breeders with a deep knowledge and experience – and love for – rabbits know that too large a hutch for some breeds, is nearly as bad as one that is too small. Often people suggest that because the domestic rabbit is so closely related to those in the wild, the conditions under which the wild rabbit lives must be perfect for the domestic. This is quite obviously a nonsense. Furthermore it is these very people who overlook the fact that the rabbit spends a very great deal of its time in extremely cramped quarters.

In the same way some welfare organisations that recommend a permanent outdoor run for the rabbit are not acting in the animal's best interests. There is a build up of disease organisms excreted by the rabbit and after a time, the run becomes a potent source of disease for the rabbit. There are many other such examples in different countries.

The best welfare of the rabbit demands that all its normal requirements are fully met, that is:

● it is kept well fed;

- it is protected from disease and dangers;
- it is kept in safety in a suitable environment;
- its normal behavioural requirements are met;
- it is protected as far as possible from stress.

An understanding of all aspects of rabbit husbandry, including the biology and life of the rabbit, its nutrition, housing and management are all necessary, if the best possible care is to be given. It should always be remembered that success can only be achieved with the fittest and best cared for stock.

An understanding of the causes of sickness and injury is equally essential. The greater the knowledge of the general principles of disease prevention and control the rabbit breeder has, the better will be his or her chances of success.

THE HEALTHY RABBIT

The starting point in the matter of the health and welfare of the domestic rabbit is a thorough understanding of the appearance, biology and behaviour of the healthy animal. The early recognition of ill health is most important, for the earlier the treatment the greater is the chance of success, not only in the case of the particular animal, but also in the prevention of contagion in other animals.

In most cases it is quite useless to commence treatment when the disease has progressed so far that the animal is obviously dying. The full benefit of veterinary advice will not be obtained unless it is obtained early, and the longer a sick animal remains in contact with others, the greater are the chances of the spread of the disease. As will be repeated many times, the prevention of disease is the most important aspect of good management.

The good stockperson will be quick to note any change in the appearance, appetite, behaviour, condition, habits, or faeces of the stock. The coat is a good indication of health. A dry, dull, harsh, staring or patchy coat indicates that something is wrong with the animal. A sleek, glossy, lustrous coat with its natural bloom indicates its well-being. Loose hairs may indicate that the rabbit is moulting, which is of course perfectly natural, but scurf should not be present.

The healthy rabbit is alert. Any sudden noise or movement will awaken its immediate interest. Its movements are easy and free and it does not sit huddled in a corner of the hutch. When resting it is relaxed, with its breathing even and not shallow. Adult rabbits have a respiration rate of from 35 to 55 breaths a minute, although youngsters may breathe nearly twice as rapidly. There should be no sound as the animal breathes.

The eyes should be bright and bold and there should be no discharge from them, nor from any other part of the body, particularly the nostrils, mouth, vent, anus or teats, which should also be free from any sores. The appetite and behaviour of the rabbit should be normal. Any animal that does not appear to be eating or behaving normally should immediately raise suspicions.

The fleshing of the rabbit also gives indication of its health. The muscles along either side of the spine should be firm and full and the rabbit should not feel 'bony'. There should be no swellings which indicate cysts, abscesses or ruptures. The healthy rabbit is full of vitality and the aim of every breeder should be to keep the stock in this condition.

For the commercial breeder, lowered production is an important indication that all is not well. The reasons for reduced rate of gain in weight, or loss of weight, or lack of appetite, should immediately be sought.

Table 12.1 gives a summary of the normal physiological and biological characteristics of the normal healthy rabbit. It must however be remembered that in some of these there is considerable variation, which occurs between breeds, strains, ages, sexes, conditions of health, environment and other factors.

Table 12.1 Physiological and biological characteristics of the rabbit

Rectal temperature	Average 39.5°C; range 38–40°C	Breed variation. Smaller animals have higher temperatures
Pulse rate	150–300 beats per minute	Very young rabbits have highest pulse rates
Respiratory rate	30–100 per minute	Average adult rate 35–50
Lactation average uninterrupted length	42 days	
Lactation peaks at	17–20 days	Depending on nutritional regime, breed of doe and size of litter
Litters number per doe per year	2–10	The lower figures are those usually in exhibition breeds, the higher figure is the maximum usually achieved in intensive farming
Litter size	2–14 young	Considerable breed, strain and individual variation. Average litter size about 5–6 for medium-sized exhibition stock, less for smaller, but 8–9 for commercial meat animals
Dental formula	$i-\dfrac{2}{1}, \quad c-\dfrac{0}{0}, \quad pm-\dfrac{3}{2}, \quad m-\dfrac{3}{3}$	
Usual life span	6–11 years	
Age of sexual maturity	16–26 weeks	The smaller breeds mature earliest
Gestation period (most common)	31–32 days	Limits for live births are usually 29–34 days
Adult weight	1–7.5 kg	Depending on breed/sex. Larger individuals have been produced (rarely) up to 12 kg
Sex ratio average	100 males to 105 females	

GENERAL PRINCIPLES OF DISEASE PREVENTION

Although a general knowledge of the symptoms, prevention and treatment of common diseases, and a knowledge of the practices and hygienic precautions necessary to avoid them, are very necessary for the successful breeder, he or she should not attempt to be his or her own veterinarian. In these days when professional post-mortem examinations and advice can be easily obtained, the breeder should be encouraged to use them to maximum benefit. A veterinarian and the MAFF

Veterinary Investigation Centres will be of assistance in this matter.

The incidence of the different diseases varies a good deal depending on the methods of housing, nutrition and management. Indeed different breeds and different strains are also subject to variations. There are also differences in the levels of mortality, and its causes, between exhibition rabbitries and commercial farms. For example, the present commercial farming of meat animals is almost invariably on wire floors with a manufactured feed, usually with a coccidiostat incorporated. Hence the amount of coccidiosis present is considerably less than in exhibition stock, where usually solid floors are used and often coccidiostats are not incorporated – or if incorporated are diluted to a dangerous level by the use of other feeds. On the other hand, the incidence of sore hocks is much more common in farmed animals than in those of the exhibitor.

It is probably true to say that in most commercial farms pasteurella is present and widespread. However, the problem with this disease may be less severe than in some exhibition breeders' establishments, because in commercial farms greater attention is paid to ventilation. Because there is a greater stress on breeding stock in commercial farming than in any other type of rabbit husbandry, diseases which may be 'triggered' by stress tend to be more common, and most certainly the mortality amongst weaned animals is higher.

The pet owner has yet different problems. First, usually the animals are more pampered than is good for them. Most, particularly those looked after by children, tend to be overfed and in some cases with foods that are not entirely suitable. Then, many are allowed free-range over a small plot of land which becomes increasingly 'rabbit sick' with a build up of disease organisms.

There is also a variation in disease with time. Thus for the 1940–50 period the disease most commonly of concern was coccidiosis. From 1953 this was replaced, not unnaturally by myxomatosis. Certainly from 1992 onwards, the disease on all rabbit breeders' lips has been viral haemorrhagic disease (VHD). It is sometimes unfortunate that concentration on a particular disease does sometimes rather blind the rabbit keeper to the presence of other diseases, which are actually of greater importance to him or her than the current fashionable disease.

Some diseases are certainly more spectacular than others and, for this reason, those that are not are usually very underrated when it comes to allotting causes to deaths or lost production. Thus it is likely that in the UK, pasteurellosis in its varied forms and enteric disorders (other than coccidiosis) contribute a great deal more to deaths, poor health and lowered production than most of the other diseases put together.

Some diseases are fairly well understood, but others are far less so. For example, a great deal is known of myxomatosis, how it is spread, and what can be done to prevent it. Its counterpart in viral haemorrhagic disease is another story. It is of course known that vaccines will prevent death, but much else as to its prevention is not yet fully understood.

In a well-managed exhibition rabbitry, diseases should be infrequent. Unfortunately, however, not all of the diseases of the rabbit are accompanied by sufficiently characteristic signs to allow the average breeder to recognise them. Accurate diagnosis is the work of veterinarians, and use should be made of their services, not only in order to attempt to treat the disease in the particular animals concerned, but in order that proper precautions can be taken to prevent further outbreaks.

Treatment of all but the most valuable stock, and animals affected with easily curable troubles, is not always to be recommended. This is because sometimes the treatment is expensive (and may cost more than the value of the animals concerned), often it requires a good deal of time and patience, and in cases of infectious diseases there is always a risk of further animals being infected. Also, in exhibition stock, animals rarely recover that richness of colour and general excellence which is so necessary, after having suffered a serious illness.

Losses due to disease are often greatly underestimated. This is true of all forms of rabbit keeping. In commercial farming, however, these losses do not arise only from actual deaths, for probably the greatest loss is occasioned by poor production and unthriftiness, causing waste of food, time and labour.

STRESS AND ITS RELATION TO WELFARE AND DISEASE

The term stress includes all those factors which impose an unusual burden on the animal. Such factors are often called stressors. The list of stressors which cause stress to the rabbit is long. It includes, but is not limited to, such things as:

● poor environment, including bad housing, poor ventilation, too high or too low a temperature, lack of adequate bedding and damp or foul bedding;
● poor, insufficient, or rapid changes in feed;
● disease, including parasites and injuries;
● the presence of dogs, cats and vermin;
● rough handling or handling by an unaccustomed handler;
● unusual or unexpected noises;
● departures from expected routines, such as lateness in feeding;
● overcrowding or insufficient space;
● bullying and fighting, particularly when animals of different ages, sexes or sizes are mixed together at the same time;
● confinement in an unsuitable box and travelling.

It must not be thought that only 'unnatural' occurrences impose stress on the rabbit. Normal functions such as kindling, pregnancy and lactation impose considerable stress on the doe.

The lack of all stress in rabbits tends to be as bad as too much stress. Some abnormal behaviour (fur chewing, for example) is undoubtedly caused by sheer boredom. The addition of some hay supplements, particularly if the animals have to be fairly active to eat them – for example, if they are placed on top of wire-mesh pens and the animal has to stretch up – often proves of value.

There are many ways in which stress can be reduced. Most of these are obvious, but that stress which occurs by the handling of the rabbits is of particular importance. If a proper programme of handling is undertaken, the stress caused by handling can be reduced considerably. In the case of the commercial farmer, contact between the stockperson and the stock is of vital importance. From about the 10th day after birth, that is to say when the eyes are fully open, the animals should be accustomed to the stockperson. Handling, in a gentle fashion, by far the best accompanied by the human voice, is the correct way. Any animal fearful of falling, or not held firmly, rapidly develops a very stressed condition. Quick movements should never occur. That area between the eyes down to just above the nostrils and up to the base of the ears is most sensitive in the rabbit, and the gentle stroking of this area produces an excellent calming effect.

Obviously on the commercial farm there is a limit to the amount of time the stockperson can spend handling the stock, but this does not apply so much to the exhibition breeder, and the pet or companion animal owner may even on occasion be thought to handle the animals rather too much!

Handling by the exhibition breeder is important, particularly of those animals which are to be shown. Not only must the breeder accustom the animals for the show bench, but he or she must train them to pose in such a way that they display their good points to the greatest advantage. It is important that this association between rabbit and man should be from an early age, for it is at this time that it is the most effective in getting rabbits accustomed to humans. From this early association they will suffer considerably less stress from later association with people.

All rabbit breeders will know how very different are the temperaments of not only different breeds of rabbit, but also different strains within those breeds, and different animals within those strains. One can have does which, even with youngsters, are of very mild temperament, whilst others are peculiarly vicious, even when she has no young. There is little that can be done to change this temperament of the animals concerned, but the progeny of such does, if correctly handled at an early enough stage (and this may sometimes be difficult) can sometimes be improved.

Not only does disease produce great stress in the rabbit but the occurrence of disease is often stimulated by the occurrence of stress. There is no doubt that many diseases are aggravated or even initiated by stress. For example, Tyzzer's disease often follows a period of unusual stress in the rabbitry, when a number of animals go down with it at the same time. In such cases the bacteria which cause the disease are normally resident in the rabbit in such small numbers that symptoms of disease do not appear, provided the animal remains in good condition. If the rabbits suffers some reverse then the disease 'flares up'. Stress triggers this development by reducing the natural powers of the body to resist the disease.

There is often a good deal of confusion between the terms 'sign' or 'symptom' and 'disease'. Many so-called diseases, for example scouring, are not diseases at all but are symptoms of one or more diseases, and should be distinguished as such. An appreciation of this point is essential to the proper understanding of disease in the rabbit.

The term 'carrier' is also sometimes misunderstood. A carrier is an animal which, whilst appearing perfectly healthy and having no signs or symptoms of a disease, can transmit that to other rabbits. Sometimes the carrier status is of temporary nature, whilst at other times the state of affairs persists. Coccidiosis in particular is a disease in which there is often found carriers and after an animal has recovered from say VHD, it may persist in shedding virus material which infects other animals for a week or two.

It is important that the rabbit breeder should have a true picture of the disease which occurs in the stock. Unless accurate records are kept the amount of disease is almost invariably understated. On many occasions the rabbit breeder totally over-looks a number of deaths. An accurate catalogue of the ages, conditions, etc. of all animals that die, including those that are 'put down' because they look like so doing, is most important. It will be of great help in the end.

In the commercial field, losses of young stock quite frequently exceed 20% of those reared to 10 weeks of age. It is true that some of these occur at birth or in the first week of life, but the majority occurs later. The figure is unacceptably high but is usually underestimated or understated by the farmer.

THE CAUSES OF DISEASE

Diseases may be caused by:

● *Bacteria* – microscopically small plants that exist in large numbers of different species. Fortunately those causing diseases are relatively few in number. Diseases of the rabbit caused by this group include pasteurellosis in its various forms, staphylococci infections, Tyzzer's disease, and others.
● *Spirochaetes* – cause 'vent disease', or to give it its proper name, rabbit *spiro-chaetosis*, which are very similar to bacteria and usually included in that group.
● *Viruses* – even smaller than bacteria. Although world wide there are some dozen or so diseases in the rabbit caused by these organisms, the only two of importance are myxomatosis and viral haemorrhagic disease (VHD).
● *Protozoa* – single-celled animals which in the rabbit cause coccidiosis.
● *Nutritional and metabolic disorders* – this group includes shortages (or occasionally excess) of vitamins, minerals and other essential items of diet, which give rise to such ailments as rickets, reproductive failures, imbalances of nutrients, poisons of various sorts and metabolic disorders such as pregnancy toxaemia, but most importantly mucoid enteritis.
● *Animal parasites* – the group includes trematodes or flukes, platyhelmynthes or flat worms, and nematodes or round worms which all give rise to worm infestations. In this group also are the external parasites such as fleas, lice, ticks and mites, etc., which can produce disease (e.g. ear canker) or can carry disease.
● *Fungus* – simple plants of cellular filaments causing ringworm and favus.
● *Inherited abnormalities* – of which the only one of importance is malocclusion of the teeth.
● *Miscellaneous conditions* – including all other conditions and ailments to which the rabbit is subject.

The most common diseases among domestic rabbits in this country are prob-ably pasteurellosis and respiratory diseases, followed by 'enteritis' in its various forms. The two viral diseases, myxomatosis and VHD have the potential for causing spectacular losses.

IMMUNITY AND THE USE OF VACCINES

The first vaccine to be generally used in this country by rabbit breeders was the vaccine against myxomatosis which became available shortly after the first outbreaks in 1953. Since the advent of VHD there has been great interest in the use of vaccines against this disease and two licences for its distribution were granted in November 1994. A knowledge of immunity and vaccination is therefore of interest and help to the rabbit breeder.

The animal body reacts immediately to the invasion of its body by any pathogen (bacteria or virus, etc.) or foreign matter by actively attempting to destroy the invader and by producing antibodies which also attempt to destroy the foreign matter. The foreign matter, which are usually bacteria, viruses, etc. are called antigens (short for antibody generating). In the case of innate or specific immunity this is always successful because the particular pathogen concerned cannot attack the rabbit with success. For example, the rabbit is innately or specifically immune to say foot and mouth disease, and the sheep is innately immune to VHD. There are numerous pathogens, however, which can attack with success the rabbit, which is not innately immune to them. If such pathogens attack the rabbit, whilst its immune system will attempt to destroy the invader, it may not succeed and the animal gets the disease.

There is another form of immunity, called acquired immunity, which will successfully prevent a disease to which the rabbit is normally susceptible because it generates the formation of antibodies. This is called acquired immunity and occurs when the animal is vaccinated. There is a second type of acquired immunity, called passive immunity, which is that acquired from the doe by the transfer of antibodies from her to her young. A doe with acquired immunity may pass on these acquired immunity antibodies but they would protect the young for only a short period.

At the present time there are only three vaccines available in this country, one for myxomatosis and two for VHD. There are many different vaccines in other parts of the world. There are three forms of vaccine. One type is prepared from organisms which normally cause the disease but which have been killed. They still, however, retain the chemicals which cause the rabbit body to produce antibodies. The second type uses live organisms whose powers to produce disease have been considerably weakened and thus whilst causing the production of antibodies they are unable to produce the disease. The third type is for use against toxins and not organisms and are not used in rabbit husbandry.

One type of vaccine, the autogenous vaccine, is produced from organisms which are producing the disease for which the vaccine is required actually obtained from one of the animals in the outbreak. This ensures that the actual strain of the bacteria causing the disease is used, usually thereby producing excellent results. Vaccines give protection for variable periods and after the appropriate period for the particular vaccine, re-vaccination is necessary. The vaccines in this country must be prescribed by a veterinary surgeon.

THE RELATIONSHIP BETWEEN THE RABBIT AND DISEASE ORGANISMS

In all animals there exists a relationship between the animal host and the disease organisms which attack it. It is important to understand the nature of this relationship. The example of myxomatosis well illustrates this relationship. The relationship relates to the fact that over a long period the host, in this case the rabbit, becomes increasingly immune to the pathogen, in this case the virus. The nature of the inheritance and increase of resistance to the disease in the rabbit, and the changes that occur in its virulence which occurs in the virus, have been demonstrated in several parts of the world.

There was always on the part of some rabbits a genetically controlled, albeit initially very low, resistance to myxomatosis. In the early days of infection in this country the case mortality was such that only about two rabbits in every thousand infected survived. Those two rabbits had a genetically controlled resistance. Gradually as these rabbits bred, it was seen that they were developing an increasing resistance to the disease with the average percentage numbers dying gradually reducing. Coupled with this were also variations in the virus itself, some strains becoming less and less virulent. Naturally the less virulent strains of the virus left those rabbits affected alive for a longer period and therefore that strain was passed on more frequently than the more virulent strains.

This relationship between the animal and the pathogen is not confined to viruses. The same is true of bacteria, worms, protozoa and the like. The same situation, for example, can be seen in different strains of *Pasteurella multocida*. Some strains of low virulence attack certain parts of the body and produce relatively little effect. More virulent strains most frequently cause the death of the host.

The same sort of relationship relates to pathogens and drugs. When a pathogen is attacked by any drug, for example an antibiotic, the dosage of that drug has to be appropriate. If the dosage given is too low, the pathogen gradually gets accustomed to the drug and builds up a resistance to it, which gives rise to the very important rule relating to the use of antibiotics: 'Hit quickly, hit hard and for the right length of time'.

THE SPREAD OF DISEASE

Disease organisms are spread, and infection therefore occurs, in various ways. There is the spread of disease by physical contact, an example being vent disease which is spread at mating. Confinement of healthy animals with diseased stock is another common cause, the disease organism passing from one animal to the next. Does will usually infect their young with coccidiosis, and many bacterial pathogens. Contamination of food will assist the spread of coccidiosis, tape worms, and other diseases, in particular those which are carried by rats and mice. Here it should be mentioned that what is called the faecal-oral route of infection is of particular importance in rabbit husbandry and must be carefully guarded against. A good deal of re-infection, and hence a build up of disease in the animal, occurs in this way. Some disease organisms may be spread through the air. Bacteria producing 'snuffles' are often carried in this way, a result of sneezing by an infected rabbit. Biting insects and fleas will efficiently spread myxomatosis. An understanding of these methods of the spread of disease organisms allows the rabbit breeder to understand the necessity for the quarantine of stock and of the precautions he must take to prevent disease spreading.

THE PROBLEM OF DISEASE

The problem of disease in the domestic rabbit is twofold. The first and most important part is prevention – which should be the first concern of all rabbit keepers or breeders; the second part concerns the elimination and treatment of disease which occurs.

The animal body, when it is healthy and in good condition should recover rapidly from minor ailments. The breeder must do everything to assist this recovery, and also to enable the rabbit to resist disease. The terms hygiene and sanitation are too often linked too closely with the term 'disease' in the rabbit breeder's mind. They should be linked with ideas of good management.

There are some diseases which are due to lack of certain essential items of diet, and there are other diseases which although caused by harmful organisms, are certainly assisted by poor nutrition; that is to say, inadequate feeding may greatly increase the susceptibility of animals to disease. As a former Director of Research on Nutrition in India has so rightly said, 'I know of nothing so potent in maintaining good health in laboratory animals as perfectly constituted food; I know of nothing so potent in producing ill health as improperly constituted food ... The greatest single factor in the acquisition and maintenance of good health is perfectly constituted food' (in R. McCarrison's Nutrition and National Health, 1944). Although these words were written 50 years ago, they remain as true today as when they were written.

Thus it can be emphatically stated that the first part of the problem of health must be tackled by good feeding, cleanliness and good hygiene, good management, and the selection of good stock. For again there is no question that different strains of rabbits resist some diseases to a greater degree than do others.

Disease prevention in the rabbitry may be complicated in several ways. The requirements of the fancier in particular are sometimes contrary to those which are necessary for strict disease prevention. For example, animals entering a rabbitry should be quarantined; stock should be allowed direct access to sunlight, for apart from its beneficial effect on them, the sun acts as a germicide; in any outbreak the affected animals should, for safety, be destroyed. But these points are opposed to the requirements of the fancier. A breeder who frequently shows would find it very difficult to separately quarantine all returning animals; sunlight will undoubtedly deteriorate the colour of the stock; and whereas in a commercial rabbitry the individual animal is of relatively little importance, and can therefore be sacrificed, in the fancier's stud the individual animals are of great importance.

These complications can only be overcome by compromise. For example, although the exhibition animals cannot be exposed to sun, the breeding stock will benefit from it, and the exhibition animals may possibly be housed separately from the remainder of the stud.

The rabbit breeder must appreciate that to attempt to overcome the problem of disease, he or she must have it in mind at all times. Prevention of disease is not a subject to which the breeder should turn only when disease appears – that is too late. It is a subject which must be an integral part of the rabbit breeder's scheme of management.

AN OUTBREAK OF AN INFECTIOUS DISEASE

There are few really serious infectious diseases in the domestic rabbit. Those that do exist, however, must be tackled immediately an outbreak occurs, in order to limit their spread.

The sick animal must be isolated, and the hutch that it occupied very thoroughly cleaned and disinfected. If the disease is one of the major infectious diseases such as haemorrhagic septicaemia, then further action must be taken. Any animals penned with the sick one should be separately isolated, and a careful eye kept on the other animals in the same rabbitry. Frequent inspection of these animals is necessary to find the first signs of any trouble. All bedding which has been in contact with sick animals must be destroyed, and burning is the only safe way. Care must be taken when removing this bedding to see that it does not contaminate other hutches or utensils such as the wheelbarrow which is used about the rabbitry, or that these are afterwards sterilised.

The source of the infection should be checked, and factors noted which helped the build up of the disease. For example, was the infection brought in by a new arrival or returning show animal? Or was it perhaps carried by rats or mice? Could it have been introduced by food? Or did flying insects come into the rabbitry? It may be that there are some predisposing factors such as bad ventilation, damp or draughts, overcrowding, or bad feeding. Such points are important and should always be checked to prevent further trouble.

THE CARE OF SICK ANIMALS

The rabbit breeder should consider what his or her plans would be if unfortunately an outbreak of disease occurred. If prepared, the problem is greatly reduced. Some diseases can spread so quickly that the most important action is immediate isolation of all sick animals. The isolation should be as complete as possible, and the hutches in which the sick animals are placed should be protected from vermin and flies.

Early treatment is really essential to success. Sometimes the breeder will be able to diagnose the disease him- or herself, but more usually professional assistance will be required. Every breeder should know of some veterinary surgeon, Veterinary Investigation Centre or laboratory where diagnosis can be made quickly.

The decision as to whether to treat a sick animal or put it down may be difficult for the exhibition breeds. In a commercial undertaking it is doubtful whether treatment for any except the most simple troubles is worthwhile, but for the fancier, for whom a single animal may be of importance, treatment is more often attempted. It should be noted that the killing of sick animals should take place away from the rabbitry to prevent any possibility of spreading the infection.

Apart from isolating the sick animal, its food, utensils and bedding must also be kept separate. The animal should be made as comfortable as possible, with plenty of good bedding, although care should be taken to use bedding which is not the slightest bit dusty. Good ventilation and plenty of fresh air are important.

In many cases there will be loss of appetite, and the animal should be tempted to eat with the best quality food. Little and often should be the rule, and no stale food should be left in front of the rabbit. Appetite may often be a sign of recovery, and indeed there is sometimes the danger of a convalescing rabbit overeating. This should of course be prevented. In all cases, except where the animal is scouring, the food should be laxative rather than the reverse. Clean fresh water should always be available, although sometimes, for example with mucoid enteritis, there is excessive thirst, and drinking should be restricted.

When handling the rabbit for treatment, it should be wrapped tightly in a towel or in sacking which will prevent struggling and injury, both to the animal and the attendant. Medicines should always be given in a little water or with food. When a wound or sore, or the ear in ear canker, is being cleaned, fresh pieces of cotton wool should be used continually, and the used pieces burnt.

MEDICINES IN THE RABBITRY

As with all animal husbandry there have been many advances in the treatment of disease in the past few years. Many of the antibiotics (although some are quite unsuitable for the rabbit) have been used with success, and there are other drugs that have proved of value. Most of these are prescription only medicines (POM) and are available therefore only from a veterinary surgeon. Table 12.2 gives a list of some of those that are of use. It should be noted that penicillin and its derivatives should only be used as a cream, it is toxic when injected. A few other antibiotics have been found to be toxic but are most unlikely to be prescribed.

Table 12.2 Some medicines used in rabbit husbandry

Name	Condition used for	Method of use
Bacitracin	Growth stimulant	Food
Chloramphenicol	Respiratory and intestinal	Injection/food/water
Clopidol	Coccidiosis	Food
Furaltadone	Intestinal	Food
Ivermectin	Parasitic and sore hocks	Injection
Neomycin	Intestinal	Food
Oxytetracycline	Respiratory	Injection/food/water
Penicillin and its derivatives	Toxic when injected	Penicillin creams are satisfactory
Robenidine	Coccidiosis	Food
Streptomycin	Respiratory	Injection
Tetracycline	Respiratory	Injection/food/water
Trimethoprim	Respiratory and intestinal	Food/water

DISINFECTANTS AND DISINFECTION

There is no universal disinfectant. Different organisms are destroyed by different preparations. For example, whilst ammonia will destroy coccidia, there is no other disinfectant which will do so. There are, however, general disinfectants and sprays against insects and parasites which can be used to kill the different types of organisms to be eliminated. Sunlight is valuable, as is heat from a blowlamp, provided that it is given time to act.

It is important that the right solution is used. For example if a wet floor is to be disinfected, then a solution above the required strength must be used as it will be diluted by the water on the floor. No disinfectant will work properly unless the items to be disinfected are *clean*. It is a true, although perhaps slightly exaggerated remark that 'a disinfectant will not work unless the cleaning is done properly, and if the cleaning is done properly there should be nothing left to disinfect'. Cleaning with a 4 or 5% solution of washing soda and hot water is satisfactory. Bad disinfection is worse than none at all, for it gives a false sense of security, and it must never be thought that all that is required for disease prevention is routine disinfection. This is part, but part only, of the matter.

The commercial meat industry has developed a technique in which each house is totally cleared in turn and, when empty, is thoroughly cleaned, disinfected and disinfested. In a perfect world this means that all infectious agents, insects and vermin are totally eliminated but this in practice is never be achieved. In principle, the system can be applied to the rabbitry of the exhibition breeders. The procedure, after the animals are removed, is to clean the house as much as possible, not forgetting walls and roof. A disinfectant as a gas, aerosol form or simple spray is then used. It must be made clear that all disinfectants are dangerous to use and the greatest care must be taken at all times. Some instruction and guidance in their use should be obtained from a knowledgeable person.

The best way of disinfecting brushes, spades, scrapers and other utensils is to stand them in a bucket of disinfectant. Feeding utensils should, of course, be cleaned with clean water afterwards. Buildings or hutches are best sprayed with disinfectant, although brushing on will often prove satisfactory. When hutches are being disinfected, care should be taken to see that corners, cracks and crevices receive attention.

In all cases the solutions and method of use recommended by the manufacturers should always be followed. It is, however, always advantageous to use disinfectants hot, as this assists their working.

Appendix

Notes on Diseases and Ailments of the Rabbit

It is impossible in a book of this kind to do more than give some general notes on the more common diseases and disorders in the rabbitry. It is also not possible to include coloured illustrations of the conditions. For those desiring further information on the subject, reference should be made to the excellent books on the subject referred to in the bibliography, especially Okerman, L. (1994) *Diseases of Domestic Rabbits*, 2nd edn., Library of Veterinary Practice Series published by Blackwell Science.

Before dealing with individual conditions, it is as well to take an overview of the disease conditions to which the domestic rabbit is subject. Table 1 lists those conditions which might be met in the UK, listed in the order in which they appear below. Very rare diseases and those that do not occur in the UK are excluded.

Table 1   Main diseases and disorders found in the domestic rabbit in Great Britain

Disease/disorder	Cause
Caused by bacteria	
Abscesses	*Staphylococcus aureus*
Enterotoxaemia	*Clostridium spiriforme* and *C. perfringens*
Mastitis	Usually *Staphylococcus aureus*, but sometimes *Pasteurella multocida*
Caused by *Pasteurella multocida*	
Chronic conjunctivitis	
Haemorrhagic septicaemia	
Reproductive tract infections (metritis, orchitis, etc.)	
Snuffles	
Torticollis (wry neck)	
Pneumonia – but also see below	
Pneumonia – other than above	Pathogens involved include *Aspergillosis, Bordetella bronchiseptica* and *Staphylococcus aureus*; inhaled matter
Pseudo-tuberculosis	*Yersinia pseudotuberculosis*
Salmonellosis	*Salmonella typhimurium* and *S. enteritidis*
Schmorl's disease	*Fusobacterium necrophorum*
Snuffles	*Pasteurella multocida*

Table 1 *continued*

Disease/disorder	Cause
Spirochaetosis	*Treponema cuniculi*
Strangles	*Streptococcus* spp.
Tuberculosis	*Mycobacterium tuberculosis*
Tyzzer's disease	*Bacillus piliformis*

Caused by viruses

Myxomatosis	Myxoma virus, a DNA virus of the pox virus family
Viral haemorrhagic disease	An RNA *Calicivirus* of the picornavirus family

Caused by protozoa

Coccidiosis	Nine species of *Eimeria* are involved, but *E. perforans* and *E. coeciola* are non-pathogenic and three other species are of low virulence and generally non-fatal
Hepatic (liver)	*E. stiedae*
Intestinal	*E. flavescens*, *E. intestinalis* and *E. piriformis* are virulent

Nutritional disorders

Constipation and scouring	Both are symptoms of other conditions
Mucoid enteritis	Unknown, possibly associated in some cases with one or more pathogens
Poisoning	Poisons/metals/excess vitamins which may occur in feeding stuffs
Pregnancy toxaemia	Almost certainly a metabolic disorder due to high nutritional requirements of the doe in later stages of pregnancy with inadequate supply of food
Rickets	Deformation due to lack of hardening of the bones
Starvation	Young unable to suckle through deformity, insufficient milk; over-bulky feed

Parasitic infestations

Ear canker	Ear mites – *Psoroptes cuniculi* and *Chorioptes cuniculi*
Insect parasites (fleas, lice, mites)	Apart from those causing ear canker and mange, include most usually: fur mites (*Cheyletiella parasitovorax*, *Listrophorus gibbus* and *Demodex cuncili*), lice (*Haemodipsus ventricosus*) and the rabbit flea *Spilopsyllus cuniculi*
Myiasis (fly strike)	Fly larvae burrowing beneath skin
Parasitic worms and flukes	Stomach worm – *Graphidium strigosum*
	Intestinal worm – *Trichostrongylus retortaeformis*
	Caecal worm – *Passalurus ambiguus*
	Liver fluke – *Fasciola hepatica*
	Tapeworms
	Cittotaenia ctenoides – found in small intestines
	Cittotaenia pectinata – found in small intestines
	Tapeworm cysts (intermediate stage of dog tapeworms)
	Taenia pisiformis – usually found in or near liver
	Taenia serialis – always found in muscle tissue
Sarcoptic mange	Mites – usually *Sarcoptes scabiei* but also *Notoedres cati*

Fungal infections

Favus	*Achorion* spp.
Ringworm	Fungal – almost invariably *Trichophyton mentagrophytes*, but occasionally other pathogenic dermatophytic fungi. Rare

Inherited abnormalities

	Lethal (e.g. spina bifida), epilepsy, hydrocephalus, dwarfism, furlessness and others. Rare except for malocclusion, see below

Disease/disorder	Cause
Malocclusion	An inherited condition where the incisors (usually, but cheek teeth too) fail to meet and thus grow to extreme lengths

Miscellaneous other conditions

Bites and other wounds	Bites and scratches from other animals, and damage occasioned by bad housing
Cancers and tumours	Rare at ages of rabbits normally encountered in commercial herds
Chilling	Poor nest boxes, badly made nest by doe, does littering on floor and not in nest, young being dragged out of nest
Congestion of the mammary glands	Lack of suckling when lactating
Desertion of young and cannibalism	In some cases undoubtedly the tendency to eat young is inherited. Lack of water, poor nutrition. Not common
Fractures	Injury, spontaneous, bad handling
Fur chewing	Cause unknown – boredom, lack of fibre and insufficient light are possible causes
Hairloss	Several causes – see notes below
Heat stroke	Excessive heat and lack of ventilation
Overgrown nails	–
Moist dermatitis (slobbers)	Excess salivation and wetting of fur
Paralysis	Most usually fractured spine, but can also result from several disease conditions
Pododermatitis, ulcerative (sore hocks)	Initially damage to the pad of the foot, followed usually by bacterial infection
Pot-belly	Enlarged liver, poor early nutrition
Ruptures of stomach	Cause unknown. Uncommon, although the incidence appears to be increasing
Trichobezoars (hair balls)	Fur chewing or swallowing on grooming. Rare, but more common in Angoras
Urine burn	Urine soaked bedding

DISEASES CAUSED BY BACTERIA

Bacteria are simple microscopic organisms which constitute an important cause of disease in the rabbit. In size they lie between the protozoan parasites, which are larger and in the rabbit cause coccidiosis, and the viruses which are considerably smaller and in the rabbit cause myxomatosis and VHD. Although other areas are affected, in general the greatest problems from bacteria occur in the respiratory tract.

Abscesses

Abscesses can be produced by several types of bacteria, but the most commonly involved is *Staphylococcus aureus*. In these cases the most common site of formation is subcutaneous, but abscesses may also occur in internal sites. These conditions are not very common, but when they are there is often a widespread incidence in the rabbitry. The tumour so formed may grow to a large size, up to that of a hen's egg and in many cases very young animals are affected as well as older. The tumour contains a thick creamy exudate. The condition is often wrongly attributed to a pasteurella problem. The only treatment is by suitable antibiotics which must be selected for their activity against the particular strain of the bacteria. See also Schmorl's disease below.

Chronic conjunctivitis

See under Pasteurella.

Enterotoxaemia

This disease, which particularly affects young rabbits, is characterised by a thin brown diarrhoea which stains the hindquarters of the animal. The onset is very rapid and the animals usually die within 24 hours. Characteristically, a number of animals in the same establishment are affected at roughly the same time. The disease is caused by bacteria of the *Clostridium* genus. Usually two species are involved, *C. spiriforme* and *C. perfringens*. Neither of these two species are normal inhabitants of the rabbit's intestines. The bacteria produce toxins which are absorbed into the blood via the intestines. The disease usually appears after some change in conditions, e.g. weaning, change of food and the like and very often the disease is present at the same time as another intestinal disease. Adults are sometimes affected. As with many intestinal disorders of the rabbit, prevention is based on good husbandry and feeding practices – reduction of stress, sufficient fibre and slow change to new diets. A second approach by the use of copper sulphate at low levels in feeding pellets and by pro-biotics has been tried with some success. Treatment can only lie in an increase in fibre by the use of a supplement.

Haemorrhagic septicaemia

See under *Pasteurella.*

Mastitis

This is an infection of the mammary glands occurring only in lactating does. It is fortunately not common. The acute form is sometimes wrongly known as milk fever or blue breast. The disease is caused by various bacteria, *Staphylococci* usually being responsible, particularly for the chronic form, whilst *Streptococci* are also concerned. The teat or teats are swollen and painful, and in the acute form there is usually a discharge. The doe has little appetite but is usually very thirsty and has a high temperature. The condition may spread until nearly all or all the teats are affected, and there is evidence that the condition is contagious. Treatment consists of bathing the affected parts with warm water containing an antiseptic. In most cases one of the antibiotics may be used to effect a cure, but veterinary advice is necessary. It is of course important to recognise that under no circumstances should the young of a doe affected by this condition be fostered to another doe.

DISEASES CAUSED BY *PASTEURELLA*

Pasteurella multocida is almost invariably present in most rabbits, and pasteurellosis is probably the cause of the greatest loss to both the rabbit breeder and farmer. The group of diseases caused by the organisms produce different disease conditions which sometimes appear to merge into each other. Finally, there appears to be little doubt that some outside influences, perhaps changes in food, other environmental changes, and the like, or perhaps a general weakness in some animals, allow the organisms a chance to build up and produce the disease conditions. Prevention and control in the earliest possible stages are therefore indicated, with every effort being made to prevent sudden changes. Different strains of rabbit and different individuals show various levels of immunity or resistance to different forms of the disease, and the strains of the bacteria are very variable in their virulence.

The organisms are usually located in the nasal cavities of the rabbit and therefore for the most usual symptoms observed are in that region. Snuffles is perhaps the most common condition produced by *P. multocida*. There are a number of strains of *P. multocida*, some of which are particularly virulent.

Chronic conjunctivitis

Chronic conjunctivitis, also known as weeping eye, is a condition in which there is a discharge from the eye. This was first seen in the UK during the 1950s. The frequency with which it has occurred has increased since that time. The condition is aggravated by poor ventilation and there is a tendency for chronic conjunctivitis to occur more frequently in some strains of rabbits than in others. It is again due to *P. multocida*. In advanced cases there may be considerable loss of fur below the eye. Treatment is sometimes successful and is by the use of an antibiotic ophthalmic cream containing either penicillin. or chloramphenicol.

Haemorrhagic septicaemia

Also known as acute pasteurellosis, haemorrhagic septicaemia was usually unrecognised in the past, but is now known to cause a good deal of loss. It is the result of infection with one of the most virulent forms of the bacteria. The symptoms are varied. In acute cases the animal may die within a few hours without much sign of the trouble. In other cases the temperature increases, as does the respiration rate, and breathing may be noisy. Haemorrhages may be found in the lungs and lymph nodes or glands, and the blood vessels are often congested with dark-coloured blood. The chest cavity usually contains a clear, yellowish fluid. Because of the variations in symptoms, diagnosis is very difficult outside the laboratory. There is a tendency for animals previously infected with another form of pasteurellosis, e.g. snuffles, to be relatively immune from this most virulent form. The prevention is again good hygiene, good ventilation, good feeding and management. On the Continent and in the USA vaccines are sometimes used to give protection, but these are not available in this country. Early injections of antibiotics have also been reported as affecting a cure. The rapidity of the disease is, however, such that treatment is usually impossible. Vaccines, not currently available in the UK, have on the Continent been found to be effective against this acute form of pasteurellosis.

Reproductive tract infections

Although not common, *P. multocida* may cause infections of the reproductive tract of both bucks and does. In does the uterus becomes infected, causing a metritis, whilst in bucks the most common form is a swelling of the testicles.

Snuffles

This disease varies from year to year in its prevalence. In some years it occurs frequently, in others less so. It is rarely present in young animals under about 10 weeks being a disease of the older rabbit. Although several other bacteria have been found to occasionally be responsible for this condition it is almost invariably caused by *P. multocida*. The main symptom is a thick, sticky, white discharge from the nose, which the animal wipes away with its forelegs. The fur on the inside of the legs becomes matted as a consequence. There is also sneezing and some coughing. The condition should not be confused with temporary irritation due to dust or dry foods (where the sneezing is temporary). The duration of the disease is very variable, some cases appearing to clear up very quickly, whilst others appear to be chronic.
Snuffles is rarely fatal, although sometimes an animal suffering from the trouble will develop a secondary infection of pneumonia, pleurisy, or acute pasteurellosis.

Poor nutrition is definitely a predisposing factor, vitamin A deficiency probably being the most important. Bad ventilation assists the development and spread of the disease, which may be very rapid. Animals which have apparently recovered are often carriers and spread the disease to other stock. Prevention therefore lies in good nutrition, good ventilation, and the elimination of all animals affected. There is unfortunately no satisfactory treatment available, although injections of various antibiotics have been claimed to effect a cure. The use of autogenous vaccines (see 'Immunity and the use of vaccines' in Chapter 12) have been used with success.

Torticollis (wry neck)

This is a condition in which the affected animal holds its head on one side. Usually deterioration occurs until the animal is unable to maintain its equilibrium and constantly falls over. The main cause of the disease is infection of the inner ear by *P. multocida*. Other minor causes, which usually produce less acute symptoms than above, are advanced ear canker, or tumours. There is no satisfactory treatment.

Pneumonia

Inflammation of the lungs is a fairly common complication of several diseases. The most common cause is *P. multocida* but other pathogens involved include *Aspergillosis, Bordetella bronchiseptica* and *Staphylococcus aureus*. A form of pneumonia is also caused by inhaled material, for example dust from food. The course of the disease is rapid and may prove fatal in three or four days. The animal usually has no appetite, and sits huddled and quiet. Temperature and respiration rate are increased, and in some cases there is a watery discharge from the eyes. The lungs after death are seen to be partly or completely darkish in colour and firm to the touch instead of pinkish and soft. The affected portions will sink in water. There is no reliable treatment for pneumonia, but the animal should be placed in a warm dry hutch where there is plenty of air. Pneumonia often arises from changed conditions such as subjection to draughts or damp. Another bacterial species *Bordetella bronchiseptica* is often found in cases of pneumonia in association with *P. multocida* and it is often suggested to be a cause of the pneumonia. However, it is often present in apparently benign form and animals normally infected with the bacteria show no signs of disease.

Pododermatitis

See under Miscellaneous conditions.

Pseudo-tuberculosis

This disease, caused by *Yersinia pseudotuberculosis*, is fortunately not common. It resembles true tuberculosis which is, however, rare in the domestic rabbit. Few symptoms of pseudo-tuberculosis are usually noticed, although there may be some loss of condition and weakness. The breathing may be laboured in the later stages if the lungs are affected. The disease is often fatal four or five weeks after infection, although the time interval varies. The rabbit dies suddenly. After death there are small, whitish-yellow nodules scattered throughout some or all of the following organs: lungs, liver, spleen, intestines and lymph glands. As the most common source of infection is from germ-contaminated food the intestines are often the first part to be affected, in particular the appendix, the contents of which are usually white and cheesy, the organ itself being spotted with nodules.

   Infection occurs from other animals or from contaminated food or water. Rats and mice carry the disease, and vermin-ridden fodder is a constant source of infection. It follows that prevention lies in protecting the rabbitry and the food and water supply (and also bedding to be used) from vermin. There is no treatment.

Salmonella infection

Salmonellosis is not often met with, but has been responsible for some outbreaks of disease causing considerable loss. The two main bacteria responsible are *Salmonella typhimurium* and *S. enteritidis*. The rabbit appears listless and dull, with quickened breathing and a rise in temperature. Loss of appetite is also sometimes accompanied by scouring and by abortion in pregnant does. The symptoms and post-mortem appearance are very variable, and diagnosis can only be made accurately by bacteriological examination. The disease is largely spread through contamination of food, water and litter, by rats and mice which carry it. These infections also occur in poultry, household pets and other animals (and occasionally in man) and may be transmitted from them. The only prevention is to eliminate contamination. Treatment is not advisable except in special cases since any animals apparently cured will remain carriers.

Schmorl's disease

Also known as necrobacillosis, this condition is caused by bacteria known as *Fusiformis necrophorus*, which can almost always be found on the skin of the rabbit. It only causes harm, however, when it enters the body through some wound. When this happens, two forms of the disease may occur. The first is a skin infection, which starts on the head, particularly the lips. The part becomes discoloured and ulcerated, the skin of the affected area dying. The second form of the disease consists of thick-walled abscesses containing yellow pus, which are extremely painful to the rabbit when touched. These abscesses form in the skin or in the internal organs, and may reach the size of a golf ball. The abscesses can be distinguished in that they are hot and cause pain when touched, as opposed to cysts which do not feel hot and which cause no pain. A frequent complication with this disease is pneumonia. With both forms, the animal may have difficulty in eating and breathing, and if the head is affected the animal usually dies within three weeks.

Early treatment with one of several types of antibiotics has on occasion proved useful. Prevention consists in ensuring that wounds are cleansed properly. Treatment is difficult in the skin type of infection but surgical removal of the abscess can be attempted by a skilled person in the case of valuable animals.

Snuffles

See under *Pasteurella*.

Spirochaetosis (vent disease)

This condition is much more common than it should be. Sometimes the percentage of infected animals in a stud is high. The disease is caused by a spirally twisted microscopic organism, *Treponema cuniculi*, closely related to bacteria. The sexual organs, and very often the anus, become crusted with sores which vary in size up to about the size of a pea or even more. The sores may run into each other to form one large mass. Although the sexual organs are first affected, the anus in the majority of cases becomes involved, and sores may spread to lips, nose and eyelids. The animal generally remains in good condition, although, in advanced cases, the desire for mating is sometimes lost. Infection occurs when a healthy animal is mated to one with the infection. The time between infection and the appearance of the sores varies, but is usually not less than about eight weeks. Whilst the usual method of infection is by mating, this appears to be not the only route, for the disease has appeared from time to time in animals that have not mated, becoming infected possibly from their dams. Nevertheless control of the disease consists in careful examination of all animals prior to mating, and examination of the parts during routine inspections. Treatment usually consists of injections of antibiotics (by a veterinarian).

Strangles

Strangles is a rare type of abscess which develops in the lower jaw, caused by streptococcal bacteria. The abscess is firm to the touch and contains a yellowish pus. The only treatment consists in lancing the cavity and swabbing with an antiseptic.

Tuberculosis

The rabbit is susceptible to all forms of tuberculosis (caused by *Mycobacterium* bacteria) of bovine, human or avian strains. The bovine form is most commonly found. Although the disease was at one time not uncommon, it has greatly decreased in incidence, due probably to the fact that milk is now much less frequently fed to domestic rabbits, and such milk as is fed is likely to be free of the bacillus. In the acute form often no symptoms are present before death, but in the chronic form there is loss of condition and appetite, weakness and usually diarrhoea. Breathing may be laboured and a cough may develop. Diagnosis is difficult and differentiation from pseudo-tuberculosis equally so. Consequently, laboratory diagnosis should be sought in cases of doubt. Infection arises from food and water contamination by tuberculan animals and birds. Control is therefore obvious, but there is no treatment.

Tyzzer's disease

This disease was only first recognised in rabbits in 1965, but since that time has been diagnosed on a number of occasions. The bacteria responsible is *Bacillus piliformis*. The disease tends to occur in many animals in the same rabbitry at the same time. It particularly affects young weaned animals up to the age of about 3 months. In some cases half or more of the animals affected die within one or two days, the only indications being a watery diarrhoea and a general apathy of the stock. There is also a chronic form in which the animals gradually lose weight and become extremely listless and weak.

The usual method of infection is from contamination of food by the discharges from sick animals. This disease occurs from a pathogen which is normally resident in the animals, with the disease developing when the bacteria are activated as it were through other causes, particularly stress. The disease can be spread by mice and rats. Some treatments with the use of antibiotics have in some cases been used with success. As treatment for the disease can be difficult and unsuccessful, the prevention is important and must consist of the removal of sick animals, the prevention of stress in any form, and the prevention of any possibility of animals eating contaminated feed, water or bedding.

DISEASES CAUSED BY VIRUSES

The rabbit in this country may suffer from only five diseases caused by viruses although world wide there are some 13. Three of those occurring in this country are extremely rare, being a particular type of tumour, encephalomyelitis, and a disease that has been termed Weybridge disease. The other two are myxomatosis and VHD.

Both of these diseases have features of interest in common. Myxomatosis was the first virus disease of animals described and so attributed and VHD is certainly amongst the last. Both have moved through the world at a quite astonishing rate. Both have attacked the wild rabbit and the domestic and both have became better known to the public in many countries, than probably any other animal disease. The case mortality in both diseases was at first very great. In the early stages of myxomatosis only two animals per thousand infected, lived. The case mortality in VHD is not so high, but the disease kills even more quickly.

Myxomatosis

Myxomatosis, caused by a poxvirus of the myxoma group, was first described in 1898 in Montevideo as a highly fatal infectious disease. Attempts were made to introduce it into Australia to kill off the wild rabbit there, but these attempts were unsuccessful until the early 1950s. In 1953 the disease was introduced into France, where vast numbers of domestic rabbits were killed, as well as wild rabbits. During October 1953 the disease appeared in England, and then spread over the entire country, killing off a very high proportion of the wild rabbits, although attacking very few domestic rabbits. The disease is spread by biting insects. The most common vector infecting the wild rabbit is the rabbit flea whilst the carrier of the disease to domestic rabbitries is the mosquito.

After a rabbit has been infected by a biting insect carrying the virus, the eyelids swell considerably, eventually completely closing over the eye. Swellings may occur on other parts of the body, particularly at the base of the ears. Death follows in almost all cases within at most some 12 days of infection, although there are some few cases of recovery. Since its arrival myxomatosis has varied in its virulence and also in the form it takes. Basically there are two forms, the first being the so-called cutaneous form, in which the symptoms are those of the original disease. The second form is known as the respiratory form, in which the incubation period is rather longer than in the cutaneous form, in some cases as long as three weeks before symptoms appear. The respiratory form, although spread by biting insects, is also spread by animal to animal contact much more frequently than the classic form. There is no treatment for myxomatosis but a vaccine is available which gives full protection. The elimination of all biting insects from the rabbitry also gives protection and the importance of removing any affected animals cannot be too strongly stressed. If these precautions are taken little trouble from this disease will arise.

Viral haemorrhagic disease (VHD)

The disease is caused by an RNA virus of the *Calicivirus* genus. It was a notifiable disease in the UK (the only one for rabbits). It first occurred in China in 1984 and then spread through many countries and most of those in Europe by 1992, when it reached England.

The disease affects only the rabbit and no other mammal or bird. It affects mainly older bucks and does and no breed seems to be more or less susceptible than any other. Animals under the age of eight weeks are rarely affected, and animals before weaning almost never. The disease is highly contagious. Direct transmission, that is from animal to animal, is the commonest form of spread. It is known that the disease can be transmitted 'mechanically' by humans and through infected food. Biting insect transmission is also likely. There is some evidence of transmission by birds. At the present time the spread of the virus by aerosol dispersion, that is simply through the air seems to be a likely method, which of course makes it a very dangerous disease. Dried virus can survive for several months. There are three basic forms of the disease:

- The peracute (hyperacute or most virulent) affects all highly susceptible rabbits. The animals die suddenly without clinical signs.
- The acute form, which is most prevalent in an epidemic, affects all animals over the age of about two months, except those vaccinated.
- The sub-acute form occurs with reduced symptoms, usually in the later stages of an epidemic. Many animals survive and become resistant to the disease.

Death usually occurs in one to two days with a maximum of three days from first infection. There are usually no outward signs of the disease, but in many cases, one or more of various inconstant signs occur, including no appetite, fever, apathy, dullness, prostration, paralysis (hind limbs), lying on side, spasms with head and lower limbs bent backwards thus arching the body with belly up, groans and cries before death, increased breathing rate, respiratory distress, nasal discharge, including blood, lacrimation and haemorrhaging around eyes, blue appearance of mucous membranes, ears and eyelids. Some animals which apparently recover from the acute form sometimes die a few weeks later.

In certain populations there appears to be an immunity of some animals to the disease, this sporadic immunity occurring in other countries. Further, after a rabbit has recovered from the disease it is immune from further infection. The only way in which it can be certain that other rabbits are immune is by vaccination. Rabbits which recover from the disease may continue to shed virus and infect other rabbits for at least a week or more.

In all countries with a substantial population of domestic rabbits, vaccination has been found to give excellent protection. Good hygiene is highly important, including the removal of litter at proper intervals. The elimination of all vermin, insects and domestic animals other than rabbits from the rabbitry is necessary, these may carry the disease. It is best to avoid contact with any rabbit breeders who during recent weeks have had sudden unexplained deaths in their rabbitries. Quarantining of all incoming stock away from all other stock for at least a week is desirable. Steps should be taken to ensure that food (hay, greenfood) comes from places where no rabbits are known.

The only disinfectants at present which have any effect are a 10% solution of formalin or a 2% solution of sodium hydroxide (undiluted bleach). Unfortunately both of these are dangerous and difficult to use. The virus withstands 60°C for at least six minutes.

Two vaccines for the disease have been licensed in the UK. Both vaccines are POM (prescription only medicines) and are obtainable only from veterinary surgeons.

DISEASES CAUSED BY PROTOZOA

Protozoa are simple, single-celled organisms some of which cause disease in both man and animals. Whilst throughout the world there are several diseases of rabbits caused by protozoa, the only disease of significance in the rabbit in the UK is coccidiosis.

Coccidiosis

This disease was probably responsible for more loss through deaths and lowered production than any other disease, (although its premier place has now been taken by diseases caused by pasteurella and by 'enteritis' complexes). By proper management it can now be reduced to negligible proportions. It is caused by several species of protozoa of the genus *Eimeria*, one species attacking the liver, the others attacking the intestines. Very often a mixed infection occurs.

The life history of the parasite is as follows. Oocysts (eggs) pass out with the faeces of an infested animal, and if the conditions are suitable, i.e. warmth and humidity, become infective within two days. These oocysts are then eaten by a rabbit and develop, liberating numbers of parasites (sporozoites), which attack the walls of the intestine or the cells of the bile ducts. These parasites then reproduce themselves and further cells are attacked and destroyed. This process continues until a sexual stage is reached when oocysts are produced and pass out with the faeces. There are two forms of the disease, one in which the intestines are attacked and one in which the liver is attacked.

The symptoms vary according to the form of the disease and the age and severity of attack, and also the condition of the animal. In the hepatic (liver) form of the disease there are often few signs and it does not often result in the death of the animal. Diarrhoea is only occasionally present and there may be some loss of condition. The liver, in advanced cases, shows a number of white or yellowish spots or streaks and, later, nodules, the contents of which vary from a thin fluid to a thick, cheesy material. The bile ducts become thickened, and in advanced chronic cases of the liver form, the liver is greatly enlarged, giving rise to 'pot-belly' in life.

In the intestinal form, the signs are more varied. There is usually loss of flesh, which is sometimes severe, and the coat becomes harsh and staring. The rabbit in severe attacks often adopts a typical huddled attitude. Sometimes there is loss of appetite, but at other times the rabbit becomes ravenously hungry and thirsty. There is often diarrhoea but not inevitably so. Internally there are small whitish spots and, later, greyish streaks on the walls of the intestine, which may be dilated. Often mucus is present, and the walls may be thickened. In both forms oocysts can be easily found with a microscope.

Infection arises from contaminated food and water. Green stuff which has been overrun by wild rabbits is a common source of infection. A great deal of re-infection occurs when food is eaten off the hutch floor, and the majority of cases in unweaned stock arise through infection from the mother.

The only way to control the disease is to prevent animals ingesting the oocysts. All contaminated food must be eliminated and in this connection it should be pointed out that the oocysts can remain dangerous for a year or more. Feeding should therefore never be allowed from the hutch floor.

Adult animals almost always act as carriers of the disease, and may do so without showing signs of infection, and thus does will often pass on the disease to their offspring. The use of wire-mesh floors through which all droppings pass has been effective in helping to control the disease, but nevertheless the vast majority of rabbits carry some of these organisms, usually of several different species. Overcrowding is a predisposing factor and should therefore be avoided.

Many compounded (pelleted) feeding stuffs now contain a coccidiostat, that is to say, a substance which assists in the control of the disease. Although it is possible, it is both unsatisfactory and rare to find coccidiostats incorporated in mixes used for rabbit feeding. With the use of pellets containing coccidiostats (ACS pellets} there is unlikely to be the need for professional prescription of sulphonamide drugs to treat outbreaks of the disease. An important point relating to coccidiostats should be made. The dosage incorporated in the pellet is such that it is at a satisfactory level for the control of the disease if only that pellet and no other food is fed to the animals. If the pellet is supplemented with other feeds then the dosage is insufficient to control the disease organisms and the disease will develop.

NUTRITIONAL DISORDERS

Prior to the introduction of complete pelleted diets for rabbits, bad feeding practice and poor nutrition were responsible for a great deal of loss, both directly through simple malnutrition, poisoning, deficiency diseases and so on, and indirectly through lowered resistance to specific diseases and waste of food by imbalance of the nutrients. The incidence of some of these nutritional problems has been reduced although there are still some cases of badly compounded foods causing loss. In addition, whilst pelleted feeds have proved of great benefit to the rabbit keeper, their use has introduced new problems. It should be borne in mind that it is not usual to find a single nutritional disorder, uncomplicated with any other and care in diagnosis is very important.

Constipation and scouring

Both these conditions are symptomatic of a variety of diseases. The breeder should make himself familiar with the normal faeces of his stock, although these will of course vary depending on the size of the animal and its food. The treatment of both conditions will always be directed toward the removal of the cause. Certain foods are undoubtedly constipative whilst others are the reverse.

In a rabbit suffering from scours, the excreta is fluid. Scouring should not be confused with the passing of faecal pellets which are softer than usual. Probably the commonest cause of scouring is an inflammation of the large intestine or the caecum. The only treatment, apart from endeavouring to trace and eliminate the cause of the trouble, is to change the food, but not suddenly, to one having the reverse effect. It is often stated that water should be withheld when an animal scours, but this is never wise.

Mucoid enteritis

This condition (today often known as mucoid enteropathy) is a most complex condition which has received much attention from research workers over the past 60 years without a final solution to its exact cause being established. One of the problems lies in the fact that some of the nutritional disorders that affect the rabbit have very variable effects and often occur in mixed forms. This disease, which has been known since the late 1920s, has, with the development of the commercial rabbit industry, become one of the most important causes of loss. During a number of years at the American Fontana Experimental Station the disease accounted for the majority of deaths (which totalled some 18%) in the pre-weaning (up to 8 weeks) stock. The situation is not the same at the present time. The highest incidence certainly occurs in post-weaned animals, but all ages up to adult may die from the disease. The condition, or a very similar one, occurs in does in very late pregnancy or in early lactation.

A number of different organisms have been suggested as causing the disease or disease complex, but none have been shown definitely to be the cause, although it is possible that toxins produced by the organisms may have some effect. The course of the disease is generally very rapid. The symptoms include an excessive thirst, rapid loss of condition, little or no appetite, and usually a thin diarrhoea. The animal sits huddled in a corner and is very inactive, often grinding its teeth and making a peculiar sound. The coat appears dull and the eye glazed and the temperature is usually subnormal. The faeces are usually associated with a good deal of mucus. On examining the alimentary tract, many different conditions may be found, but always some mucous is present, together with gases and watery fluids. In the colon there is almost invariably a thick gelatinous, mucous plug. Usually there is some drier than usual digested remains and this may be so extensive that much of the caecal contents is dry and impacted. In some cases there are varying degrees of enteritis but this is thought to be unrelated to the mucoid enteritis complex.

Outbreaks of this disease often follow changes in feeding, for example, a rapid change to a new batch of compounded feeding stuffs, an excessively hot period in a badly ventilated house, and so on. Certainly it seems that some prevention results from removing such possibilities.

The condition, or at least one form of it, may be produced by changing the feed rapidly to an excessive amount of fresh young lucerne or clover, and it has been suggested that young white clover will almost always produce the condition, although this is not proven. An inherited predisposition to the condition appears to occur in different strains.

The use of antibiotics has in some cases been said to reduce the amount of mucoid enteritis, on occasions by as much as 75% and the use of antibiotic supplemented feeds for weaning stock is fairly common practice on the Continent and is said to be very effective.

One of the suggestions as to a likely cause relates to the too rapid change of feed from a mainly milk diet to an adult diet with excess carbohydrate and lack of fibre. This accords well with a common preventative measure of ensuring that the diet of young stock should be supplemented with additional fibre. Prevention of mucoid enteritis certainly partly lies in good feed practices and the selection of the correct feeds at the right time.

Poisoning

There are a number of other deficiency diseases, which require specialist diagnosis, but apart from these, the breeder may be faced with cases of poisoning. These may arise from zinc poisoning (sometimes due to badly galvanised hutch fittings), phosphorus poisoning (generally through rat poisons being given inadvertently to stock), mercurial poisoning through the feeding of seed corn which has been dressed, and other forms. The diagnosis of poisoning is again a specialist task, and the only prevention is to ensure that food given is definitely free from such harmful ingredients.

Pregnancy toxaemia

This is a complex condition, the cause, or causes, of which have not been finally confirmed. It occurs in does in advanced pregnancy or during lactation, less often in does with their first litters but increasingly in does with their subsequent litters. The most likely explanation would seem to be a lack of nutrient supply at a time when this is most needed. Some does completely recover without ill effects, whilst others die. There is no treatment. Prevention lies in ensuring the correct nutrition of the doe with the prevention of excessive fatness.

Rickets

Rickets is a condition in which the bones fail to ossify (i.e. 'harden') and become deformed. The condition, at one time quite common, is due to a lack of calcium and phosphorous in the diet. Vitamin D assists the bones to ossify, and proper levels in the food are important, and sunlight (in the presence of which the animal can form its own vitamin D requirement) assists in preventing rickets. An adequate mineral content in the diet is of course necessary, and on a good diet the animals will not suffer from this disease.

Starvation

Death from simple starvation is not so rare as might be supposed. Very young stock may die from starvation because they are unable to suckle through some deformity such as a cleft palate, or because the doe gives insufficient milk. Other cases occur when the rations are of such a bulky nature that the rabbit cannot eat sufficient to satisfy its nutritional needs.

PARASITIC INFESTATIONS

Ear canker

Ear canker was at one time very prevalent, but is much less so today, albeit that the incidence is still unacceptably high. It is caused by one of two types of mite, usually *Psoroptes cuniculi* but sometimes *Chorioptes cuniculi*. The adult mites are about 0.5 mm long, and can be seen in scrapings from an affected ear. The mites attack the inside of the ear and cause inflammation and severe irritation, yellow or brown scabs being produced. The rabbit scratches its ear and shakes its head constantly. Infestation occurs by the transmission of mites from one animal to the other, and the condition is very contagious. The mites can live up to three or four weeks away from a rabbit. Signs of the trouble appear about two or three weeks after the animal is first attacked. The complete life cycle of the mite from birth to egg-laying takes about three weeks.

Prevention is assisted by careful examination of the ears of all stock at regular intervals, and particularly of new arrivals to the rabbitry. When an animal is attacked, the bedding from its hutch should be burned and the hutch carefully disinfected. The old form of treatment, which is still effective, consists in removing all crusts or scabs with cottonwool wrapped round a thin stick and dipped in hydrogen peroxide. After the removal of the scabs one of the proprietary ear canker preparations should be applied, or liquid paraffin containing 1% phenol, or any benzyl benzoate preparation, or any proprietary acaricide. Modern treatment consists of the subcutaneous injection of ivermectin at the rate of 400 µg per kg of liveweight of the animal. One of the benefits of this treatment is that other parasites which exist are dealt with at the same time. The treatment does not kill the eggs of the mite and should therefore be repeated some three weeks later.

Fleas, lice and mites

Apart from mange-producing mites, the domestic rabbit may occasionally be infested with several species of fleas, lice, red mites, ticks, and non-mange-producing mites. Infestations of these are rare in properly kept animals, but a dressing of any good vermin powder, brushed into the coat, will deal effectively with the infestation as will the subcutaneous injection of ivermectin mentioned above.

Myiasis (fly strike)

This is a rare condition in well-kept stock, but is more common in the animals of inexperienced keepers, when care is not taken to see that the hindquarters are kept clean. It may also, much less frequently, occur in other circumstances. Keeping hutches clean assists in its prevention. The condition usually occurs in hot weather when flies (normally greenbottle flies of *Lucilia* species but also bluebottle flies) are hatched. These flies, usually carrion eaters, lay their eggs in the fur around the anus. They are attracted to this when it is matted with faeces and/or urine, but they may also be attracted by secretions from the inguinal glands in that area. The eggs hatch into larvae (maggots) within about 24 hours and the larvae burrow into and under the skin. Secondary types of flies may also attack the fly-struck areas, and following the initial damage, bacterial infection may occur.

If veterinary advice is not sought, then the only treatment is to cut away the fur and remove the maggots, bathing thereafter with an antiseptic fluid. The application of a good insecticide helps. As with the other parasitic conditions of this nature, ivermectin injections (at 400 µg per kg of body weight) have been used with success.

Parasitic worms and flukes

At one time, when greenfeeds were collected for rabbits, the presence of parasitic worms and flukes were fairly common. Today these are much less so. Also unless a severe infestation occurs, and this is unusual, little harm results to the animal.

Round worms
Round worms, with the exception of the stomach worm (*Graphidium strigosum*), the intestinal worm (*Trichostrongylus retortaeformis*) and the caecal worm (*Passalurus ambiguus*), are very rare. The stomach worm is about 12 mm long, and pinkish in colour. It sucks blood from, and may perforate, the stomach wall. A reliable treatment consists of the use of tetrachloroethylene in capsule form, the dosage being 0.55 cc/kg liveweight. The life cycle of this worm is direct, that is, no intermediate host is

necessary and eggs passed out can infect a rabbit directly.

The intestinal worm is found in the small intestine, is hair-like and whitish in colour and about 6 mm long. It may cause inflammation of the intestine and diarrhoea, if present in large numbers. Treatment consists of dosing with oil of chenopodium in capsule form at the rate of 1 cc/kg liveweight.

The caecal worm is the most common worm found in the rabbit, but it is relatively harmless and rarely causes any damage. The worm is white, about 12.7 mm long, with the tail tapering to a fine point.

Flukes

Two species of flukes may be found in the bile ducts of the liver of the rabbit. The main host of the flukes, which are leaf-like and about 25 mm long, or 8 mm long, depending on species, is the sheep, and consequently prevention rests in not feeding herbage which has been overrun by sheep. There is no reliable treatment for fluke in the domestic rabbit.

Tapeworms

Various species occur. These consist of head with suckers and a flat, segmented body. They vary between 2 and 30 cm in length. The eggs produced by these particular worms must pass through an intermediate host (a mite) before they can re-infect a rabbit. Treatment consists of dosing with a taeniacide or 'worm powder', or again with ivermectin.

Tapeworm cysts

Two types of tapeworm cysts are found in the rabbit. Both are the intermediate stages of the dog tapeworms. The first species (the intermediate stage of *Taenia pisiformis* sometimes known as *Cysticercus pisiformis*) occurs in the abdomen, attached to various parts of the intestine. It is a pea-sized bladder within which is a small white head. The second type is the intermediate stage of *Taenia serialis* (sometimes known as *Cysticercus serialis*) and is found in the muscles of the rabbit, immediately below the skin. This cyst, which may be as large as a golf ball, is filled with fluid and contains a number of white heads (each being the size of a pinhead) attached to the inside of the cyst wall.

The adult tapeworms of which these are the intermediate stage are found in the intestines of the dog. The eggs are passed out and contaminate feed or water which is eaten by the rabbit. The parasite is liberated from the egg by the digestive juices and, passing through the wall of the intestine and the liver, finally reaches its permanent site.

Whilst, quite often, large numbers of the small abdominal type are found in the domestic rabbit, it is rare to find more than one or two of the muscle types in the same animal. The large cyst in the muscle is not painful when touched. Neither of the cysts cause much damage, although the passage of the parasite through the liver to its final site may cause some harm, particularly in severe infestations.

Prevention can only be accomplished by taking care that no food or water given to the stock has been contaminated in any way by dogs, and if a dog is kept by the breeder, then steps should be taken to see that it is 'wormed' when need arises. There is no treatment for the abdominal cyst, but the muscle cyst can be removed surgically.

It is essential that all the heads on the wall of the cyst are removed, or the cyst will reform.

Sarcoptic mange

Body or skin mange is relatively rare. It is caused by one of two species of mites (*Sarcoptes scabiei* and *Notoedres cati*). The mites burrow into the skin causing intense irritation. The fur comes off from the infected area, scabs form, and the scratching of the rabbit may cause open sores. The condition usually starts on the head, but may spread to any part of the body. If unchecked, the animal may die in a few weeks in an emaciated condition, for the intense irritation does not allow it to feed properly. For a positive diagnosis it is necessary to examine scrapings from the affected parts under the microscope for the presence of the mites.

When an animal is attacked, its isolation, the burning of the bedding, and disinfection of the hutch are essential. If the condition is caught in the early stages the treatment consists of clipping away the fur from the affected region, removing scabs formed by bathing in a weak disinfectant solution, and applying a good mange preparation containing either benzyl benzoate or benzene hexachloride, or any proprietary acaricide. Treatment does not usually kill the eggs and must therefore be repeated 7 to 10 days later.

DISEASES CAUSED BY FUNGI

There are several rather rare conditions caused by attacks of fungi in the rabbit but being so uncommon are of little significance. This does not however apply to ringworm and favus. The most important fungal infections are ringworm and favus. Both are transmissible to man and therefore great care should be taken in the unlikely event of a case appearing and professional advice sought.

Favus

This is caused by a fungus of the genus *Achorion* and is very similar to ringworm, although the crusts are cup-shaped and give off a characteristic odour. Permanent baldness results from an attack of favus. The same precautions and treatment as for ringworm should be used.

Ringworm

This is caused by a species of fungus known as *Trichophyton mentagrophytes* which attacks the skin and hair follicles and shafts, usually starting on or near the head but then spreading. Circular bald patches appear together with reddish spots which later form yellow crusts. These crusts fall off and the skin becomes ulcerated. The disease may spread rapidly, and bad cases should therefore be destroyed. In mild cases treatment consists in the application of any reliable fungicide.

INHERITED ABNORMALITIES

There are a number of inherited abnormalities in the rabbit, including: furlessness, spina bifida, dwarfism, epilepsy, acrobatic (when the rabbit walks on its front feet), shaking palsy (when the animal suffers varying effects, but mainly tremors), hydrocephalus, enlargement of the eye, absence or additional incisors, yellow fat, abnormal ear carriage, and many others. Most of these are never seen in normal stocks of rabbits and are therefore, to the rabbit breeder, of little significance. The most important condition, and one which is being found with increasing frequency, is malocclusion of the teeth.

Malocclusion of the teeth

With increasing frequency rabbits are found in which the upper and lower incisors do not meet, and the teeth, continuing to grow, reach several inches in length and prevent the animal from eating. The condition may be produced by an accident but the great majority of cases are inherited as a simple recessive factor. The teeth in such a condition may be clipped and filed to the correct length, which may result in a permanent cure if the problem arose from accident, but usually repeated clipping is necessary. This is laborious treatment and unless the animal is particularly valuable, it should be destroyed. Less frequently the molars and premolars ('cheek teeth') suffer the same deformity, and in this case the tongue and cheeks are often damaged. The animal must then be destroyed. As the condition is usually inherited action should be taken to eliminate such stock. If only those animals which show the condition are eliminated from the breeding programme, the condition will remain in the strain. The only reliable and quick way to eliminate the condition is by mating all animals to be bred to an animal actually having the condition. In this way half of the animals born will have malocclusion if the animal being checked has the condition in a recessive state. It should then not be used for breeding.

MISCELLANEOUS DISORDERS AND CONDITIONS

Bites, injuries and wounds

These may be caused by fighting, particularly amongst bucks, or by laceration on nails or wire. The fur should be clipped away and the wound cleansed with a diluted antiseptic solution. After thorough cleansing an antiseptic ointment or tincture of iodine should be applied. In some cases of extensive wounds, stitching may be necessary. If abscesses form these must be lanced and cleaned. Abscesses should be lanced in such a way that further drainage from them is possible. Occasionally an eye may be severely injured during fighting. A veterinary surgeon may be able to repair some of the damage, but blindness often results.

Cancers and tumours

These are a good deal more common in the older rabbit than is generally supposed. However, usually the animals, particularly in commercial herds, do not live long enough for sufficient development to take place to cause any problems. No preventative measures or treatment are possible.

Chilling

Chilling undoubtedly causes some deaths for which there appears to be no other explanation. Young rabbits still in the nest are particularly susceptible. Very young rabbits often die overnight, whilst older ones may appear sick for a day or two and then die. Symptoms vary a good deal but generally scouring is present as well as slobbering. There is congestion of the lungs. No treatment is available but prevention lies in giving adequate protection to stock. When a doe does not line her nest sufficiently with fur, then additional fur should be given.

Congestion of the mammary glands

This condition, often referred to as 'caked udder', may occur when a doe loses her whole litter at an early stage. The mammary glands become congested, inflamed and painful. In severe cases the glands may become hard and split. The condition can be prevented by gradual weaning or by fostering young to a doe when she loses her own. The doe should be put on a laxative diet and fluids should be restricted.

Desertion of young and cannibalism

A fairly common complaint is that does neglect their newly born young or eat them. These vices may be due to several causes. The temperament of the doe is important, and a doe may neglect her first litter. If she destroys or neglects her second, she should be eliminated. Lack of maternal instinct is a familial tendency, and does should be selected which do not show these characteristics. Bad nutrition, particularly the lack of B group vitamins, has been shown to be a cause, and lack of water another. Undoubtedly some does will destroy their young if they have injured them whilst panicking. A doe will consume the afterbirth which is attached to the youngsters and may, inadvertently, eat part of the youngster as well. By selection of does having a quiet temperament and by supplying adequate food and water, these troubles can largely be eliminated.

Fractures

Fractures of limbs may infrequently occur, particularly amongst young stock. Simple fractures may be treated by placing the limb in a splint, but in the case of multiple or extensive fractures, the animal is best destroyed. Spontaneous fractures of the spine occur particularly in the more mature doe with a number of previous litters. Some spinal fractures also occur when an animal is lying half in and half out of a small hole in a partition and is suddenly startled and leaps up. Bad handling of a rabbit may also cause a fracture of the spine and the condition only becomes obvious when a paralysis of the hind legs occurs, usually when the spine is fractured. There is no treatment for the condition.

Fur chewing

This mostly occurs when young meat rabbits are penned together. Small mouthfuls of fur are bitten off and eventually swallowed completely. Small bald patches are seen and the coat appears 'ragged'. Several animals in a pen may be so attacked, usually the dominant animal in the pen being the attacker. The cause is unknown. Insufficient light and boredom have both been put forward as causes, but the condition can usually be prevented by giving a supplement of hay.

Hair loss

There are numerous causes of hair loss (mostly rare) which can be summarised here but reference should be made elsewhere for fuller details. The causes include:

- bacterial, e.g. chronic conjunctivitis and Schmorl's disease;
- fungal diseases, e.g. ringworm;
- mite induced, e.g. sarcoptic mange;
- genetic, e.g. hairlessness;
- nutritional, e.g. magnesium deficiency; fur pulling by pregnant does;
- some severe moults;
- induced moults producing almost complete hairlessness;
- fur chewing; and
- constant rubbing by an animal.

Heat stroke

Pregnant does are most often affected, but heat stroke occurs with other classes of rabbits as well. The condition is caused by excessive heat and inadequate ventilation. Temperatures over about 30°C with inadequate ventilation are the limits above which trouble may occur. These conditions may be found in a poorly made travelling box on hot days or when they are left in cars. Often, the condition is fatal and the only treatment consists of giving shade and good ventilation with water to drink. Sprinkling with cold water may also assist.

Overgrown nails

The nails of the rabbit constantly grow, but are usually kept relatively short by wear. This is particularly the case on wooden floors, but occasionally, particularly on mesh floors, they become too long and should be clipped back to within approximately 6 mm of the quick, which may be seen by holding the nail over a light. They should not be cut too short otherwise pain and bleeding may result.

Moist dermatitis (slobbers)

A condition in which the rabbit has an excessive flow of saliva from the mouth, which wets the fur down the jaw and chest. It may be due to a sore mouth such as inflamed gums, or to overgrown teeth, and also sometimes occurs after chilling. Poor watering facilities which keep the skin and fur wet is also a predisposing factor. The constant wetness in slobbers sometimes leads to bacterial invasion, itself leading to a form of dermatitis, causing hair loss, inflammation and ulceration. Having removed the cause of the wetness, treatment of the dermatitis is by a broad spectrum antibiotic ointment or injection.

Paralysis

This may be due to a number of factors, such as fracture of the spine, muscular paralysis through excess cod liver oil feeding, a very rare nervous condition known as syringomyelia, poisoning, and sometimes as a result of chilling. Usually the animal will be somewhat constipated. There is no satisfactory treatment but the animal may recover if placed in a warm, dry hutch and carefully fed.

Pododermatitis (sore hocks)

Under this general heading are included those conditions affecting the pad of the rabbit's foot in which ulceration occurs. In exhibition animals a bare pad (an area devoid of fur) is considered a fault, whilst a sore hock (where the skin is broken) is considered a disqualification at shows. Certain breeds, being less well-furred on the pad of the foot, have a greater tendency to sore hocks than other breeds.

The pad of the foot becomes ulcerated (usually with *Staphylococcus aureus* infection) and inflamed. Almost always the hind feet are affected, but very occasionally the front feet also become involved. The condition may make the animal so uncomfortable that it often loses flesh, a doe will not usually mate or attend to her young, and the animal generally loses its vitality. The affected animal can often be seen shaking and licking its feet.

Nervous stock, which continually stamp their feet or move about all the time, are more likely to develop the condition, but the most general cause is damp bedding, or a rough floor. In the case of mesh floors the condition is produced when a poor quality mesh with rough or damaged surfaces is used. The whole secret of successful treatment lies in keeping the pad of the foot dry. The bedding must be clean and dry and renewed frequently to keep it so. Leaves or peat moss are both excellent bedding materials for this purpose. Allowing the animal a run on dry soil is also beneficial. The affected parts should be carefully washed in a warm water and mild antiseptic. After thorough drying, a dressing of iodine ointment should be applied and repeated daily until the condition clears up. When the abrasions have become infected, penicillin cream may be of value. If abscesses form, as they may do in very severe cases, they must be lanced, the pus squeezed out, and the cavity which is left cleansed with iodine. A second treatment is the application of boracic powder after cleaning, the pad then being bandaged. Some difficulty may be experienced in keeping the bandage on, but a canvas lace-up 'boot' can be used to keep the bandage in place. There are some reports that ivermectin, at suitable dosages, injected subcutaneously has produced excellent results.

There is a certain amount of evidence that a tendency to sore hocks is inherited, and therefore only under exceptional circumstances should animals developing the condition be used for the production of future breeding stock. In a commercial rabbitry it is probably best to cull the animals affected. The rabbit exhibitor can go some way to preventing the problem by not breeding from very soft-coated animals, especially of the Rex variety.

Pot-belly

This term refers to a chronic condition in which the abdomen becomes permanently enlarged. It is sometimes used wrongly in reference to bloat. The chronic enlargement generally results from a severe attack of liver coccidiosis as described above but may also be seen in badly reared young rabbits which have been given excessive amounts of bulky food. There is no treatment, but the condition can be largely prevented by good husbandry.

Rupture

Very infrequently a rupture of the abdominal wall occurs, and part of the intestines protrude. Surgical treatment by a veterinary surgeon is usually satisfactory. Some cases of rupture of the stomach have been reported and the incidence of this condition appears to be increasing. Generally the cause is unknown although the presence of trichobezoars (see below) have been suggested as one cause. In many cases, however, these are not present. In some rare cases the stomach may rupture in severe cases of bloat.

Trichobezoars or fur/hair balls

This is a complaint in which a ball of wool or fur is formed, usually in the stomach, with the eventual obstruction to the passage of food. It is only when an obstruction occurs that the trichobezoar is dangerous and many animals live for a considerable period with one. The condition is more common in Angoras although it occurs in other breeds. It results from the rabbit licking or nibbling its own fur or that of another animal in the hutch (see Fur chewing). In general there is no treatment for a hair ball. Several treatments have been tried, including pineapple juice (which apparently contains an enzyme which helps breaks down the mass), the use of a good purgative such as castor oil, and others. Surgical removal is expensive and may be dangerous. Prevention lies in the feeding of sufficiently fibrous foods.

Urine burn

This is a condition similar in appearance to vent disease but caused by inflammation of the anus and sexual organs by urine-soaked bedding. Treatment consists of ensuring dry bedding, bathing the affected parts with an antiseptic solution and applying tincture of iodine or preferably a good antiseptic ointment.

Selected Further Reading
and References

The following books are recommended for more detailed treatment of their special subjects. Some are now, however, out of print but can usually be borrowed from libraries, or contact the British Rabbit Council, Purefoy House, 7 Kirkgate, Newark, Nottinghamshire, NG24 1AD.

BREEDS

Birch, P. (in press) *The Beginner's Guide to the Netherland Dwarf*. Coney Press, Chattisham, Ipswich. (This began as a series in *Fur & Feather* and has been praised worldwide, and endorsed by the leading Netherland Dwarf clubs.)

British Rabbit Council (1995) *Breed Standards*, 1996–2000. British Rabbit Council, Newark. (Current breed standards for all the recognised breeds.

Brown, M. (1982) *Exhibition and Pet Rabbits* 2nd edn. Triplegate, Hindhead. (Contains details and standards of many breeds including foreign, with some interesting historical notes.)

Cornish, W. (1943) *The Havana and Havana-Rex Rabbit*. Fur & Feather, Ipswich.

Cumpsty, D. (1978) *Book of the Netherland Dwarf*. Spur Publications, Hindhead.

Hodgkiss, J. (1996) *The Rex Rabbit*. Coney Press, Chattisham, Ipswich. (The most comprehensive and best treatment of the Rex rabbit yet published.)

Howden, A. S. (1984) *The Book of the Tan Rabbit*. (Revised by G. Waite.) Fur & Feather, Ipswich.

Prior, P. E. (1994) *The English Rabbit*, 2nd edn. Coney Press, Chattisham, Ipswich.

Ralphes, P. (1983) *Read About Rabbits – French and Dwarf Lops*. Winckley Publishing, Preston.

Read, J. (1966) *The Dutch Rabbit*. Fur & Feather, Ipswich.

Scott, A. and Bush, H. (1983) *Read About Rabbits – Rex*. Winckley Publishing, Preston.

Smith, E. (1981) *Read About Rabbits – Chinchilla*. Winckley Publishing, Preston.

Wilkins, E. (1942) *The Book of the Belgian Hare*, 4th edn. Fur & Feather, Ipswich.

Wolstenholme, J. (1995) *The Beginner's Guide to the Cashmere Lop*. Coney Press, Chattisham, Ipswich. (This is also recommended and sold by the National Cashmere Club.)

Woodgate, F.G. (1942) *The Complete Book of the Rabbit*. Fur & Feather, Ipswich. (A detailed description of breeds existing in the UK in the 1940s.)

Woodward, C. (1982) *Read About Rabbits – New Zealand*. Winckley Publishing, Preston.

GENETICS AND BREEDING

Bowman, J. C. (1984) *An Introduction to Animal Breeding*, 2nd edn. Edward Arnold, London. (Somewhat advanced but excellent discussion of the basic principles of genetics in relation to breeding.)

Hammond, J. (1925) *Reproduction in the Rabbit*. Oliver and Boyd, Edinburgh. (A classic monograph and the first detailed description of the subject.)

Hammond, J., Jr., Bowman, J. C. and Robinson, T. J. (1983) *Hammond's Farm Animals*, 5th edn. Edward Arnold, London. (A detailed discussion on fertility, growth, genetics and breeding of farm animals, but of great value to the serious rabbit breeder.)

Lush, J. L. (1945) *Animal Breeding Plans*, 3rd edn. Iowa State College Press, Ames. (One of the earliest American textbooks on the subject but nonetheless one of the best, if allowances are made for progress in genetics since then. The book has been reprinted a number of times.)

Nicholas, F. W. (1993) *Veterinary Genetics*. Clarendon Press, Oxford. (Certainly one of the best texts available on the subject.)

Pickard, J. N. and Crew, F. A. E. (1931) *The Scientific Aspects of Rabbit Breeding*. Fur & Feather, Ipswich. (The first book on this subject with considerable emphasis on the genetics of the rabbit.)

Robinson, R. (1957) *Genetic Studies of the Rabbit*. Bibliographia Genetica XVII. The Hague. (The classic and still the most detailed review of the genetics of the rabbit.)

Robinson, R. (1978) *Colour Inheritance in Small Livestock*. Fur & Feather, Ipswich. (A review of colour inheritance in small animals including the rabbit, covering everything of interest in colour inheritance.)

Searle, A. G. (1968) *Comparative Genetics of Cost Colour in Mammals*. Logos Press, with Elek Books, London. (An advanced text dealing with colour inheritance.)

Willis, M.B. (1991) *Dalton's Introduction to Practical Animal Breeding*. Blackwell Science, Oxford. (A most useful and clear introduction to the subject.)

MISCELLANEOUS

Arrington, L. R. and Kelley, K. C. (1976) *Domestic Rabbit Biology and Production*. University Presses of Florida. (An interesting American treatment of the biology, nutrition, disease and general management of commercial rabbits.)

Blount, W. P. (1957) *Rabbits' Ailments*, Rev. edn. Fur & Feather, Ipswich. (The first detailed examination of the diseases of the rabbit and, although out-of-date, most interesting.)

Cheeke, P. R., Patton, N. M., Lukefahr, S. D., and McNitt, J. I. (1987) *Rabbit Production*, 6th edn. Interstate Printers & Publishers, Illinois. (A very fully revised textbook on the domestic rabbit, first published by the then Director, G. S. Templeton, of the US Rabbit Experiment Station, by two Directors of the Oregon State University Rabbit Research Centre, and two other authorities on the subject.)

Cheeke, P. R. (1987) *Rabbit Feeding and Nutrition*. Academic Press, London. (The most detailed treatment of the subject yet published.)

Dowle, H. D. H. (1992) (Revised by J. C. Sandford and J. Potter), *Rabbit Judgeship*. Coney Press, Chattisham, Ipswich. (The only book to treat the subject in detail, by one of the greatest judges ever.)

Lang, J. (1981) *The Nutrition of the Commercial Rabbit*. In: *Nutrition Abstracts and Reviews – Series B*, **51**, Commonwealth Bureau of Nutrition, Aberdeen. pp. 197–225 and 287–302.

Lebas and Colin. (1992) Proceedings of the 5th World Rabbit Science Association (WRSA) Congress, Oregon State University.

Lebas, F., Coudert, P., Rouvier, R. and de Rochambeau, H. (1986) *The Rabbit: Husbandry, Health and Production*. FAO Animal Production and Health Series, No. 21. Food and Agriculture Organization, Rome. (An excellent production dealing with utilitarian rabbit husbandry, by four scientists from several rabbit research stations in France.)

Lockley, R. M. (1964) *The Private Life of the Rabbit. An Account of the Life History and Social Behaviour of the Wild Rabbit*. Andre Deutsch, London. (Whilst this book, by a leading naturalist, who once tried commercial chinchilla rabbit farming, relates to the wild rabbit it gives an excellent account of social behaviour in rabbits generally.)

McDonald, P., Edwards, R.A. and Greenhalgh, J. F. D. (1995) *Animal Nutrition*, 5th edn. Longman, London. (Although rather advanced, an extremely useful discussion of the nutrition of animals, including detailed examination of the nature and evaluation of foods.)

Manning, P.J., Ringler, D. H. and Newcomer, C. E. (Editors) (1994) *The Biology of the Laboratory Rabbit*, 2nd edn. Academic Press, London. (A new edition of the work edited by Weisbroth *et al.* (see below). Incorporates much new material, but both editions are of value.)

Okerman, L. (1994) *Diseases of Domestic Rabbits*, 2nd edn., Library of Veterinary Practice Series. Blackwell Science, Oxford.

Weisbroth, S. H., Flatt, R. E. and Kraus, A.L.(Editors) (1974) *The Biology of the Laboratory Rabbit*. Academic Press, New York. (A highly technical and very detailed account of the anatomy, physiology, biochemistry, genetics and diseases of the rabbit and its use in research.)

Index

(Entries in **bold** denote tables and summaries)